Pocket
MEDICINE

Third Edition

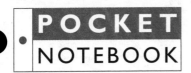

POCKET
NOTEBOOK

Pocket
MEDICINE

Third Edition

Edited by
MARC S. SABATINE, M.D., M.P.H.

The Massachusetts General Hospital
Handbook of Internal Medicine

Wolters Kluwer | Lippincott Williams & Wilkins
Health

Philadelphia · Baltimore · New York · London
Buenos Aires · Hong Kong · Sydney · Tokyo

Acquisitions Editor: Sonya Seigafuse
Managing Editor: Ryan Shaw
Project Manager: Jennifer Harper
Manufacturing Coordinator: Kathleen Brown
Marketing Manager: Kimberly Schonberger
Creative Director: Doug Smock
Production Services: Aptara, Inc.

Third Edition
© 2008 by Lippincott Williams & Wilkins, a Wolters Kluwer business
530 Walnut Street
Philadelphia, PA 19106
LWW.com

Second edition, © 2004 Lippincott Williams & Wilkins
First edition, © 2000 Lippincott Williams & Wilkins

Printed in the USA

Library of Congress Cataloging-in-Publication Data

Pocket medicine / [edited by] Marc S. Sabatine.–3rd ed.
    p. ; cm.
  Includes bibliographical references and index.
    ISBN-13: 978-0-7817-7144-3
    ISBN-10: 0-7817-7144-7
  1. Internal medicine–Handbooks, manuals, etc. I. Sabatine, Marc S.
  [DNLM: 1. Internal Medicine–Handbooks. 2. Clinical Medicine–Handbooks.
WB 39 P7395 2008]
  RC55.P63 2008
  616–dc22

                                                        2007022013

DISCLAIMER

Care has been taken to confirm the accuracy of the information presented and to describe generally accepted practices. However, the authors, editors, and publisher are not responsible for errors or omissions or for any consequences from application of the information in this book and make no warranty, expressed or implied, with respect to the currency, completeness, or accuracy of the contents of the publication. Application of this information in a particular situation remains the professional responsibility of the practitioner.

The authors, editors, and publisher have exerted every effort to ensure that drug selection and dosage set forth in this text are in accordance with current recommendations and practice at the time of publication. However, in view of ongoing research, changes in government regulations, and the constant flow of information relating to drug therapy and drug reactions, the reader is urged to check the package insert for each drug for any change in indications and dosage and for added warnings and precautions. This is particularly important when the recommended agent is a new or infrequently employed drug.

Some drugs and medical devices presented in this publication have Food and Drug Administration (FDA) clearance for limited use in restricted research settings. It is the responsibility of health care providers to ascertain the FDA status of each drug or device planned for use in their clinical practice.

The publishers have made every effort to trace copyright holders for borrowed material. If they have inadvertently overlooked any, they will be pleased to make the necessary arrangements at the first opportunity.

To purchase additional copies of this book, call our customer service department at (800) 639–3030 or fax orders to (301) 824–7390. International customers should call (301) 714–2324. Lippincott Williams & Wilkins customer service representatives are available from 8:30 am to 6:00 pm, EST, Monday through Friday, for telephone access. Visit Lippincott Williams & Wilkins on the Internet: http://www.lww.com.

10 9 8 7 6 5 4 3

CONTENTS

NEPHROLOGY

Eugene Rhee, Ishir Bhan, Hasan Bazari

HEMATOLOGY-ONCOLOGY

*David B. Sykes, David T. Ting, David A. Barbie, Yi-Bin Chen,
   Daniel J. DeAngelo, David P. Ryan*

INFECTIOUS DISEASES

Rachel P. Simmons, Meghan A. Baker, Nesli Basgoz

ENDOCRINOLOGY

Leigh H. Simmons, Michael Mannstadt, F. Richard Bringhurst

RHEUMATOLOGY

Katherine P. Liao, Robert P. Friday, Margaret Seton

NEUROLOGY

Tracey A. Cho, Keith A. Vossel, Timothy W. Yu, David M. Greer

APPENDIX

ABBREVIATIONS

SUBJECT INDEX

CONTRIBUTING AUTHORS

Aaron L. Baggish, MD
Cardiology Fellow, Massachusetts General Hospital

Ednan K. Bajwa, MD
Pulmonary and Critical Care Fellow, Massachusetts General Hospital

Meghan A. Baker, MD
Infectious Diseases Fellow, Massachusetts General Hospital

David A. Barbie, MD
Hematology-Oncology Fellow, Dana-Farber/Partners Oncology Program

Nesli Basgoz, MD
Attending Physician, Infectious Diseases Unit, Massachusetts
    General Hospital
Associate Professor of Medicine, Harvard Medical School

Hasan Bazari, MD
Attending Physician, Nephrology Unit, Massachusetts General Hospital
Program Director, Internal Medicine Residency, Massachusetts
    General Hospital
Assistant Professor of Medicine, Harvard Medical School

Alexander Benson, MD
Internal Medicine Resident, Massachusetts General Hospital

Ishir Bhan, MD
Nephrology Fellow, BWH/MGH Joint Nephrology Fellowship Program

F. Richard Bringhurst, MD
Physician, Endocrine Unit and Senior Vice President for Medical Services,
    Massachusetts General Hospital
Associate Professor of Medicine, Harvard Medical School

Ti-Bin Chen, MD
Hematology-Oncology Fellow, Dana-Farber/Partners Oncology Program

Tracey A. Cho, MD, MA
Neurology Resident, Partners Neurology Residency

Daniel J. DeAngelo, MD, PhD
Adult Leukemia Program, Dana-Farber Cancer Institute &
    Brigham and Women's Hospital
Assistant Professor of Medicine, Harvard Medical School

Robert P. Friday, MD, PhD
Rheumatology Fellow, Massachusetts General Hospital

Lawrence S. Friedman, MD
Chair, Department of Medicine, Newton-Wellesley Hospital
Assistant Chief of Medicine, Massachusetts General Hospital
Professor of Medicine, Harvard Medical School
Professor of Medicine, Tufts University School of Medicine

David M. Greer, MD, MA
Director, Neurological Consultation Service, Massachusetts
    General Hospital
Associate Program Director, Partners Neurology Residency Program
Assistant Professor of Neurology, Harvard Medical School

Katherine P. Liao, MD
Internal Medicine Resident, Massachusetts General Hospital

Atul Malhotra, MD
Associate Physician, Divisions of Pulmonary and Critical Care and Sleep
    Medicine, Brigham and Women's Hospital
Medical Director of the Brigham Sleep Disorders Research Program
Assistant Professor of Medicine, Harvard Medical School

Rajeev Malhotra, MD
Internal Medicine Resident, Massachusetts General Hospital

Michael Mannstadt, MD
Endocrinology Fellow, Massachusetts General Hospital

Michelle O'Donoghue, MD
Cardiology Fellow, Massachusetts General Hospital

Sahil A. Parikh, MD
Cardiology Fellow, Brigham and Women's Hospital

Eugene Rhee, MD
Nephrology Fellow, BWH/MGH Joint Nephrology Fellowship Program

David P. Ryan, MD
Attending Physician, Cancer Center, Massachusetts General Hospital
Clinical Director, Tucker Gosnell Center for Gastrointestinal Cancers
Assistant Professor of Medicine, Harvard Medical School

Marc S. Sabatine, MD, MPH
Associate Physician, Cardiovascular Division, Brigham and Women's Hospital
Affiliate Physician, Cardiology Division, Massachusetts General Hospital
Assistant Professor of Medicine, Harvard Medical School

Paul S. Sepe, MD
Internal Medicine Resident, Massachusetts General Hospital

Margaret Seton, MD
Director, Rheumatology Fellowship Program, Massachusetts
    General Hospital
Assistant Professor of Medicine, Harvard Medical School

Leigh H. Simmons, MD
Internal Medicine Resident, Massachusetts General Hospital

Rachel P. Simmons, MD
Internal Medicine Resident, Massachusetts General Hospital

David B. Sykes, MD, PhD
Internal Medicine Resident, Massachusetts General Hospital

David T. Ting, MD
Internal Medicine Resident, Massachusetts General Hospital

Keith A. Vossel, MD, MSc
Neurology Resident, Partners Neurology Residency

Patrick S. Yachimski, MD
Gastroenterology Fellow, Massachusetts General Hospital

Timothy W. Yu, MD, PhD
Neurology Resident, Partners Neurology Residency

To the 1st Edition

It is with the greatest enthusiasm that I introduce *Pocket Medicine*. In an era of information glut, it will logically be asked, "Why another manual for medical house officers?" Yet, despite enormous information readily available in any number of textbooks, or at the push of a key on a computer, it is often that the harried house officer is less helped by the description of differential diagnosis and therapies than one would wish.

Pocket Medicine is the joint venture between house staff and faculty expert in a number of medical specialties. This collaboration is designed to provide a rapid but thoughtful initial approach to medical problems seen by house officers with great frequency. Questions that frequently come from faculty to the house staff on rounds, many hours after the initial interaction between patient and doctor, have been anticipated and important pathways for arriving at diagnoses and initiating therapies are presented. This approach will facilitate the evidence-based medicine discussion that will follow the workup of the patient. This well-conceived handbook should enhance the ability of every medical house officer to properly evaluate a patient in a timely fashion and to be stimulated to think of the evidence supporting the diagnosis and the likely outcome of therapeutic intervention. *Pocket Medicine* will prove to be a worthy addition to medical education and to the care of our patients.

DENNIS A. AUSIELLO, MD
Physician-in-Chief, Massachusetts General Hospital
Jackson Professor of Clinical Medicine, Harvard Medical School

PREFACE

For Matteo with love

Written by residents, fellows, and attendings, the mandate for *Pocket Medicine* was to provide, in a concise a manner as possible, the information a clinician needs to know to approach and manage the most common inpatient medical problems.

The tremendous response to the pevious editions suggests we were able to help fill an important need for clinicians. With this third edition come several major improvements including: a thorough updating of every topic; the addition of several new topics (intracardiac devices, interpretation of CXRs, fungal infections, tick-borne infections, and hypothermia for anoxic brain injury); incorporation of references to the most recent reviews and important studies published through the start of 2007; and the use of color. We welcome any suggestions for further improvement.

Of course medicine is far too vast a field to ever summarize in a textbook of any size. Whole textbooks have been devoted to many of the topics discussed herein. *Pocket Medicine* is meant only as a starting point to guide one during the initial phases of diagnosis and management until one has time to consult more definitive resources. Although the recommendations herein are as evidence-based as possible, medicine is both a science and an art. As always, sound clinical judgment must be applied to every scenario.

I am grateful for the support of the house officers, fellows, and attendings at the Massachusetts General Hospital. It is a privilege to work with such a knowledgeable, dedicated, and compassionate group of physicians. I always look back on my time there as Chief Resident as the best job I have ever had. I am grateful to several outstanding mentors, including Hasan Bazari, Denny Ausiello, Larry Friedman, Nesli Basgoz, Mort Swartz, Eric Isselbacher, Bill Dec, Mike Fifer, Peter Yurchak, and Roman DeSanctis. Special thanks to my parents for their perpetual encouragement and love and, of course, to my wife, Jennifer Tseng, who, despite being a surgeon, is my closest advisor, my best friend, and the love of my life.

I hope that you find *Pocket Medicine* useful throughout the arduous but incredibly rewarding journey of practicing medicine.

MARC S. SABATINE, MD, MPH

Approach *(a systematic approach is vital)*
- **Rate** and **rhythm**
- **Intervals** (PR, QRS, QT) and **axis** (? LAD or RAD)
- **Chamber enlargement** (? LAE and/or RAE, ? LVH and/or RVH)
- **QRST changes** (? Q waves, poor R wave progression, ST Δ, or T wave inversions)

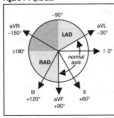

Figure 1-1 QRS axis

Left axis deviation (LAD)
- **Definition:** axis beyond −30° (S > R in lead II)
- **Etiologies:** LVH, LBBB, inferior MI, elevated diaphragm, WPW
- **Left anterior hemiblock:** LAD (often < −45°) *and* qR in I & rS in II, III, aVF *and* QRS <120 msec *and* no other cause of LAD

Right axis deviation (RAD)
- **Definition:** axis beyond +90° (S > R in lead I)
- **Etiologies:** RVH, PE, COPD (usually not > +110°), septal defects, lateral MI, WPW
- **Left posterior hemiblock:** RAD (often > +110°) *and* rS in I & qR in III *and* QRS <120 msec *and* no other cause of RAD

		Bundle Branch Blocks
Normal	V_1 V_6	Initial depol. is left-to-right across septum (r in V_1 & q in V_6; nb, absent in LBBB) followed by LV & RV free wall, with LV dominating (nb, RV depol. later and visible in RBBB).
RBBB		1. QRS ≥120 msec (100–119 = incomplete) 2. rSR′ in R precordial leads (V_1,V_2) 3. Wide S wave in I,V_5, and V_6 4. ± ST↓ or TWI in R precordial leads
LBBB		1. QRS ≥120 msec (100–119 = incomplete) 2. Broad, slurred, monophasic R in I & V_6 (± S if cardiomeg) 3. Absence of Q in I,V_5, and V_6 4. Displacement of ST & Tw opposite major QRS deflection 5. ± PRWP, LAD, Q's in inferior leads

Bifascicular block: RBBB + LAHB/LPHB;Trifascicular: 1° AVB + RBBB + LAHB/LPHB

Prolonged QT interval *(JAMA 2003;289:2120; NEJM 2004;350:1013; www.torsades.org)*
- QT measured from beginning of QRS complex to end of T wave
- QT varies w/ HR, correct w/ Bazett formula: $QTc = QT/\sqrt{RR}$ (nl QTc ≤440 msec)
- Etiologies:
  Antiarrhythmics: class IA and class III
  Psychiatric drugs: antipsychotics (phenothiazines, haloperidol, atypicals), lithium
  Antimicrobials: macrolides, quinolones, voriconazole, pentamidine, atovaquone, chloroquine, amantadine, foscarnet
  Other drugs: antiemetics (droperidol, 5-HT_3 antagonists), alfuzosin, methadone
  Electrolyte disturbances: hypoCa, ? hypoK, ? hypoMg
  Autonomic dysfxn: ICH (deep TWI), stroke, carotid endarterectomy, neck dissection
  Congenital (Long QT Syndrome): K/Na channelopathies, may be assoc w/ deafness
  Misc: CAD, CMP, bradycardia, high-grade AVB, hypothyroidism, hypothermia

ECG P wave Criteria	Left Atrial Enlargement (LAE)		Right Atrial Enlargement (RAE)	
	>120 msec	>40 msec		
	II	or V_1 >1 mm	II >2.5 mm	or V_1 >1.5 mm

Left ventricular hypertrophy (LVH)
- Etiologies: HTN, AS/AI, HCMP, coarctation of aorta
- Criteria (all w/ Se <40%, Sp >85%)
  Romhilt-Estes point-score system: 4 points = probable, 5 points = definite
  ↑ Amplitude (any of the following): largest R or S in limb leads ≥20 mm or S in V_1 or V_2 ≥30 mm or R in V_5 or V_6 ≥30 mm (3 points)

ST displacement opposite to QRS deflection: w/o dig (3 points); w/ dig (1 point)
LAE (3 points); LAD (2 points); QRS duration ≥90 msec (1 point)
Intrinsicoid deflection (QRS onset to peak of R) in V_5 or V_6 ≥50 msec (1 point)
Sokolow-Lyon: S in V_1 + R in V_5 or V_6 ≥35 mm
Cornell: R in aVL + S in V_3 >28 mm in men or >20 mm in women
Other: R in aVL ≥11 mm (or, if LAD, ≥13 mm and S in III ≥15 mm)

Right ventricular hypertrophy (RVH)
- Etiologies: cor pulmonale, congenital (tetralogy, TGA, PS, ASD, VSD), MS, TR
- Criteria (all tend to be insensitive, but highly specific, except in COPD)
  R>S in V_1 or R in V_1 ≥7 mm, S in V_5 or V_6 ≥7 mm, drop in R/S ratio across precordium
  RAD ≥ +110° (LVH + RAD → biventricular hypertrophy)

Ddx of dominant R wave in V_1 or V_2
- Ventricular enlargement: RVH (RAD, RAE, deep S waves in I, V_5, V_6); HCMP
- Myocardial injury: True posterior MI (often IMI); Duchenne muscular dystrophy
- Abnormal depolarization: RBBB (QRS >120 msec, rSR'); WPW (↓ PR, δ wave, ↑ QRS)
- Other: dextroversion; lead misplacement; normal variant

Low voltage
- QRS ampltude (R+S) <5 mm in all limb leads & <10 mm in all precordial leads
- Etiologies: COPD (precordial leads only), pericardial effusion, myxedema, obesity, pleural effusion, restrictive or infiltrative CMP, diffuse CAD

Pathologic Q waves
- Definition: ≥40 msec or >25% height of the R wave in that complex
- Small (septal) q waves in I, aVL, V_5 & V_6 are normal, as can be isolated Qw in III, aVR, V_1
- "Pseudo-infarct" pattern may be seen in LBBB, infiltrative disease, HCMP, COPD, PTX, WPW

Poor R wave progression (PRWP) (Archives 1982;142:1145)
- Definition: loss of anterior forces w/o frank Q waves (V_1-V_3); R wave in V_3 ≤3 mm
- Etiologies:
  old anteroseptal MI (usually R wave V_3 ≤1.5 mm, ± persistent ST ↑ or TWI V_2 & V_3)
  cardiomyopathy
  LVH (delayed RWP with prominent left precordial voltage)
  RVH/COPD (small R wave and prominent S wave in lead I)
  LBBB; WPW; clockwise rotation of the heart; lead misplacement

ST elevation (STE) (NEJM 2003;349:2128)
- **Acute MI** (upward convexity ± TWI) or prior MI with persistent STE
- **Coronary spasm** (Prinzmetal's angina; transient STE in a coronary distribution)
- **Pericarditis** (diffuse, upward concavity STE; associated with PR ↓; Tw usually upright; **myocarditis; cardiac contusion;** ventricular aneurysm
- **Pulmonary embolism** (occ. STE V_1-V_3; typically associated TWI V_1-V_4, RAD, RBBB)
- **Repolarization abnormalities**
  LBBB (↑ QRS duration, STE discordant from QRS complex)
    dx of STEMI in setting of LBBB: ≥1 mm STE concordant w/ QRS (Se 73%, Sp 92%)
    or ≥5 mm discordant (Se 31%, Sp 92%) (NEJM 1996;334:481)
  LVH (↑ QRS amplitude)
  Hyperkalemia (↑ QRS duration, tall Ts, no Ps)
  Brugada syndrome (rSR', downsloping STE V_1-V_2)
- **Normal early repolarization:** most often seen in leads V_2-V_5 and in young adults
  J point ↑ 1-4 mm; notch in downstroke of R wave; upward concavity of ST; large Tw; ratio of STE / T wave amplitude <25%; pattern may disappear with exercise

ST depression
- **Myocardial ischemia** (± T wave abnormalities) or acute true posterior MI (V_1-V_3)
- **Digitalis effect** (downsloping ST± T wave abnormalities, does not correlate with dig levels)
- **Hypokalemia** (± U wave)
- Repolarization abnl in association with LBBB or LVH (usually in leads V_5, V_6, I, aVL)

T wave inversion (TWI)
- Myocardial ischemia or infarct; peri/myocarditis; cardiomyopathy; mitral valve prolapse
- Repolarization abnl in association with LVH/RVH ("strain pattern"), BBB
- Post-tachycardia or post-pacing
- Electrolyte, digoxin, PaO_2, $PaCO_2$, pH, or core temperature disturbances
- Intracranial bleed ("cerebral T waves," usually with ↑ QT)
- Normal variant in children (V_1-V_4) and leads in which QRS complex predominantly ⊖

Cardiac Causes		
Disorder	**Typical characteristics**	**Other S/S; Dx studies**
Angina	substernal pressure → neck, jaw, arm duration < 30 min ± dyspnea, diaphoresis, N/V ↑ w/ exertion; ↓ w/ NTG or rest however, relief by NTG in ED not reliable indicator *(Annals EM 2005;45:581)*	± ECG Δs (ST ↓/↑, TWI)
MI	same as angina but ↑ intensity duration ≥30 min	± ECG Δs (ST ↑/↓, TWI) ⊕ troponin or CK-MB
Pericarditis	sharp pain radiating to trapezius aggravated by respiration relieved by sitting forward	± pericardial friction rub ECG Δs (diffuse ST ↑ & PR ↓) ± pericardial effusion
Myocarditis	same as above	same as above, ±↑ Tn & CHF
Aortic dissection	sudden onset tearing, knifelike pain anterior or posterior mid-scapular	hyper- or hypotension asymmetric BP/pulses; new AI widened mediastinum on CXR false lumen on imaging

Pulmonary Causes		
Disorder	**Typical characteristics**	**Other S/S; Dx studies**
Pneumonia	pleuritic dyspnea, fever, cough, sputum	fever, tachypnea, crackles infiltrate on CXR
Pleuritis	sharp, pleuritic	± pleural friction rub
Pneumothorax	unilateral, sharp, pleuritic sudden onset	unilateral hyperresonance, ↓ BS, PTX on CXR
PE	pleuritic sudden onset	tachypnea, tachycardia, hypoxemia TWI V_1–V_4, RAD, RBBB, occ STE V_1–V_3 ⊕ CTA, V/Q scan or angiogram
Pulmonary HTN	dyspnea, exertional pressure	hypoxemia, loud P_2, right-sided S_3 & S_4

GI Causes		
Disorder	**Typical characteristics**	**Other S/S; Dx studies**
Esophageal reflux	substernal burning acid taste in mouth; water brash ↑ by meals, recumbency; ↓ by antacids	esophageal pH probe Bernstein acid perfusion test EGD
Esophageal spasm	intense substernal pain ↑ by swallowing, ↓ by NTG or CCB	upper GI series manometry
Mallory-Weiss tear	precipitated by vomiting	EGD
Boerhaave's syndrome	precipitated by vomiting severe pain, ↑ with swallowing	palpable SC emphysema mediastinal air on chest CT
Peptic ulcer disease	epigastric pain relieved by antacids ± hematemesis, melena	EGD ± H. pylori test
Biliary disease	RUQ pain, nausea/vomiting aggravated by fatty foods	RUQ U/S, LFTs rarely inferior STE
Pancreatitis	epigastric/back discomfort	↑ amylase & lipase, abd CT

Musculoskeletal and Miscellaneous Causes		
Disorder	**Typical characteristics**	**Other S/S; Dx studies**
Costochondritis	localized sharp or dull pain	tenderness to palpation
Cervical spine disease/OA	precipitated by motion, lasts sec to h	x-rays
Herpes zoster	intense unilateral pain	dermatomal rash & sensory findings
Anxiety	"tightness"	

Pretest Likelihood of CAD						
Sx	Nonanginal ≤1 of 3 sx		Atypical = 2 of 3 sx		Typical = 3 of 3 sx	
Age	Men	Women	Men	Women	Men	Women
30–39	5%	1%	22%	4%	70%	26%
40–49	14%	3%	46%	13%	87%	55%
50–59	22%	8%	59%	32%	92%	80%
60–69	28%	19%	67%	54%	94%	91%

sx: (1) substernal chest pain, (2) provoked by exertion, (3) relieved by rest or NTG (*NEJM* 1979;300:1350)

Exercise tolerance test ("stress test") (*NEJM* 2001;344:1840)
- **Indications**: dx CAD, evaluate Pts w/ known CAD & Δ in clinical status, risk stratify Pts s/p ACS, evaluate exercise tolerance, localize ischemia (radionuclide imaging required)
- **Contraindications**:
  Absolute: AMI w/in 48 h, high-risk UA, acute PE, severe AS, uncontrolled CHF, uncontrolled arrhythmias, myopericarditis, acute aortic dissection
  Relative: LM CAD, mod valvular stenosis, severe HTN, HCMP, high-degree AVB, severe electrolyte abnl, inability to exercise
- **Exercise**: standard Bruce (Se ~60%; Sp ~75%; Se <50% for 1VD, >85% for 3VD or LM), modified Bruce (begins w/o treadmill incline), submax (if <3 wks post-MI), or sx-limited hold antianginal meds if trying to dx CAD; give if assessing if Pt is ischemic on meds
- **Pharmacologic**: if unable to exer. or low exer. tol. (Se & Sp ≈ exercise; better if LBBB) coronary vasodilators (will reveal CAD, but will *not* tell you if Pt *ischemic*): dipyridamole or adenosine (may precipitate bradycardia and bronchospasm) chronotropes/inotropes (~physiologic): dobutamine (may precipitate tachyarrhythmias)
- **Imaging**: used for Pts w/ uninterpretable baseline ECG, after indeterminate ECG test, pharmacologic tests, or localization of ischemia
  uninterpretable ECG: paced, LBBB, resting ST↓ >1 mm, dig., LVH (= Se, ↓ Sp), WPW
  SPECT (thallium-201 or ^{99m}Tc-sestamibi; usually w/ pharm test):
  ↑ Se (~85%) and Sp (~75%); can ECG-gate to assess LV systolic fxn; ↑↑ cost
  echocardiography: ↑ Se (~85%) and Sp (~75%); operator-dependent; ↑ cost

Test results
- **HR** (must achieve ≥85% of max predicted HR (220-age) for *exercise* test to be dx), **BP** response, peak **double product** (HR × BP), HR recovery (HR$_{peak}$–HR$_{1\ min\ later}$; nl >12)
- **Max exercise capacity** achieved (METS or mins)
- Occurrence of **symptoms** (at what level of exertion and similarity to presenting sx)
- **ECG changes**: *downsloping* or *horizontal* ST ↓ predictive of CAD (but distribution of ST ↓ do *not* localize ischemic territory); ST ↑ highly predictive
- Duke treadmill score = exercise mins − (5 × max ST dev) − (4 × angina index) [0 none, 1 nonlimiting, 2 limiting]; score ≥5 → <1% 1-y mort; −10 to +4 → 2–3%; ≤ −11 → ≥5%
- **Imaging**: radionuclide defects or echocardiographic wall motion abnormalities
  reversible defect = ischemia; fixed defect = infarct
  false ⊕: breast → ant "defect" and diaphragm → inf "defect"
  false ⊖ may be seen if balanced ischemia

High-risk test results (PPV ~50% for LM or 3VD, ∴ consider coronary angiography)
- ECG: ST ↓ ≥2 mm or ≥1 mm in stage 1 or in ≥5 leads *or* ≥5 min in recovery; ST ↑; VT
- Physiologic: ↓ BP, exercise <4 METS, angina during exercise, Duke score ≤ −11; EF <35%
- Radionuclide: ≥1 lg or ≥2 mod. reversible defects, transient cavity dilation, ↑ lung uptake

Myocardial viability
- Goal: identify hibernating myocardium that could regain fxn after revascularization
- Options: **MRI** (Se >95%, Sp ~70%), **PET** (Se ~90%, Sp ~75%), **dobutamine stress echo** (Se ~70%, Sp ~85%); **rest-redistribution thallium** (Se ~90%, Sp ~55%)

Coronary calcium score (*JAMA* 2004;291:210)
- Quantitative evaluation of extent of calcium and thus estimate of plaque burden
- *Not* able to assess % narrowing; ? risk stratification if intermed. Framingham risk score

CT & MR coronary angiography (*NEJM* 2001;345:1863; *JAMA* 2006;296:403; *JACC* 2006;48:1475)
- Assess for significant stenoses: Se & Sp >85% (for 64-slice CT)
- Up to 30% of segments nonevaluable (w/ 16-slice CT, fewer w/ newer generation CT) and calcium generates artifact
- Image quality best at slower & regular HR (give β-blockers if possible, goal HR 55-60)
- High NPV → most useful to rule out CAD

Indications for coronary angiography in stable CAD or asymptomatic Pts

- CCS class III-IV angina despite medical Rx or angina + systolic dysfxn
- High-risk stress test findings (see prior topic)
- Uncertain dx after noninvasive testing (& compelling need to determine dx), occupational need for definitive dx (eg, pilot), or inability to undergo noninvasive testing
- Systolic dysfxn with unexplained cause
- Survivor of SCD, polymorphic VT, sustained monomorphic VT
- Suspected spasm or nonatherosclerotic cause of ischemia (eg, anomalous coronary)

Pre-cath checklist

- Document peripheral arterial exam (femoral, DP, PT pulses; femoral bruits)
- √ CBC, PT, & Cr; give IVF (± bicarb, acetylcysteine; see "CIARF"); blood bank sample
- NPO >6 h
- ASA 325 mg; consider clopidogrel pretreatment (300-600 mg ≥2-6 h before PCI)

Coronary revascularization in stable CAD (JACC 2006;47:e1; JACC 2004;44:e213)

- CABG ↓ mortality c/w med Rx (albeit before statins & ACEI/ARB) in Pts w/ 3VD, left main, or 2VD w/ critical prox LAD, and espec. if ↓ EF (but viable myocardium)
- PCI ↓ angina c/w med Rx; does not ↓ D/MI (COURAGE, NEJM 2007;356:1503)
- PCI comparable to CABG in Pts w/o 3VD, w/o DM, and nl EF
- In general, for stable CAD w/o critical anatomy and w/o ↓ EF, initial focus should be on optimal medical therapy
- If revasc deemed necessary, PCI preferred if limited # of discrete lesions, nl EF, no DM, poor operative candidate; CABG preferred if extensive or diffuse disease, ↓ EF, DM, or concomitant valvular heart disease

PCI

- **Balloon angioplasty**: effective, but c/b dissection and by elastic recoil & neointimal hyperplasia → restenosis; now reserved for small lesions, ? some SVG lesions
- **Bare metal stents (BMS)**: ↓ elastic recoil → 33-50% ↓ restenosis & repeat revasc (to ~10% by 12 mos) c/w balloon angioplasty; requires ASA lifelong & clopidogrel x ≥ 4 wks
- **Drug-eluting stents (DES)** (NEJM 2006;354:483): ↓ neointimal hyperplasia → ~75% ↓ restenosis, ~50% ↓ clinical need for repeat revasc (to <5% by 12 mos), & no Δ death/MI over 1 y c/w BMS (Circ 2007;115:813); requires ASA lifelong & clopidogrel x ≥ 1 y (Circ 2007;115:813)

Post-PCI complications

- Postprocedure √ vascular access site, distal pulses, ECG, CBC, Cr, CK-MB
- **Bleeding**
  hematoma/overt bleeding: manual compression, reverse/stop anticoag
  retroperitoneal bleed: may present with ↓ Hct ± back pain; ↑ HR & ↓ BP late;
  Dx: abd/pelvic CT (I−); Rx: reverse/stop anticoag, IVF/PRBC as required
  if bleeding uncontrolled, consult performing interventionalist or surgery
- **Vascular damage**
  pseudoaneurysm: triad of pain, expansile mass, systolic bruit; Dx: U/S; Rx: manual compression, U/S-directed compression or thrombin injection, or surgical repair
  AV fistula: continuous bruit; Dx: U/S; Rx: surgical repair
  ↓ perfusion to LE (embolization, dissection, thrombus): loss of distal pulse; Dx: angio; Rx: percutaneous or surgical repair
- Other local: nerve injury, infection
- **MI**: >3× ULN of CK-MB occurs in 5-10%; Qw MI in <1%
- **Renal failure**: contrast-induced manifests w/in 24 h, peaks 3-5 d (see "CIARF")
- **Cholesterol emboli syndrome** (typically in middle-aged & elderly and w/ Ao atheroma)
  renal failure: late and progressive, eos in urine
  mesenteric ischemia, abd pain, LGIB, pancreatitis
  intact distal pulses but livedo pattern and toe necrosis
  Hollenhorst plaques in retinal arteries
- **Stent thrombosis**: p/w acute chest pain & STE; requires urgent return to cath lab. Acute thrombosis often due to mechanical complication (underexpansion of stent or unrecognized dissection) or d/c of antiplt Rx (JAMA 2005;293:2126). Risk of late stent thrombosis may be higher w/ DES than BMS (JACC 2006;48:2584).
- **In-stent restenosis**: mos after PCI, gradual return of typical anginal sx (10% p/w ACS) Due to combination of elastic recoil (↓ w/ stenting vs. balloon angioplasty) and neointimal hyperplasia (↓ w/ DES vs. BMS) and not recurrent atherosclerosis.

ACUTE CORONARY SYNDROMES

Myocardial ischemia typically due to atherosclerotic plaque rupture → coronary thrombosis

Spectrum of Acute Coronary Syndromes			
Dx	**UA**	**NSTEMI**	**STEMI**
Coronary thrombosis	Subtotal		Total
History	angina that is new-onset, crescendo, or at rest; usually <30 min		angina at rest usually ≥30 min
ECG	± ST depression and/or TWI		ST elevations
Troponin/CK-MB	⊖	⊕	⊕ ⊕

Ddx (causes of myocardial ischemia/infarction other than atherosclerotic plaque rupture)
- Nonatherosclerotic coronary artery disease
  Spasm: Prinzmetal's variant, cocaine-induced (6% of CP + cocaine use r/i for MI)
  Vasculitis: Kawasaki's syndrome, Takayasu's arteritis, PAN, Churg-Strauss, SLE, RA
  Aortic dissection w/ retrograde extension involving coronary (usually RCA → IMI)
  Spontaneous coronary artery dissection (often in setting of pregnancy)
- Coronary artery embolism: endocarditis, prosthetic valve, mural thrombus, myxoma
- Fixed CAD but ↑ myocardial O_2 demand (eg, ↑ HR, anemia, AS) → "demand" ischemia
- Myocarditis (myocardial necrosis, but not caused by CAD)

Clinical manifestations (JAMA 2005;294:2623)
- **Typical angina**: retrosternal pressure/pain/tightness ± radiation to neck, jaw, or arms
  precip. by exertion, relieved by rest or NTG; in ACS, new-onset, crescendo, or at rest
- **Associated symptoms**: dyspnea, diaphoresis, N/V, palpitations, or lightheadedness
- ~23% of MIs are initially unrecognized b/c silent or atypical sx (AJC 1973;32:1)

Physical exam
- Signs of ischemia: S_4, new MR murmur 2° papillary muscle dysfxn, paradoxical S_2
- Signs of heart failure: ↑ JVP, crackles in lung fields, ⊕ S_3
- Signs of other areas of atherosclerotic disease: carotid or femoral bruits, ↓ distal pulses

Diagnostic studies
- **ECG**: ST dev., TWI, LBBB not known to be old
  Qw or PRWP suggests prior MI and ∴ CAD
  ✓ ECG at presentation, with Δ in sx, and at 6-12 h; c/w baseline
  dx of STEMI in setting of LBBB: ≥1 mm STE concordant w/ QRS (Se 73%, Sp 92%)
  or ≥5 mm discordant (Se 31%, Sp 92%) in any lead (NEJM 1996;334:481)

Localization of MI		
Anatomic area	**ECG Leads w/ STE**	**Coronary Artery**
Septal	V_1-V_2	Proximal LAD
Anterior	V_3-V_4	LAD
Apical	V_5-V_6	Distal LAD, LCx, or RCA
Lateral	I, aVL	LCx
Inferior	II, III, aVF	RCA (~85%), LCx (~15%)
RV	V_1-V_2 & V_4R (most Se)	Proximal RCA
Posterior	ST depression V_1-V_2	RCA or LCx

If ECG non-dx and suspicion high, consider additional lateral leads (V_7-V_9) to further assess LCx territory.
STE in III >STE in II and lack of STE in I or aVL suggest RCA rather than LCx culprit in IMI.

- **Cardiac biomarkers**: serial testing at presentation, 6-12 h after sx onset
  troponin (I or T): most Se & Sp marker; rise & fall in approp. clinical setting is dx of MI
  detectable 4-6 h after injury, peaks 24 h, may remain elevated for 7-10 d in STEMI
  "false ⊕" (non-ACS myonecrosis): myocarditis, toxic CMP, severe CHF, PE or severe
  resp. distress, cardiac trauma or cardioversion, sepsis, SAH, "demand" ischemia
  renal failure: ? false ⊕ (↓ clearance, skeletal myopathy) vs. true microinfarctions;
  in Pts w/ ACS & ↓ CrCl, ↑ Tn → poor prognosis (NEJM 2002;346:2047)
  CK-MB: less Se & Sp (skel. muscle, tongue, diaphragm, intestine, uterus, prostate)
- **Echocardiogram**: new wall motion abnormality (operator & reader dependent)
- **Myocardial perfusion**: inject sestaMIBI during sx (no stress); image later

Likelihood of ACS			
Feature	**High** (any of below)	**Intermediate** (no high features, any of below)	**Low** (no high/inter. features, may have below)
History	chest or L arm pain like prior angina h/o CAD	chest or L arm pain age >70 y male, diabetes	atypical sx (eg, pleuritic, sharp, or positional pain)
Exam	hypotension, CHF, transient MR	PAD or CVD	pain reproduced on palp.
ECG	new STD (≥0.5 mm) TWI (≥2 mm)	old Q waves old ST or T wave abnl	TWF/TWI (in leads w/ Rw) normal
Biomarkers	⊕ Tn or CK-MB	normal	normal

(Adapted from ACC/AHA 2002 Guideline Update for UA/NSTEMI)

Approach to triage
- If hx and initial ECG & biomarkers non-dx, repeat ECG & biomarkers 6-12 h later
- If remain normal and low likelihood of ACS, search for alternative causes of chest pain
- If remain normal and Pt is pain-free, have ruled out MI, *but* if clinical suspicion remains for ACS based on hx, then still need to r/o UA w/ stress test to assess for inducible ischemia;
  if low risk (age ≤70; ∅ prior CAD, CVD, PAD; ∅ rest angina) can do as outPt w/in 72 h (0% mortality, <0.5% MI, *Ann Emerg Med* 2006;47:427);
  if not low risk, admit and evaluate for ischemia (stress test or cath)
- If ECG or biomarker abnl or high likelihood of ACS based on hx, then admit and Rx as per below

---

UA/NSTEMI (NSTE ACS)

Anti-Ischemic Treatment	
Nitrates (SL, PO, topical, or IV)	↓ anginal sx, no ↓ in mortality
β-blockers metoprolol 5 mg IV q5 min × 3 then 25 mg PO q6h titrate to HR 55-60	13% ↓ in progression to MI (*JAMA* 1988;260:2259) *Contraindicated* if HR <55, SBP <100, moderate or severe CHF, 2°/3° AVB, severe bronchospasm
Calcium channel blockers (nondihydropyridines)	Consider in Pts who cannot tolerate β-blockers due to bronchospasm
Morphine	Consider if persistent sx or pulmonary edema Should not be used to mask persistent CP
Oxygen	Use if necessary to keep S_aO_2 >90%

(Adapted from ACC/AHA 2002 Guideline Update for UA/NSTEMI)

Antiplatelet Therapy	
Aspirin 162-325 mg PO (1st dose crushed/chewed) then 75-162 mg PO qd	50-70% ↓ D/MI (*NEJM* 1988;319:1105) If ASA allergy, use clopidogrel instead (and desensitize to ASA)
Clopidogrel (ADP receptor blocker) 300 mg PO × 1 → 75 mg PO qd (requires ~6 h to steady-state) 600 mg load may be superior (faster and greater plt inhib; *Circ* 2005;111:2099)	Give in addition to ASA if conservative strategy or if PCI planned. 20% ↓ CVD/MI/stroke (CURE, *NEJM* 2001;345:494) ↑ benefit if given upstream *prior* to PCI (PCI-CURE, *Lancet* 2001;358:527), although need to wait >5 d after d/c clopidogrel prior to CABG
GP IIb/IIIa inhibitors (GPI) abciximab: 0.25 mg/kg IVB → 0.125 μg/kg/min eptifibatide: 180 μg/kg IVB (×2 q10' if w/ PCI) → 2 μg/kg/min (1 if CrCl <50) tirofiban: 0.4 μg/kg/min × 30 min → 0.1 μg/kg/min (1/2 dose if CrCl <30) infusions given 18-24 h post-PCI	Given in addition to oral antiplt Rx(s) In setting of PCI, ~ 50% ↓ D/MI (CAPTURE, *Lancet* 1997;349:1429; ESPRIT, *Lancet* 2000;356:2037) Consider upstream eptifibatide or tirofiban (not abciximab) if high-risk (⊕ Tn, TRS ≥4) or refractory sx. 10-20% ↓ D/MI (PURSUIT, *NEJM* 1998;339:436; PRISM-PLUS, *NEJM* 1998;338:1488), although most benefit peri-PCI (*Circ* 1999;100:2045).

Anticoagulant Therapy	
UFH 60 U/kg IVB (max 4000 U) 12 U/kg/h (max 1000 U/h)	24% ↓ D/MI (JAMA 1996;276:811) titrate to aPTT 50-70 sec
Enoxaparin (low-molecular-weight heparin) 1 mg/kg SC bid × 2-8 d (±30 mg IVB) (qd if CrCl <30)	Consider instead of UFH. ~10% ↓ D/MI (JAMA 2004;292:89). Benefit greatest if conservative strategy. Can perform PCI on enoxaparin.
Bivalirudin (direct thrombin inhibitor) 0.1 mg/kg IVB → 0.25 mg/kg/h at time of PCI: additional 0.5 mg/kg IVB (0.75 if not already on bival) → 1.75 mg/kg/h	Use instead of heparin for Pts w/ HIT With invasive strategy, bival alone noninferior to heparin + GPI (non-signif 8% ↑ D/MI/UR) w/ 47% ↓ bleeding (ACUITY, NEJM 2006;355:2203)
Fondaparinux (Xa inhibitor) 2.5 mg SC qd	C/w enox, 17% ↓ mortality & 38% ↓ bleeding by 30 d (OASIS-5; NEJM 2006;354:1464). However, ↑ risk of cath thromb.; ∴ must supplement w/ UFH if PCI.

Coronary angiography (JACC 2002;40:1366)
- **Conservative approach** = selective angiography
  medical Rx with pre-d/c stress test; angio only if recurrent ischemia or strongly ⊕ ETT
- **Early invasive approach** = routine angiography w/in 24-48 h
  Indicated if high risk: recurrent ischemia, ⊕ Tn, ST∆, TRS ≥3, CHF, ↓ EF, recent PCI <6 mos, sustained VT, prior CABG, hemodynamic instability
  25% ↓ MI, 34% ↓ rehosp for ACS, & nonsignif 8% ↓ D c/w cons. (JAMA 2005;293:2908)
  ↑ peri-PCI MI counterbalanced by ↓↓ in spont. MI
  Long-term mortality benefit likely only if c/w cons. strategy with low rate of angio/PCI
  Early invasive approach not found to be superior in ICTUS trial (NEJM 2005;353:1095), but results dominated by peri-PCI MI; post-d/c benefits of INV c/w prior data

TIMI Risk Score for UA/NSTEMI (JAMA 2000;284:825)				
Calculation of Risk Score		**Application of Risk Score**		
Characteristic	Point	Score	D/MI/UR by 14 d	
Historical		0-1	5%	
Age ≥65 y	1	2	8%	
≥3 Risk factors for CAD	1	3	13%	
Known CAD (stenosis ≥50%)	1	4	20%	
ASA use in past 7 d	1	5	26%	
Presentation		6-7	41%	
Severe angina (≥2 episodes w/in 24 h)	1	Higher risk Pts (TRS ≥3) derive ↑ benefit from ASA, GP IIb/IIIa inhibitors, and early angiography (JACC 2003;41:89S)		
ST deviation ≥0.5 mm	1			
⊕ cardiac marker (troponin, CK-MB)	1			
RISK SCORE = Total points	**(0-7)**			

Figure 1-2 Approach to UA/NSTEMI

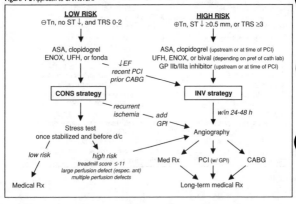

Prinzmetal's (variant) angina
- Coronary spasm → transient STE usually w/o MI (*but* MI, AVB, VT can occur)
- Pts usually young, smokers, ± other vasospastic disorders (eg, migraines, Raynaud's)
- Tends to occur in morning; precipitated by hyperventilation or cold, *not* exertion
- Angiography → nonobstructive CAD, focal spasm w/ hyperventilation, acetylcholine
- Treatment: high-dose CCB, nitrates (+SL NTG prn), ? α-blockers; d/c smoking
- Cocaine-induced vasospasm: avoid βB as unopposed α-stimulation can worsen spasm
  Cocaine also associated with premature atherosclerosis (*NEJM* 2001;345:351)

STEMI

Fibrinolysis
- Indications: sx <12 h and either STE ≥0.1 mV (≥1 mm) in ≥2 contig. leads or LBBB not known to be old; benefit if sx >12 h less clear; reasonable if persistent sx & STE
- Door-to-needle time should be ≤30 mins
- ~20% ↓ in mortality in anterior MI or LBBB; ~10% ↓ in mortality in IMI
- Prehospital lysis: further 17% ↓ in mortality (*JAMA* 2000;283:2686)
- ~1% risk of ICH; high-risk groups include elderly (~2% if >75 y), women, low wt
- Advanced age not contraindic., ↑ risk of ICH in elderly (>75 y) makes PCI more attractive
- Fibrin-specific lytic (front-loaded TPA) 14% ↓ mort. c/w SK (1% abs Δ; GUSTO, *NEJM* 1993;329:673) although ↑ ICH (0.7% vs. 0.5%); 3rd gen. bolus lytics easier to administer, but no more efficacious

Contraindications to Fibrinolysis	
Absolute Contraindications	**Relative Contraindications**
• Any prior ICH	• Hx of severe HTN or SBP >180 or DBP >110 on presentation (? absolute contra. if low-risk MI)
• Intracranial neoplasm, aneurysm, AVM	• Ischemic stroke >3 mos prior
• Nonhemorrhagic stroke or closed head trauma w/in 3 mo	• Prolonged CPR (>10 min)
• Active internal bleeding or known bleeding diathesis	• Trauma or major surgery w/in 3 wk
• Suspected aortic dissection	• Recent internal bleed (w/in 2-4 wk); active PUD
	• Noncompressible vascular punctures
	• Prior SK exposure (if considering SK)
	• Pregnancy
	• Current use of anticoagulants

Primary PCI (*NEJM* 2007;356:47)
- Should be performed **w/in 90 mins** of arrival by skilled operator at high-volume center
- Superior to lysis: 27% ↓ death, 65% ↓ reMI, 54% ↓ stroke, 95% ↓ ICH (*Lancet* 2003;361:13)
- *Transfer* to center for 1° PCI may also be superior to lysis (DANAMI-2, *NEJM* 2003;349:733) *if* can achieve acceptable door-to-balloon times (see below)

Fibrinolysis vs. Primary PCI	
Assess Time and Risk	
1. Time to presentation (efficacy of lytics ↓ w/ ↑ time from sx onset)	
2. Risk from STEMI (high-risk Pts fare better with mechanical reperfusion)	
3. Risk of fibrinolysis (if high risk of ICH, PCI safer option)	
4. Time required for transport to skilled PCI lab (benefit of PCI over lytic time-dependent)	
If sx <3 h and no delay to invasive strategy, no pref. for either strategy	
Fibrinolysis preferred	**Primary PCI preferred**
Early presentation (<3 h) *and* **delay to invasive strategy** (see time goals in next column)	**Skilled PCI lab available w/o delay** Door-to-balloon <90 min (Door-to-balloon)-(door-to-needle) <1 h
Invasive strategy not an option (skilled lab unavailable or difficult vasc. access)	**High-risk STEMI** (shock, Killip class ≥3)
	Contraindic. to lysis (incl ICH risk >4%)
	Late presentation (sx onset >3 h ago)
	Dx of STEMI in doubt

PCI lab should have surgical backup. Adapted from ACC/AHA 2004 STEMI Guidelines (*Circ* 2004;110:e82). Do not let decision regarding *method* of reperfusion delay *time* to reperfusion. Mort. ↑ w/ time to reperfusion ("time = muscle").

Nonprimary PCI
- Facilitated PCI: lytic before PCI *harmful* (*Lancet* 2006;367:569); upstream GPI under study
- Rescue PCI: beneficial if <50% ST segment resolution by 90 mins (*NEJM* 2005;353:2758)
- Routine angio ± PCI w/in 24 h of successful lysis: ↓ D/MI/Revasc (*Lancet* 2004;364:1045)
- *Late* PCI (median day 8) of occluded infarct-related artery: no benefit (*NEJM* 2006;355:2395)

Antithrombotic Therapy	
Aspirin 162-325 mg PO (crushed/chewed)	23% ↓ in death (ISIS-2, Lancet 1988;ii:349)
UFH 60 U/kg IVB (max 4000 U) 12 U/kg/h (max 1000 U/h)	No demonstrated mortality benefit ↑ patency with fibrin-specific lytics Titrate to aPTT 50-70 sec
Enoxaparin 30 mg IVB × 1 → 1 mg/kg SC bid (>75 y: no bolus, 0.75 mg/kg SC bid) (CrCl < 30 ml/min: 1 mg/kg SC qd)	Lysis: 17% ↓ D/MI w/ ENOX × 7 d vs. UFH × 2 d (ExTRACT-TIMI 25, NEJM 2006;354;1477) PCI: acceptable alternative to UFH (age & CrCl adjustments untested in 1° PCI)
Fondaparinux 2.5 mg SC QD	Lysis: superior to placebo & to UFH, with less bleeding (OASIS-6, JAMA 2006;295;1519) PCI: risk of cath thromb.; should not be used
Clopidogrel 300 mg load → 75 mg qd (>75 y: no load with fibrinolytic) ? 600 mg load if PCI	Lysis: 41% ↑ in patency, 7% ↓ mort., no Δ in major bleed or ICH (CLARITY-TIMI 28, NEJM 2005;352:1179; COMMIT, Lancet 2005;366:1607) PCI: should be administered to all
GP IIb/IIIa inhibitors abciximab, eptifibatide, ? tirofiban	Lysis: no indication (GUSTO V, Lancet 2001;357:1905) PCI: 60% ↓ D/MI/urg TVR (NEJM 2001;344:1895)

Immediate Adjunctive Therapy	
β-blockers metoprolol 5 mg IV q5min × 3 then 25 mg PO q6h titrate to HR 55-60	~20% ↓ arrhythmic death or reMI, 30% ↑ cardiogenic shock, & no Δ overall mortality when given to Pts incl. those w/ mod CHF (COMMIT, Lancet 2005;366:1622) Contraindicated if HR <60, SBP <100, moderate or severe CHF, 2°/3° AVB, severe bronchospasm
Nitrates SL or IV	? ~5% ↓ mortality (Lancet 1994;343:1115; 1995;345:669) Use for relief of sx, control of BP, or Rx of CHF Contraindic. in hypovolemia, sx RV infarcts, sildenafil
Oxygen	Use if necessary to keep S_aO_2 >90%.
Morphine	Relieves pain, ↓ anxiety, venodilation → ↓ preload
ACE inhibitors captopril 6.25 mg tid, titrate up as tolerated	~10% ↓ mortality (Lancet 1994;343:1115 & 1995; 345:669) Greatest benefit in ant. MI, EF <40%, or prior MI Contraindicated in severe hypotension or renal failure
ARBs	Appear ≈ ACEI (VALIANT, NEJM 2003;349:20)
Insulin	Consider insulin infusion in 1st 48 h to normalize glc

LV failure (~25%)
- Diurese to achieve PCWP 15-20 → ↓ pulmonary edema, ↓ myocardial O_2 demand
- ↓ Afterload → ↑ stroke volume & CO, ↓ myocardial O_2 demand
  can use IV NTG or nitroprusside (risk of coronary steal) → short-acting ACEI
- Inotropes if CHF despite diuresis & ↓ afterload; use dopamine, dobutamine, or milrinone
- **Cardiogenic shock** (~7%) = MAP <60 mmHg, CI <2 L/min/m², PCWP >18 mmHg inotropes, IABP,VAD to keep CI >2; pressors (eg, norepinephrine) to keep MAP >60; coronary revascularization ASAP (NEJM 1999;341:625)

IMI complications (Circ 1990;81:401; Annals 1995;123:509)
- **Heart block** (~20%, occurs because RCA typically supplies AV node)
  40% on present., 20% w/in 24 h, rest by 72 h; high-grade AVB can develop abruptly
  Rx: atropine, epi, isoproterenol, aminophylline (100 mg/min × 2.5 min), temp wire
- **Precordial ST** ↓ (15-30%): anterior ischemia vs. true posterior STEMI vs. reciprocal Δs
- **RV infarct** (30-50%, but only 1/2 of these clinically significant)
  hypotension; ↑ JVP, ⊕ Kussmaul's; 1 mm STE in V₄R; RA/PCWP ≥0.8; prox RCA occl.
  Rx: optimize preload (RA goal 10-14, BHJ 1990;63:98); ↑ contractility (dobutamine);
  maintain AV synchrony (pacing as necessary); reperfusion (NEJM 1998;338:933);
  mechanical support (IABP or RVAD); pulmonary vasodilators (eg, inhaled NO)

Mechanical complications (incid. <1% for each; typically occur a few days post-MI)
- **Free wall rupture**: large MI in elderly, tear at jxn w/ nl myocardium; p/w PEA or hypoTN, pericardial sx, tamponade; Rx: volume resusc., ? pericardiocentesis, inotropes, surgery
- **VSD**: lg MI in elderly; AMI → apical VSD, IMI → basal septum; 90% w/ harsh murmur ± thrill (NEJM 2002;347:1426); Rx: diuretics, vasodil., inotropes, IABP, **surgery**, perc. closure
- **Papillary muscle rupture**: small MI; more likely in IMI → PM pap. muscle (supplied by PDA) than AMI → AL pap. muscle (supplied by diags & OMs); 50% w/ new murmur, rarely a thrill, ↑ v wave in PCWP tracing; Rx: diuretics, vasodilators, IABP, **surgery**

Arrhythmias post-MI

- Treat as per ACLS for unstable or symptomatic bradycardias & tachycardias
- **AF** (10-16% incidence): β-blocker, amiodarone, digoxin (particularly if CHF), heparin
- **VT/VF**: lido or amio × 6-24 h, then reassess; ↑ βB as tol., replete K & Mg, r/o ischemia; early monomorphic (<48 h post-MI) does *not* carry bad prognosis
- Accelerated idioventricular rhythm (AIVR): slow VT (<100 bpm), often seen after successful reperfusion; typically self-terminates and does not require treatment
- Consider *backup* transcutaneous pacing (TP) if: 2° AVB type I, BBB
- **Backup TP or initiate transvenous pacing** if: 2° AVB type II; BBB + AVB
- **Transvenous pacing (TV)** if: 3° AVB; new BBB + 2° AVB type II; alternating LBBB/RBBB
  (can bridge w/ TP until TV, which is best accomplished under fluoroscopic guidance)

Other Post-MI Complications		
Complication	**Clinical features**	**Treatment**
LV thrombus	~30% incid. (esp. lg antero-apical MI)	Anticoagulate × 3-6 mo
Ventricular aneurysm	Noncontractile outpouching of LV; 8-15% incid.; persistent STE.	Surgery if recurrent CHF, thromboemboli, arrhythmia
Ventricular pseudoaneurysm	Rupture → sealed by thrombus and pericardium	Surgery
Pericarditis	10-20% incid.; 1-4 d post-MI ⊕ pericardial rub; ECG Δs rare	High-dose aspirin, NSAIDs Minimize anticoagulation
Dressler's syndrome	<4% incid.; 2-10 wk post-MI Fever, pericarditis, pleuritis	High-dose aspirin, NSAIDs

Prognosis

- In registries, in-hospital mortality is 6% w/ reperfusion Rx (lytic or PCI) and ~20% w/o
- Predictors of mortality: age, time to Rx, anterior MI or LBBB, heart failure (*Circ* 2000;102:2031)

Killip Class		
Class	**Definition**	**Mort.**
I	no CHF	6%
II	⊕ S₃ and/or basilar rales	17%
III	pulmonary edema	30-40%
IV	cardiogenic shock	60-80%

(Am J Cardiol 1967;20:457)

Forrester Class Mortality			
		PCWP (mmHg)	
		<18	>18
CI	>2.2	3%	9%
	<2.2	23%	51%

(NEJM 1976;295:1356)

PREDISCHARGE CHECKLIST AND LONG-TERM POST-ACS MANAGEMENT

Risk stratification

- Stress test if anatomy undefined or significant residual CAD after PCI of culprit vessel
- Echocardiogram to assess EF

Medications (barring contraindications)

- **Antiplatelet Rx**: ASA 81-162 mg indefinitely; clopidogrel × 9-12 mos (? longer if DES)
- **β-blocker**: 23% ↓ mortality after acute MI
- **Statin**: high-intensity lipid-lowering (eg, atorvastatin 80 mg, *NEJM* 2004;350:1495)
- **ACEI**: life-long if CHF, ↓ EF, HTN, DM; 4-6 wks or at least until hosp. d/c in all STEMI ? long-term benefit in CAD w/o CHF (*NEJM* 2000;342:145 & 2004;351:2058; *Lancet* 2003;362:782)
- Aldosterone antagonist: if EF <40% & signs of HF (see "Heart Failure")
- Nitrates: standing if symptomatic; SL NTG prn for all
- **Warfarin**: beyond indic. for AF and LV thrombus, comb. of warfarin (goal INR 2-2.5) + ASA ↓ D/MI/CVA c/w ASA alone, but ↑ bleeding (WARIS-II, *NEJM* 2002;347:969)

ICD

- If sust. VT/VF >2 d post-MI not due to reversible ischemia
- No benefit solely for EF ≤35% in 1st 40 d after MI (DINAMIT, *NEJM* 2004;351:2481)

Risk factors and lifestyle modifications

- Low chol. (<200 mg/d) & low fat (<7% saturated) diet; LDL goal <70 mg/dl
- BP <140/90 mmHg, <130/80 if diabetes or chronic kidney disease, consider <120/80
- Smoking cessation
- If diabetic, HbA1c <7% (avoid TZDs if CHF)
- Exercise (≥30 mins 3-4 × per wk)
- Weight loss with BMI goal 18.5-24.9 kg/m²
- Influenza vaccination (*Circ* 2006;114:1549)

PA CATHETER AND TAILORED THERAPY

Theoretical considerations

- Cardiac output (CO) = SV × HR; SV depends on LV end-diastolic volume (LVEDV) ∴ manipulate LVEDV to optimize CO while minimizing pulmonary edema
- Balloon at tip of catheter inflated → floats into "wedge" position. Column of blood extends from tip of catheter, through pulmonary circulation, to a point just proximal to LA. Under conditions of no flow, PCWP ≈ LA pressure ≈ LVEDP, which is proportional to LVEDV.
- Situations in which these basic assumptions fail:
  1) Catheter tip not in West lung zone 3 (and ∴ PCWP = alveolar pressure ≠ LA pressure)
  2) PCWP > LA pressure (eg, mediastinal fibrosis, pulmonary veno-occlusive disease)
  3) Mean LA pressure > LVEDP (eg, MR, MS)
  4) Altered LVEDP-LVEDV relationship (ie, abnormal compliance, ∴ normal LVEDP may not be optimal in that Pt)

Indications (JACC 1998;32:840)

- **Diagnosis and evaluation**
  Ddx of shock (cardiogenic vs. distributive) and of pulmonary edema (cardiogenic vs. not)
  Evaluation of CO, intracardiac shunt, pulmonary HTN, MR, cardiac tamponade
- **Therapeutics**
  Tailored therapy to optimize PCWP, SV, S_vO_2 in heart failure/shock
  Guide to vasodilator therapy (eg, inhaled NO, nifedipine) in pulmonary HTN
  Guide to perioperative management in high-risk patients
- **Contraindications**
  Absolute: right-sided endocarditis, thrombus, or mechanical R-sided valve
  Relative: coagulopathy (reverse), recent PPM or ICD (place under fluoroscopy), LBBB (~3% risk of CHB, place under fluoro), bioprosthetic R-sided valve

Efficacy concerns

- No benefit to PAC in high-risk surgery or ARDS (JAMA 2005;294:1664)
- No benefit in decompensated CHF (JAMA 2005;294:1625); untested in cardiogenic shock
- Clinical estim. of CO & PCWP incorrect 1/2 the time (Chest 1991;99:1451), ∴ may use PAC to (a) manage cardiogenic shock, or (b) answer hemodynamic question, then remove

Placement

- Insertion site: **right internal jugular vein** or the **left subclavian vein** to facilitate "anatomic" catheter tip flotation into the pulmonary artery
- **Inflate** the balloon when **advancing** and to **measure PCWP**
- Use resistance to inflation and pressure tracing to avoid overinflation
- **Deflate** the balloon when **withdrawing** and at all other times
- CXR should be obtained after bedside placement to assess for catheter position and PTX
- If catheter cannot be successfully floated (typically if severe TR or RV dilatation) or if another relative contraindication exists, consider fluoroscopic guidance

Complications

- **Central venous access**: pneumo/hemothorax (1-3%), art. puncture, air embolism
- **Catheter advancement**: atrial or ventricular arrhythmias, RBBB (∴ CHB in ~3% of Pts w/ preexisting LBBB), catheter knotting, cardiac perforation and tamponade, PA rupture
- **Catheter maintenance**: infection (especially if catheter left in place for >3 d), thrombus, pulmonary infarction (≤1.3%), PA rupture, balloon rupture

Pressures in relation to respiratory cycle

- Intrathoracic pressure (usually slightly ⊖) is transmitted to vessels and heart
- Transmural pressure (=preload) = measured intracardiac pressure-intrathoracic pressure
- **Always take measurements at end-expiration,** when intrathoracic pressure closest to zero ("high point" in spont. breathing Pts; "low point" in Pts on ⊕ pressure vent.)
- When intrathoracic pressures are ↑ (lung disease, PEEP, auto-PEEP), measured PCWP will overestimate true transmural pressures. Can approximate by subtracting ½ PEEP.

Cardiac output

- **Thermodilution**: saline injected in RA. Δ in temp. over time measured at thermistor (in PA) used to calculate CO. May be inaccurate if low CO, severe TR, or intracardiac shunt.
- **Fick method**: O_2 consumption (L/min) = CO (L/min) × arteriovenous O_2 difference. CO derived by dividing O_2 consumption by observed AV O_2 difference [10×1.34 ml O_2/g Hb × Hb g/dl × ($S_aO_2 - S_vO_2$)]. O_2 consumption commonly estimated by weight-based algorithm. May be inaccurate in distributive shock (sepsis).

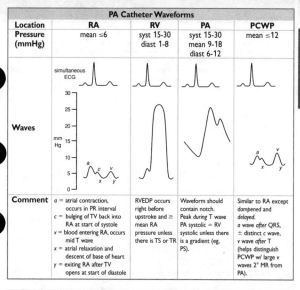

PA Catheter Waveforms				
Location	**RA**	**RV**	**PA**	**PCWP**
Pressure (mmHg)	mean ≤6	syst 15-30 diast 1-8	syst 15-30 mean 9-18 diast 6-12	mean ≤12
Waves				
Comment	a = atrial contraction, occurs in PR interval c = bulging of TV back into RA at start of systole v = blood entering RA, occurs mid T wave x = atrial relaxation and descent of base of heart y = exiting RA after TV opens at start of diastole	RVEDP occurs right before upstroke and ≥ mean RA pressure unless there is TS or TR	Waveform should contain notch. Peak during T wave. PA systolic = RV systolic unless there is a gradient (eg, PS).	Similar to RA except dampened and delayed. a wave after QRS, ≥ distinct c wave, v wave after T (helps distinguish PCWP w/ large v waves 2° MR from PA).

Hemodynamic Profiles of Various Forms of Shock				
Type of shock	**RA** (JVP)	**PCWP** (CXR)	**CO** (UOP)	**SVR** (Cap refill)
Hypovolemic	↓	↓	↓	↑
Cardiogenic	nl or ↑	↑	↓	↑
Septic – hyperdynamic	variable	variable	↑	↓
Septic – hypodynamic	variable	variable	↓	nl or ↑
RV Infarct	↑	nl or ↓	↓	↑
Massive PE	↑	nl or ↓	↓	↑
Tamponade	↑	↑	↓	↑

(Surrogates for hemodynamic parameters shown below parameter in parentheses.)

Tailored therapy
- **Goals**: optimize both MAP and CO while ↓ risk of pulmonary edema
  MAP = CO × SVR; CO = HR × SV (which depends on preload, afterload, and contractility)
  pulmonary edema when PCWP >20-25 (higher levels may be tolerated in chronic CHF)
- **Optimize preload** = LVEDV ≈ LVEDP ≈ LAP ≈ PCWP (NEJM 1973;289:1263)
  in MI, LVEDP of 20-25 optimal → **PCWP of 15-20 optimal** (a wave boosts LVEDP)
  can optimize in individual Pt by measuring SV w/ different PCWP (create Starling curve)
  give NS or diurese (eg, furosemide) to achieve optimal filling pressures
  4% albumin more potent volume expander than NS, but no improvement in mortality, except possibly in severe sepsis (SAFE, NEJM 2004;350:2247)
- **Optimize afterload** = [(peak pressure × radius) / (2 × wall thick.)] and ∴ ∝ MAP & SVR
  if SVR too high (→ ↓ SV & ↓ CO): vasodilators (eg, nitroprusside, NTG, hydral.,ACEI)
  if SVR too low (→ ↓ MAP): vasopressors (eg, norepinephrine [α, β], phenylephrine [α], or vasopressin [V₁] if septic shock or refractory to catecholamines, NEJM 2001;345:588)
- **Optimize contractility** (no direct measure; SV ∝ CO for a given preload & afterload)
  if too low despite optimal preload & afterload: ⊕ inotropes (eg, dobutamine, milrinone)

Early goal-directed therapy in septic shock (in first 6 h; NEJM 2001;345:1368)
- Arterial & central venous lines (no PAC) and measure central venous (not mixed) O₂ sat
- Target CVP 8-12, MAP ≥65, & UOP ≥0.5 ml/kg/h using fluid & vasopressors as needed
- Target S_cvO₂ ≥70% using PRBCs and inotropes (dobutamine)

Definitions (*Braunwald's Heart Disease*, 7th ed., 2004)
- Failure of heart to pump blood forward at sufficient rate to meet metabolic demands of peripheral tissues or ability to do so only at abnormally high cardiac filling pressures
- Low-output (↓ cardiac output) vs. high-output (↑ stroke volume ± ↑ cardiac output)
- Left-sided (pulmonary edema) vs. right-sided (↑ JVP, hepatomegaly, peripheral edema)
- Backward (↑ filling pressures, congestion) vs. forward (impaired systemic perfusion)
- Systolic (inability to expel sufficient blood) vs. diastolic (failure to relax and fill normally)

Figure 1-3 Approach to left-sided heart failure

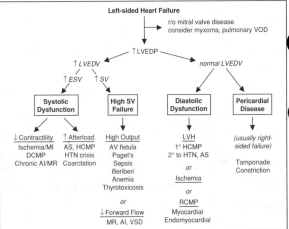

History
- Low output: fatigue, weakness, exercise intolerance, Δ MS, anorexia
- Congestive: left-sided → dyspnea, orthopnea, paroxysmal nocturnal dyspnea
  right-sided → peripheral edema, RUQ discomfort

Functional classification (New York Heart Association)
- Class I: symptomatic only with greater than ordinary activity
- Class II: symptomatic with ordinary activity
- Class III: symptomatic with minimal activity
- Class IV: symptomatic at rest

Physical exam (*JAMA* 2002;287:628)
- Hemodynamic profile
  Congestion ("dry" vs. "wet"):
  ↑ JVP (~80% of the time JVP >10 → PCWP >22; *J Heart Lung Trans* 1999;18:1126)
  ⊕ hepatojugular reflux = >1 cm ↑ in JVP for ≥15 sec with abdominal pressure
    73% Se & 87% Sp for RA >8 and 55% Se & 83% Sp for PCWP >15 (*AJC* 1990; 66:1002)
  Valsalva square wave (↑ SBP thru strain) (*JAMA* 1996;275:630)
  S_3 (in Pts w/ HF → ~40% ↑ risk of HF hosp. or pump failure death; *NEJM* 2001;345:574)
  rales, dullness at base 2° pleural effus. (often absent due to lymphatic compensation)
  ± hepatomegaly, ascites and jaundice, peripheral edema
  Perfusion ("warm" vs. "cold"):
  narrow pulse pressure (<25% of SBP), cool & pale extremities, ↓ UOP, muscle atrophy
- Other signs: ± Cheyne-Stokes respirations, abnormal PMI (diffuse, sustained, or lifting depending on cause of heart failure), ± S_4 (diastolic dysfunction), ± murmurs (valvular disease, distorted MV annulus, displaced papillary muscles)

Evaluation for the presence of heart failure
- CXR: pulm edema, pleural effusions (usually R > L), ± cardiomegaly, Kerley B-lines
- Natriuretic peptides (BNP & NT-proBNP) to exclude HF as cause of dyspnea (see "Dyspnea"); also to predict risk of rehosp. (*Circ* 2003;107:1278)
- Evidence of ↓ perfusion to vital organs: ↑ BUN, ↑ Cr, ↓ serum Na, abnormal LFTs
- Echocardiogram: ↓ EF and ↑ chamber size → systolic dysfxn
  hypertrophy, abnormal MV inflow, tissue Doppler abnormalities → ? diastolic dysfxn
  valvular abnormalities; pericardial abnormalities
- PA catheterization: ↑ PCWP, ↓ CO and ↑ SVR (low-output failure)

Evaluation of the causes of heart failure
- ECG: evidence for CAD, LVH, LAE, heart block (? infiltrative CMP), low voltages (? DCMP)
- Coronary angiography (or ? CT coronary angiography)
- If no CAD, w/u for nonischemic DCMP, HCMP, or RCMP (see "Cardiomyopathies")

Treatment of Chronic Heart Failure	
Diet, exercise	Na <2g/d, fluid restriction, exercise training in ambulatory Pts
ACEI	40% ↓ mort. in NYHA IV (CONSENSUS, *NEJM* 1987;316:1429) 16% ↓ mort. in NYHA II/III (SOLVD-T, *NEJM* 1991;325:293) 20% ↓ mort. in asx, post-MI, EF ≤40% (SAVE, *NEJM* 1992;327:669) 20% ↓ reMI; 20-30% ↓ rehosp for HF (↑ amt of benefit w/ ↓ EF) 30% ↓ HF in asx Pts w/ EF ≤35% (SOLVD-P, *NEJM* 1992;327:685) High-dose ACEI (>30 mg/d of lisinopril) more efficacious than low-dose (<5 mg/d) (ATLAS, *Circ* 1999;100:2312) Watch for azotemia, ↑ K (can ameliorate by low-K diet, diuretics, kayexalate), cough, angioedema
ATII receptor blockers (ARBs)	*Consider in Pts with ↓ EF and sx, in addition to ACEI or as alternative if cannot tolerate ACEI (eg, b/c cough)* Non-inferior to ACEI (VALIANT, *NEJM* 2003;349:1893) Good alternative if ACEI intol (CHARM-Alternative, *Lancet* 2003;362:772) 25% ↓ HF (Val-HeFT, *NEJM* 2001;345:1667) and 15% ↓ mort. when added to ACEI (CHARM-Added, *Lancet* 2003;362:767)
Hydralazine + nitrates	*Consider if cannot tolerate ACEI/ARB or in blacks w/ Class III/IV* 25% ↓ mort. c/w placebo (V-HeFT I, *NEJM* 1986;314:1547) Inferior to ACEI (V-HeFT II, *NEJM* 1991;325:303) 40% ↓ mort. in blacks on standard Rx (A-HeFT, *NEJM* 2004;351:2049)
β-blocker (data for carvedilol, metoprolol, bisoprolol)	*EF will transiently ↓, then ↑. Contraindic in decompensated HF.* 35% ↓ mort. & 40% ↓ rehosp. in NYHA II-IV (*JAMA* 2002;287:883) Carvedilol superior to metoprolol tartrate (COMET, *Lancet* 2003;362:7)
Aldosterone antagonists	*Consider if HF severe or post-MI, adeq. renal fxn; watch for ↑ K* 30% ↓ mort. in NYHA III/IV & EF ≤35% (RALES, *NEJM* 1999;341:709) 15% ↓ mort. in post-MI, EF ≤40% (EPHESUS, *NEJM* 2003;348:1309)
Biventricular pacing	*Consider if refractory HF, EF ≤35%, and QRS ≥120 ms, and especially if also evid. of dyssynchrony on echocardiography* 36% ↓ mortality and improved EF (CARE-HF, *NEJM* 2005;352:1539)
ICD	*Consider in 1° prevention if ↓ EF or for 2° prevention* ↓ mort. in Pts w/ MI & EF ≤ 30% (MADIT II, *NEJM* 2002;346:877) (but no Δ mort. 6-40 d post-MI; DINAMIT, *NEJM* 2004;351:2481) 23% ↓ mort. in all DCMP, EF ≤35% (SCD-HeFT, *NEJM* 2005;352:225) ↓ arrhythmic death in nonisch DCMP (DEFINITE, *NEJM* 2004;350:2151)
Diuretics	Loop ± thiazides diuretics (sx relief; no mortality benefit)
Digoxin	23% ↓ HF hosp., no Δ mortality (DIG Trial, *NEJM* 1997;336:525) ? ↑ mort. in women, ? related to ↑ levels (*NEJM* 2002;347:1403) ? optimal dig concentration 0.5-0.8 ng/ml (*JAMA* 2003;289:871)
Anticoagulation	*Consider if AF, LV thrombus, large akinetic LV segment, EF <30%*
Restoration of sinus rhythm	Catheter ablation of AF → 21% ↑ in EF, improvement in sx, exercise capacity, & QoL (*NEJM* 2004;351:2373)

(*Circ* 2002;105:2099, 2223; *NEJM* 2003;348:2007)

Recommended Therapy by CHF Stage			
Stage (Not NYHA Class)		**Pt Characteristics**	**Therapy**
A	High risk for HF ⊖ Structural heart dz Asx	HTN, DM, CAD Cardiotoxin exposure FHx of CMP	Treat HTN, lipids, DM, SVT D/c smoking, EtOH Encourage exercise ACEI if HTN, DM, CVD, PAD
B	⊕ Structural heart dz Asx	Prior MI, ↓ EF, LVH Or Asx valvular dz	All measures for stage A ACEI & βB if MI/CAD or ↓ EF
C	⊕ Structural heart dz ⊕ Symptoms of HF (prior or current)	Overt HF	All measures for stage A ACEI, βB, diuretics, Na restrict Consider aldactone, ICD, BiV Consider nitrate/hydral, digoxin
D	Refractory HF requiring specialized interventions	Sx despite maximal medical Rx	All measures for stage A-C Mechanical assist devices Transplant, IV inotropes

(*JACC* 2005;46:e1)

Precipitants of acute heart failure
- **Myocardial ischemia or infarction**
- **Renal failure** (acute, progression of CKD, or insufficient dialysis) → ↑ preload
- **Hypertensive crisis** (incl. from RAS), worsening AS → ↑ L-sided afterload
- **Dietary indiscretion** or medical **noncompliance**
- **Drugs** (βB, CCB, NSAIDs, TZDs) or **toxins** (EtOH, anthracyclines)
- Myocarditis, infective endocarditis, arrhythmias
- COPD or PE → ↑ R-sided afterload
- Anemia, systemic infection, thyroid disease

Treatment of acute pulmonary edema (LMNOP)
- **L**asix
- **M**orphine (↓ sx of dyspnea + venodilator + afterload reduction)
- **N**itrates (venodilator)
- **O**xygen & non-invasive ventilation (↓ mort.; *JAMA* 2005;294:3124; *Lancet* 2006;367:1155)
- **P**osition (sit Pt up & have legs dangling over side of bed → ↓ preload)

Treatment of advanced heart failure (*JAMA* 2002;287:628)
- Tailored Rx w/ PA catheter (qv): goals of MAP >60, CI >2.2, SVR <800, PCWP <18
- **IV vasodilators**: NTG, nitroprusside (risk of coronary steal in Pts w/ CAD) nesiritide ↓ PCWP & sx (*JAMA* 2002;287:1531), but may ↑ Cr & mortality (*JAMA* 2005;293:1900)
- **Inotropes** (properties in addition to ↑ inotropy listed below) dobutamine: vasodilation at doses ≤5 μg/kg/min; mild ↓ PVR; desensitization over time dopamine: splanchnic vasodil. → ↑ GFR & natriuresis; vasoconstrict. at ≥5 μg/kg/min milrinone: prominent systemic & pulmonary vasodilation; ↓ dose by 50% in renal failure
- **Ultrafiltration**: ~1 L greater fluid loss at 48 h and ~50% ↓ in rehosp. (*JACC* 2007;49:675)
- **Mechanical circulatory support** intraaortic balloon pump (IABP): ↓ afterload & ↑ coronary perfusion ventricular assist device (LVAD): can use as a bridge to transplantation; as destination therapy (48% ↓ mort. c/w med Rx; REMATCH, *NEJM* 2001;345:1435), or possibly as platform for recovery (*NEJM* 2006;355:1873); percutaneous VAD under study
- Cardiac transplantation: 15-20% mort. in 1st year, median survival 10 y

Heart failure with preserved EF (*Circ* 2002;105:1387, 1503 & 2003;107:659; *NEJM* 2004;351:1097)
- 40-60% of Pts w/ HF have normal or only min. impaired systolic fxn (EF ≥40%) (*NEJM* 2006;355:251, 260). Mortality rates similar to those w/ systolic dysfxn.
- ~30% of population over age 45 w/ diastolic dysfxn on echo, ~20% mild, <10% mod/sev, but only 50% of severe and 5% of moderate cases were symptomatic (*JAMA* 2003;289:194)
- Etiologies causes of impaired relaxation: ischemia, LVH, HCMP, aging, hypothyroidism causes of ↑ passive stiffness: prior MI, LVH, RCMP
- Diagnosis: clinical s/s of HF w/ preserved systolic *and* impaired diastolic fxn: abnormal MV inflow: E/A reversal and Δs in E wave deceleration time ↓ myocardial relax.: ↑ isovolumic relax. time and ↓ early diastole tissue Doppler velocity LV hypertrophy, LA dilatation
- Treatment: diuresis for volume overload, Na/fluid restriction HR & BP control w/ βB, CCB, ACEI, ARB (↓ rehosp., CHARM-Preserved, *Lancet* 2003;362:777) relief of ischemia, statins

CARDIOMYOPATHIES

Diseases with mechanical and/or electrical dysfunction of the myocardium

DILATED CARDIOMYOPATHY (DCMP)

Definition and epidemiology (Circ 2006;113:1807)
- Ventricular dilatation, normal to ↓ wall thickness, and ↓ contractility
- Incidence: 5-8 cases/100,000 population per y; prevalence: 1 in 2500

Etiologies (NEJM 1994;331:1564 & 2000;342:1077)
- **Ischemia:** systolic dysfxn & dilation out of proportion to CAD (poor remodeling post-MI)
- **Valvular disease:** systolic dysfxn due to chronic volume overload in MR & AI
- **Familial** (~25%): mutations in cytoskeletal, nuclear, and filament proteins
- **Idiopathic** (~25% of DCMP, ? undiagnosed infectious, alcoholic, or genetic cause)
- **Infectious myocarditis** (10-15%, often due to immune rxn to infxn; NEJM 2000;343:1388)
  Viruses (coxsackie, adeno, echovirus, CMV): subacute (dilated LV w/ mod dysfxn) to fulminant (nondilated, thickened, edematous LV w/ severe dysfxn)
  Bacterial, fungal, rickettsial, TB, Lyme (mild myocarditis, often with AVB)
  HIV: ~8% of asx HIV ⊕; due to HIV vs. other viruses vs. meds (NEJM 1998;339:1093)
  Chagas: apical aneurysm ± thrombus, RBBB, megaesophagus or colon (NEJM 1993;329:639)
- **Toxic**
  Alcohol (5%) typically 7-8 drinks/d × >5 y, but much interindividual variability
  Anthracyclines (risk ↑ as dose >550 mg/m^2, may manifest late); cyclophosphamide
  Cocaine, antiretrovirals, lead, CO, radiation
- **Infiltrative** (5%): often mix of DCMP + RCMP (qv) with thickened wall, amyloidosis, sarcoidosis, hemochromatosis
- **Autoimmune**
  Collagen vascular disease (3%): polymyositis, SLE, scleroderma, PAN, RA, Wegener's
  Peripartum (last month → 5 mos postpartum): <0.1% of preg.; ↑ risk w/ multiparity & ↑ age; ~50% will improve; ? ↑ risk w/ next preg. (JAMA 2000;283:1183)
  Idiopathic giant cell: avg age 42 y, fulminant myocarditis, VT (NEJM 1997;336:1860)
  Eosinophilic (variable peripheral eosinophilia): hypersensitivity (mild CHF) or acute necrotizing (STE, effusion, severe CHF)
- **Stress-induced** ("Takotsubo," apical ballooning): mimics MI with pain, ± STE, ± ↑ Tn; deep TWI & ↑ QT; mid/apical dyskinesis; usually improve over 1-2 wks (NEJM 2005;352:539)
- **Tachycardia-induced:** likelihood proportional to rate and duration
- **Metabolic & other:** hypothyroidism, acromegaly, pheo, thiamine, sleep apnea

Clinical manifestations
- **Heart failure:** both congestive & poor forward flow sx; signs of L- & R-sided HF
  diffuse, lat.-displaced PMI, S$_3$, ± MR or TR (annular dilat., displaced pap. muscle)
  Embolic events (~10%), arrhythmias & palpitations
  Chest pain on exertion seen in up to one-third (even with no CAD)

Diagnostic studies and workup
- CXR: moderate to marked cardiomegaly, ± pulmonary edema & pleural effusions
- ECG: may see PRWP, Q waves, or BBB; low voltage; AF (20%)
- Echocardiogram: LV dilatation, ↓ EF, regional or global LV HK, ± RV HK, ± mural thrombi
- Laboratory evaluation: TFTs, iron studies, HIV, SPEP, ANA; others per clinical suspicion
- Stress test: completely ⊖ test useful to r/o ischemic etiology (low false ⊖ rate), but ⊕ test does not rule in ischemic etiology (high false ⊕ rate, even w/ imaging)
- Coronary angiography to r/o CAD if risk factors, h/o angina, Qw MI on ECG, equivocal ETT
- ? Endomyocardial biopsy (Circ 1989;79:971; Clin Res Card 2006;95:569)
  yield 10% (of these, 75% show myocarditis, 25% show evidence of systemic disease)
  40% false ⊖ rate (patchy disease) and false ⊕ (necrosis → inflammation)
  no proven Rx for myocarditis; ∴ biopsy for prognosis or if suspect systemic disease
- Cardiac MRI: detect myocarditis or infiltrative disease, but nonspecific (EHJ 2005;26:1461)

Treatment
- Standard HF therapy (see "Heart Failure")
- Implantation of devices may be tempered by possibility of reversibility of CMP
- Immunosuppression: used for giant-cell myocarditis (prednisone + AZA), collagen vascular disease, peripartum (? IVIg), and eosinophilic; no proven benefit for viral myocarditis

HYPERTROPHIC CARDIOMYOPATHY (HCMP)

Definition and epidemiology
- LV (usually ≥15 mm) and/or RV hypertrophy disproportionate to hemodynamic load
- Prevalence: 1 case/500 population; 50% sporadic, 50% familial
- Differentiate from 2° LVH: hypertension (espec. elderly women; *NEJM* 1985;312:277), AS, elite athletes (wall thickness usually <13 mm & symmetric and nl/↑ rates of tissue Doppler diastolic relaxation; *NEJM* 1991;324:295)

Pathology
- Autosomal dominant mutations in genes encoding cardiac sarcomere proteins
- Myocardial fiber disarray with hypertrophy
- Morphologic hypertrophy variants: asymmetric septal; concentric; mid-cavity; apical

Pathophysiology
- Subaortic outflow obstruction: narrowed tract 2° hypertrophied septum + systolic anterior motion (SAM) of ant. MV leaflet 2° Venturi forces (may be fixed, variable, or nonexistent) and papillary muscle displacement. Gradient (∇) worse w/ ↑ contractility (digoxin, β-agonists), ↓ preload, or ↓ afterload.
- Mitral regurgitation: due to SAM (mid-to-late, post.-directed regurg. jet) and abnormal mitral leaflets and papillary muscles (pansystolic, ant.-directed regurg. jet)
- Diastolic dysfunction: ↑ chamber stiffness + impaired relaxation
- Ischemia: small vessel dz, perforating artery compression (bridging), ↓ coronary perfusion
- Syncope: Δs in load-dependent CO, arrhythmias

Clinical manifestations (70% are asymptomatic at dx)
- **Dyspnea** (90%): due to ↑ LVEDP, MR, and diastolic dysfunction
- **Angina** (25%) even in absence of epicardial CAD; microvasc. dysfxn (*NEJM* 2003;349:1027)
- **Arrhythmias** (AF in 20-25%; VT/VF) → palpitations, syncope, sudden cardiac death

Physical exam
- Sustained PMI, S_2 paradox. split if severe outflow obstruction, ⊕ S_4 (occ. palpable)
- **Systolic crescendo-decrescendo murmur** at LLSB: ↑ w/ **Valsalva** & standing
- ± mid-to-late or holosystolic murmur of MR at apex
- Bisferiens carotid pulse (brisk rise, decline, then 2nd rise); JVP w/ prominent *a* wave
- Contrast to AS, which has murmur that ↓ w/ Valsalva and ↓ carotid pulses

Diagnostic studies
- CXR: cardiomegaly (LV and LA)
- ECG: LVH, anterolateral and inferior pseudo-Qw, ± apical giant TWI (apical variant)
- **Echocardiogram**: no absolute cutoffs for degree of LVH but $\frac{septum}{post\ wall} \geq 1.3$ suggestive

  as is septum >15 mm; other findings include dynamic outflow obstruction, SAM, MR
- Cardiac cath: subaortic pressure ∇; *Brockenbrough sign* = ↓ pulse press. postextrasystole (in contrast to AS, in which pulse pressure ↑ postextrasystole)
- Annual echo, 48-h Holter, & exercise testing for risk stratification once dx is made

Treatment (*NEJM* 2004;350:1320)
- Heart failure
  - ⊖ **inotropes/chronotropes**: β-blockers, CCB (verapamil), disopyramide. Careful use of diuretics. Vasodilators only if systolic dysfxn. Avoid digoxin.
  If refractory to drug therapy and there is *obstructive* physiology (∇ >50 mmHg):
  a) Alcohol septal ablation (*NEJM* 2002;347:1326)
     triphasic ∇ response: acute ↓ → ± partial ↑ back to 50% of baseline → ↓ over mos by 6-12 mos achieve resting ∇ ~16 mmHg & stress-induced ∇ ~45 mmHg
     complications: RBBB; transient 3° AVB w/ 10-20% req. PPM; VT
  b) Surgical myotomy-myectomy: long-term sx improvement in 90% (*Circ* 2005;112:482)
  c) ? Dual-chamber pacing, but large placebo effect (*JACC* 1997;29:435; *Circ* 1999; 99:2927)
  If refractory to drug therapy and there is *nonobstructive* pathophysiology: transplant
- AF: rate control with β-blockers, maintain SR with disopyramide, amiodarone, sotalol
- Sudden cardiac death: ICD (*JACC* 2003;42:1687). Major risk factors include history of VT/VF; ⊕ FHx SCD, unexplained syncope, NSVT, hypotension w/ exercise, LV wall ≥30 mm; ∇ ≥30 mmHg; high-risk mutations
- Counsel to avoid dehydration, extreme exertion
- Endocarditis prophylaxis
- First-degree relatives: periodic screening w/ echo (as timing of HCMP onset variable)

RESTRICTIVE CARDIOMYOPATHY (RCMP)

Definition
- Impaired ventricular filling due to ↓ compliance

Etiology (NEJM 1997;336:267)
- **Myocardial processes**
  autoimmune (scleroderma, polymyositis-dermatomyositis)
  infiltrative diseases (see primary entries for extracardiac manifestations, Dx, Rx)
    amyloidosis: age at present. ~60 y; male:female = 3:2
      AL (MM, light-chain disease, WM); familial (transthyretin, TTR); senile (TTR, ANP)
      ECG: ↓ QRS amplitude (70%), pseudoinfarction pattern (Qw), AVB (10-20%),
        hemiblock (20%), BBB (5-20%)
      Echo: biventricular hypertrophy, granular sparkling texture (65%), biatrial
        enlargement, valve thickening (65%), small effusion
      normal voltage & normal septal thickness has NPV ~90%
    sarcoidosis: age at present. ~30 y; more common in blacks, N. Europeans, women
      5% of those with sarcoid w/ overt cardiac involvement; cardiac w/o systemic in 10%
      ECG: AVB (75%), RBBB (20-60%), VT
      Echo: regional WMA (particularly basal septum) with thinning or mild hypertrophy
      nuclear imaging: gallium uptake in areas of sestaMIBI perfusion defects
    hemochromatosis: presents in middle-aged men (particularly N. European)
  storage diseases (Gaucher's, Fabry's, Hurler's, glycogen storage diseases)
  diabetes mellitus
  idiopathic fibrosis
- **Endomyocardial processes**
  chronic eosinophilic: Löffler's endocarditis (temperate climates; ↑ eos.; mural thrombi
    that embolize); endomyocardial fibrosis (tropical climates; var. eos.; mural thrombi)
  toxins (radiation, anthracyclines)
  serotonin (carcinoid, serotonin agonists, ergot alkaloids)
  metastatic cancer

Pathology & pathophysiology
- Normal or ↑ wall thickness ± infiltration or abnormal deposition
- ↓ myocardial compliance → nl EDV but ↑ EDP → ↑ systemic & pulm. venous pressures
- ↓ ventricular cavity size → ↓ SV and ↓ CO

Clinical manifestations
- **Right-sided > left-sided heart failure** with peripheral edema > dyspnea
- **Diuretic "refractoriness"**
- **Thromboembolic events**
- Poorly tolerated tachyarrhythmias

Physical exam
- ↑ JVP, ± Kussmaul's sign (classically seen in *constrictive pericarditis*)
- Cardiac: ± S₃ and S₄, ± murmurs of MR and TR
- Congestive hepatomegaly, ± ascites and jaundice, peripheral edema

Diagnostic studies
- CXR: normal ventricular chamber size, enlarged atria, ± pulmonary congestion
- ECG: low voltage, pseudoinfarction pattern (Qw), ± arrhythmias
- Echo: symmetric wall thickening, biatrial enlarge., ± mural thrombi, ± cavity obliteration
    diastolic dysfxn: ↑ early diastolic (E) and ↓ late atrial (A) filling, ↑ E/A ratio, ↓ decel. time
- Cardiac MRI: may reveal inflammation or evidence of infiltration (although nonspecific)
- Cardiac catheterization
  atria: **M's** or **W's** (prominent x and y descents)
  ventricles: **dip & plateau** (rapid ↓ pressure at onset of diastole, rapid ↑ to early plateau)
    concordance of LV and RV pressure peaks during respiratory cycle (vs. discordance in
    constrictive pericarditis; Circ 1996;93:2007)
- Endomyocardial biopsy if suspect infiltrative process
- Restrictive cardiomyopathy vs. constrictive pericarditis: see "Pericardial Disease"

Treatment (in addition to Rx'ing underlying disease)
- Gentle diuresis
- Control HR and maintain SR (important for filling). Dig pro-arrhythmic in amyloid.
- Anticoagulation (particularly with AF or low CO)
- Transplantation for refractory cases

VALVULAR HEART DISEASE

AORTIC STENOSIS (AS)

Etiology
- **Calcific:** predominant cause in Pts >70 y; risk factors include HTN and ↑ chol.
- **Congenital heart disease** (ie, bicuspid AoV): cause in 50% of Pts <70 y
- **Rheumatic heart disease** (AS usually accompanied by AI and usually w/ MV disease)
- AS mimickers: hypertrophic obstructive CMP; subAo membrane

Clinical manifestations (usually indicates AVA <1 cm² or concomitant CAD)
- **Angina:** ↑ O_2 demand (hypertrophy) + ↓ O_2 supply (↓ cor perfusion pressure) ± CAD
- **Syncope** (*exertional*): peripheral vasodil. w/ fixed CO → ↓ MAP → ↓ cerebral perfusion
- **Heart failure:** dyspnea due to pulmonary edema; can be precip. by AF (loss of LV filling)
- Acquired von Willebrand disease (~20% of sev. AS): destruction of vWF (*NEJM 2003;349:343*)

Physical examination
- High-pitched, **mid-systolic crescendo-decrescendo murmur** at RUSB
  radiates to sternal notch, carotids, apex (often holosystolic = Gallavardin effect)
  ↑ w/ passive leg raise, ↓ w/ standing & Valsalva, but not specific
- In contrast, dynamic outflow obstruction ↓ w/ passive leg raise & ↑ w/ standing & Valsalva
- Ejection click sometimes heard with *bicuspid* AoV
- Signs of severity: *late-peaking* murmur, paradoxically split S_2 or inaudible A_2, small and
  delayed carotid pulse ("*pulsus parvus et tardus*"), LV heave, ⊕ S_4 (occasionally palpable)

Diagnostic studies
- ECG: LVH, LAE, LBBB
- CXR: cardiomegaly, post-stenotic dilation of Ao, AoV calcif., pulmonary congestion
- **Echo:** valve morphology, estimated pressure gradient (∇), calculated AVA, EF
- **Cardiac catheterization:** ∇ from simultaneous LV & Ao pressures, calculated AVA,
  but primarily to *r/o concomitant CAD* (seen in ~50% of calcific AS)
- **Dobutamine challenge** during echo or cath if low EF and ∇ <30 to differentiate:
  afterload mismatch (↑ SV & ↑ ∇; implies good contractile reserve & ↑ EF post-AVR) vs.
  pseudostenosis (↑ SV, no change in ∇, ↑ AVA; implies low AVA artifact of LV dysfxn) vs.
  fixed CMP (no change in SV, ∇, or AVA; implies EF prob. will not improve w/ AVR)

Classification of Aortic Stenosis				
Stage	Mean Gradient (mmHg)	Jet Vel. (m/s)	AVA (cm²)	LVEF
Normal	0	1	3-4	normal
Mild	<25	<3	1.5-2	normal
Moderate	25-40	3-4	1.0-1.5	normal
Severe, compensated	>40	4	<1.0	normal
Severe, decompensated	Variable	Variable	<1.0	↓

Treatment (*JACC 2006;48:e1*)
- **AVR: symptomatic AS** (almost invariably severe; if not look for another cause of sx)
  asx sev. AS + EF <50%; also consider if *asx sev. AS and AVA <0.6 cm²*, **mean
  gradient >60 mmHg, aortic jet >5 m/s, ↓ BP w/ exercise** (can *carefully* exercise
  asx AS to uncover sx, do *not* exercise sx AS), **or high likelihood of rapid prog.**
  asymptomatic mod.-sev. AS *and* undergoing CABG, valvular or aortic surgery
- Medical therapy: used in symptomatic Pts who are not operative candidates
  careful diuresis, control HTN, maint. SR; dig; ? statin (*NEJM 2005;352:2389; JACC 2007;49:554*)
  avoid venodilators (nitrates) and ⊖ inotropes (β-blockers & CCB) in severe AS
  nitroprusside if sev. AS, EF <35%, CHF w/ CI <2.2, but normotensive (*NEJM 2003; 348:1756*)
- IABP: stabilization, bridge to surgery
- Balloon valvuloplasty: 50% ↑ in AVA & 50% ↓ peak ∇, *but* 50% restenosis by 6-12 mos &
  risk of peri-PAV stroke (*NEJM 1988;319:125*), ∴ use as bridge to AVR or if not surgical cand.
- Percutaneous AVR remains under study (*Circ 2006;114:1616*)
- Endocarditis prophylaxis; avoid vigorous physical exertion once AS moderate-severe

Natural history (*Circulation 1968;38(Suppl.V):61*)
- Usually *slowly progressive* until symptoms develop
- Echo q1-2 y if mod., q3-5 y if mild, or if Δ sx
- AVA ↓ ~0.1 cm² per y (*Circ 1997;95:2262*), but marked interindividual variability
- Angina → 5 y mean survival; syncope → 3 y mean survival; CHF → 2 y mean survival

AORTIC INSUFFICIENCY (AI)

Etiology
- **Valve disease**
  rheumatic heart disease (usually mixed AS/AI and concomitant MV disease)
  bicuspid AoV: natural hx: 1/3 → normal, 1/3 → AS, 1/6 → AI, 1/6 → endocarditis → AI
  infective endocarditis
  valvulitis: RA, SLE
  amphet. & DA agonists that stimulate 5-HT receptors (*NEJM* 1998;339:719 & 2007;356:29, 39)
- **Root disease**
  HTN
  aortic aneurysm or dissection, annuloaortic ectasia, Marfan syndrome
  aortic inflammation: giant cell, Takayasu's, ankylosing spond., reactive arthritis, syphilis

Clinical manifestations
- Acute: sudden ↓ forward SV and ↑ LVEDP (noncompliant ventricle) → pulmonary edema
  ± hypotension and cardiogenic shock
- Chronic: clinically silent while LV dilates (↑ compliance to keep LVEDP low) → chronic
  volume overload → LV decompensation → CHF

Physical examination
- **Early diastolic decrescendo murmur at LUSB** (RUSB if dilated aortic root)
  ↑ with sitting forward, expiration, handgrip
  severity of AI proportional to duration of murmur (except in acute and severe late)
  Austin Flint murmur: diastolic rumble at apex (AI jet interfering w/ mitral inflow)
- **Wide pulse pressure** due to ↑ stroke volume → many of classic signs (see table)
  (pulse pressure narrows in late AI with ↓ LV function)
- PMI diffuse and laterally displaced; soft S_1, (early closure of MV); ⊕ S_3 (≠ ↓ EF in AI)
- Bisferiens (twice-beating) arterial pulse

Classic Eponymous Signs in Chronic AI	
Sign	**Description**
Corrigan's pulse	"water hammer" pulse (ie, rapid rise and fall or collapsing)
Hill's sign	(popliteal SBP - brachial SBP) >60 mmHg
Duroziez's sign	gradual pressure over femoral artery → systolic and diastolic bruits
Traube's sound	double sound heard at femoral artery when compressed distally
de Musset's sign	head-bobbing with each heartbeat (low Se)
Müller's sign	systolic pulsations of the uvula
Quincke's pulses	subungual capillary pulsations (low Sp)

(*Southern Medical Journal* 1981;74:459)

Diagnostic studies
- ECG: LVH, LAD; CXR: cardiomegaly ± aortic dilatation
- **Echocardiogram**: severity of AI (severe AI = width of regurgitant jet >65% LVOT or
  presence of flow reversal in descending aorta) and LV size & fxn
- Cardiac MRI (severity of AI, aortic root size, LV size & fxn); aortography (severity of AI)

Treatment (*NEJM* 2004;351:1539; *JACC* 2006;48:e1)
- **Surgery (AVR)**
  symptomatic severe AI (if AI *not* severe, unlikely to be cause of sx)
  asx severe AI *and* **EF <50%** or **LV dilation** (syst. diam. >55 mm or diast. diam.
  >75 mm) or undergoing cardiac surgery
- Medical therapy: **vasodilators** (nifedipine, ACEI, hydralazine) if severe AI w/ sx or LV
  dysfxn & Pt not operative cand.; benefit in asx severe AI w/ nl LV fxn controversial
  (*NEJM* 1994;331:689 & 2005;353:1342); diuretics and digoxin if CHF
- Acute decompensation (consider ischemia and endocarditis as possible precipitants)
  IV afterload reduction (nitroprusside) and inotropic support (dobutamine)
  ± chronotropic support (↑ HR → ↓ diastole → ↓ time for regurgitation)
  pure vasoconstrictors and IABP contraindicated
  surgery usually needed for acute severe AI which is poorly tolerated by LV

Natural history
- *Variable* progression (unlike AS, can be fast or slow)
- Once decompensation begins, prognosis poor w/o AVR (mortality ~10%/y)

MITRAL STENOSIS (MS)

Etiology
- **Rheumatic heart disease** (RHD): *fusion of the commissures* → "fish mouth" valve due to autoimmune rxn to beta strep infxn; seen largely in developing world today
- Functional MS due to severe mitral annular calcific. (MAC) → encroachment upon leaflets
- Congenital, myxoma, thrombus, large endocarditis lesions
- Valvulitis (eg, SLE, amyloid, carcinoid) or infiltration (eg, mucopolysaccharidoses)

Clinical manifestations
- **Dyspnea** and **pulmonary edema** (if due to RHD, sx usually begin in 30's) precipitants: tachycardia, volume overload (incl. pregnancy), AF, fever, anemia
- **Atrial fibrillation**: often precipitates heart failure in Pts w/ MS
- **Embolic events** (especially in atrial fibrillation or endocarditis)
- Pulmonary symptoms: hemoptysis, frequent bronchitis (due to congestion), PHT

Physical examination
- **Low-pitched mid-diastolic rumble at apex** w/ presystolic accentuation (if not in AF) appreciated best when Pt in left lateral decubitus position, ↑ w/ exercise severity of MS proportional to *duration* of murmur (not intensity)
- **Opening snap** (high-pitched early diastolic sound at left sternal border and apex) MVA proportional to S_2-OS interval (tighter valve → ↑ LA pressure → shorter interval)
- Loud S_1 (unless MV calcified), occasionally palpable

Diagnostic studies
- ECG: **LAE** ("P mitrale"), ± atrial fibrillation, ± RVH
- CXR: **dilated left atrium** (straightening of left heart border, double density on right, left mainstem bronchus elevation)
- **Echo**: estimated pressure gradients (∇), RVSP, calculated valve area, valve echo score (based on leaflet mobility, leaflet thickening, subvalvular thickening, calcification); exercise TTE if discrepancy between sx and severity of MS at rest; TEE to assess for LA thrombus before percutaneous valvuloplasty
- **Cardiac cath**: ∇ from simultaneous PCWP & LV pressures, calculated MVA (Gorlin formula); LA pressure tall *a* wave and blunted *y* descent; ↑ PA pressures

Classification of Mitral Stenosis			
Stage	Mean gradient (mmHg)	MV area (cm^2)	PA Systolic (mmHg)
Normal	0	4-6	<25
Mild	<5	1.5-2	<30
Moderate	5-10	1-1.5	30-50
Severe	>10	<1	>50

Treatment (*Circ* 2005;112:432; *JACC* 2006;48:e1)
- Medical: Na restriction, cautious diuresis, β-blockers
- Anticoagulation if AF, prior embolism, LA thrombus, or large LA
- Indications for mechanical intervention: heart failure sx w/ MVA ≤1.5 or heart failure sx w/ MVA >1.5 but ↑ PASP, PCWP, or MV ∇ w/ exercise, or asx Pts w/ MVA ≤1.5 and PHT (PASP >50 mmHg or >60 mmHg w/ exercise), or ? new onset AF
- **Percutaneous mitral valvuloplasty** (PMV): preferred Rx if RHD; MVA doubles, ∇ ↓ by 50%; ≈MVR if valve score <8, ≤mild MR, Ø AF or LA clot (*NEJM* 1994;331:961; *Circ* 2002;105:1465)
- Surgical (MV repair if possible, o/w replacement): consider in sx Pts w/ MVA ≤1.5 if PMV not available or valve morphology not suitable

MITRAL REGURGITATION (MR)

Etiology
- **Leaflet abnormalities**: **myxomatous degeneration (MVP)**, **endocarditis**, **rheumatic heart disease**, valvulitis (collagen-vascular disease), congenital, trauma
- **Ruptured chordae tendinae**: myxomatous, spontaneous, endocarditis, trauma
- **Papillary muscle dysfunction**: ischemia/MI (usually *posteromedial* papillary m. b/c supplied by PDA alone while anterolateral papillary m. supplied by diags. & OMs), displacement due to CMP, infiltration
- **Annulus**: any cause of LV dilatation; calcific. (typically seen w/ HTN, ↑ chol., DM, CKD)
- HCMP (see "Cardiomyopathy")

Clinical manifestations
- Acute: **pulmonary edema**, hypotension, cardiogenic shock (NEJM 2004;351:1627)
- Chronic: typically asx for y, then as LV fails → progressive DOE, fatigue, AF, PHT

Physical examination
- **High-pitched, blowing, holosystolic murmur** at apex; radiates to axilla; ± thrill
  ↑ w/ handgrip (Se 68%, Sp 92%), ↓ w/ Valsalva (Se 93%) (NEJM 1988;318:1572)
  ant. leaflet abnl → post. jet heard at spine; post. leaflet abnl → ant. jet at sternum
- Lat. displ. hyperdynamic PMI, obscured S_1, widely split S_2 (A_2 early b/c ↓ afterload); ± S_3
- Carotid upstroke brisk (vs. in AS where it is diminished and delayed)

Diagnostic studies
- ECG: LAE, LVH, ± atrial fibrillation
- CXR: dilated LA, dilated LV, ± pulmonary congestion
- **Echocardiogram**: MV anatomy (ie, cause of MR), degree of MR via jet area (can underestimate eccentric jets), jet at origin ("vena contracta"), or effective regurgitant orifice (ERO; predicts survival, NEJM 2005;352:875), and LV function (EF supranormal in compensated states, ∴ EF <60% with severe MR = LV impairment)
  TEE used if TTE inconclusive or pre/intra-op to assess prob. of repair vs. replacement
- **Cardiac cath**: prominent PCWP cv waves (not spec. for MR), LVgram for MR severity & EF

Classification of Mitral Regurgitation				
Severity	Regurg fraction	Jet Area (% of LA)	Jet width (cm)	ERO (cm²)	Angio (see footnote)
Mild	<30%	<20	<0.3	<0.2	1+
Moderate	30-49%	20-40	0.3-0.69	0.2-0.39	2+
Severe	≥50%	>40	≥0.70	≥0.40	3/4+

1+ = LA clears w/ each beat; 2+ = LA does not clear, faintly opac. after several beats; 3+ = LA & LV opac. equal

Treatment (Circ 2003;108:2432; JACC 2006;48:e1)
- **Surgery** (repair preferred over replacement as preserves LV fxn and lower mort.)
  symptomatic severe MR
  asx severe MR and **EF 30-60%** or **LV systolic diam. >40 mm**, ? AF or PHT
  ? MV repair (not replacement) for asx severe MR w/ preserved LV fxn or
  sx severe MR w/ severe LV dysfxn (EF <30% or systolic diam. >55 mm)
- Medical: indicated if Pt not an operative candidate
  ↓ **preload** (↓ CHF and ↓ amount of MR by ↓ MR orifice): diuretics, nitrates
  ↓ afterload (ACEI, hydralazine/nitrates): benefits unproven; indicated only if LV dysfxn
  maintain sinus rhythm
- Percutaneous MV repair: edge-to-edge clip (JACC 2005;46:2134) and annuloplasty band placed in coronary sinus (Circ 2006;113:851) remain under study
- Acute decompensation (consider ischemia and endocarditis as possible precipitants)
  IV afterload reduction (nitroprusside), inotropic support (dobutamine), IABP
  vasoconstrictors contraindicated
  surgery usually needed for acute severe MR as prognosis is poor w/o MVR

Prognosis
- 5-y survival w/ medical therapy 80% if asx, but 45% if sx

MITRAL VALVE PROLAPSE (MVP)

Etiology
- Definition: displacement of any part of either MV leaflet or their coaptation point ≥2 mm above mitral annulus in parasternal long axis echocardiographic view
- Myxomatous involvement of the MV apparatus with proliferation of the spongiosa
- Idiopathic, familial, and assoc. w/ connective tissue diseases (eg, Marfan's, Ehlers-Danlos)
- Prevalence 1-2.5% of general population (NEJM 1999;341:1)

Clinical manifestations
- Asymptomatic
- MR due to prolapse of the leaflet or ruptured chordae
- Endocarditis; embolic events
- ? Atypical chest pain, arrhythmias

Physical exam
- Midsystolic click ± mid-to-late systolic murmur
  - ↓ LV volume (standing, strain phase of Valsalva) → click & murmur heard earlier
  - ↑ LV volume or ↑ impedance to LV ejection → click & murmur heard later & softer

Treatment
- Endocarditis prophylaxis no longer recommended (*Circ* 2007;115:epub)
- Aspirin or anticoagulation if prior neurologic event or atrial fibrillation

PROSTHETIC HEART VALVES

Mechanical valves
- **Bileaflet-tilting disk** (eg, St. Jude Medical); single-tilting disk; caged-ball
- Characteristics: very durable but thrombogenic and ∴ require anticoagulation
  consider if age <60-65 y or if already need for anticoagulation

Bioprosthetic
- **Heterograft** (eg, Carpentier-Edwards) or **pericardial**
- Characteristics: less durable, but minimally thrombogenic
  consider if age >60-65 y, lifespan <20 y, or contraindication to anticoagulation

Physical examination
- Normal: **crisp sounds**, ± soft murmur during forward flow (normal to have small ∇)
- Abnormal: regurgitant murmurs, absent mechanical valve closure sounds

Anticoagulation with Prosthetic Valves			
	Warfarin		ASA
Valve	INR 2-3	INR 2.5-3.5	75-100 mg
Mechanical valves			
1st 3 mo		⊕	
After 3 mo			
Aortic valve	⊕		
Aortic valve + risk factor		⊕	
Mitral valve ± risk factor		⊕	
Bioprosthetic valves			⊕ for all
1st 3 mo			
No risk factors	±		
+Risk factor	⊕		
After 3 mo			
No risk factors			
Aortic valve + risk factor	⊕		
Mitral valve + risk factor		⊕	
Risk factors: AF, ↓ EF, prior embolic event, hypercoagulable state, mechanical valve other than bileaflet or Medtronic Hall, ? multiple valves			

(*JACC* 2006;48:e1)

Management of Anticoag. Peri-Procedure in Pts with Mech. Valve	
AVR and no risk factors	d/c warfarin 48-72 h before surgery restart 24 h after surgery
Risk factors for thromboembolism (incl. mechanical mitral valve)	Preop: d/c warfarin, start UFH when INR <2 4-6 h preop: d/c UFH Postop: restart UFH & warfarin ASAP

Procedures include noncardiac surgery, invasive procedures, and major dental work (*JACC* 2006;48:e1)

Endocarditis prophylaxis

Complications
- Valve thrombosis: treat w/ surgery (severe sx, L-sided, large clot burden) or lytic or UFH
- Pannus formation (typically forms on inferior surface of valve)
- Embolization (r/o endocarditis); risk of thromboembolism 1-2%/y even w/ warfarin Rx
- Structural failure (r/o endocarditis as cause)
  mechanical valves: rare except for Bjork-Shiley
  bioprosthetic valves: 30% fail rate w/in 10-15 y
- Hemolysis (especially with caged-ball valves)
- Paravalvular leak (r/o endocarditis); small *central* jet of regurg normal in mechnical valves
- Endocarditis

PERICARDIAL DISEASE

GENERAL PRINCIPLES

Anatomy
- Two-layered (parietal & visceral) tissue sac surrounding heart & proximal great vessels

Disease states
- Inflammation (w/ or w/o fluid accumulation) → pericarditis
- Fluid accumulation (usually in setting of inflammation) → effusion or tamponade
- Change in compliance (sequela of inflammation) → constriction

---

PERICARDITIS AND PERICARDIAL EFFUSION

Etiologies of Pericarditis	
Infectious (50%)	Viral: coxsackievirus, echovirus, adenovirus, EBV, VZV, HIV Bacterial (from endocarditis, pneumonia, or s/p cardiac surgery): S. pneumococcus, N. meningitidis, S. aureus Tuberculous (extension from lung or hematogenous); Lyme disease Fungal: Histo, Coccidio, Candida; Protozoal: Entamoeba, Echino
Neoplastic (35%)	Common: metastatic (lung, breast, lymphoma, leukemia, renal cell) Rare: primary cardiac & serosal tumors (mesothelioma)
Autoimmune	Connective tissue diseases (SLE, RA, scleroderma, Sjögren's) Vasculitides (PAN, Churg-Strauss, Wegener's) Drug-induced (procainamide, hydralazine, INH, CsA)
Uremia	Develops in ~20% of Pts, especially if on HD. May be transudative.
Cardiovascular	Acute transmural MI (5-20%) Late post-MI (Dressler's syndrome) Proximal aortic dissection (up to 45%) Chest trauma or s/p cardiac procedure / surgery Postirradiation (>4000 cGy to mediastinum; may be acute or delayed; may be transudative)
Idiopathic	Most presumed to be undx viral
Effusions w/o pericarditis	CHF, cirrhosis, nephrotic syndrome, hypothyroidism, amyloidosis. Transudative.

(Lancet 2004;363:717)

Clinical manifestations (NEJM 2004;351:2195)
- **Pericarditis**: chest pain that is pleuritic, positional (↓ by sitting forward), radiates to trapezius; may be *absent* in tuberculous, neoplastic, post-XRT, and uremic pericarditis; ± fever; ± s/s of systemic etiologies
- **Effusion**: ranges from asymptomatic to tamponade (see below)

Physical exam
- **Pericarditis**: multiphasic friction rub (leathery sound w/ up to 3 components: atrial contraction, ventricular contraction, ventricular relaxation) that is notoriously variable and evanescent
- **Effusion**: distant heart sounds, dullness over left posterior lung field due to compressive atelectasis from pericardial effusion (Ewart's sign), PMI *not* displaced (in contrast to DCMP)

Diagnostic studies (EHJ 2004;25:587)
- ECG: may show evidence of pericarditis w/ diffuse STE (*concave up*), PR depress., TWI; classically and in contrast to STEMI, TWI do not occur until ST segments normalize; may show evidence of large effusion w/ low voltage and electrical alternans
- CXR: large effusion (>250 cc of fluid) → cardiomegaly w/ "water-bottle" heart and epicardial halo
- Echocardiogram: presence, size, & location of *effusion*; presence of *tamponade physiology*; pericarditis itself w/o spec. abnl, although can see pericardial stranding (fibrin or tumor) can also detect asx myocarditis
- CT will reveal pericardial effusions, often appearing larger than on echocardiography
- CK-MB or troponin (⊕ in ~30%, JACC 2003;42:2144) if myopericarditis

Workup for effusion

- r/o infxn: usually apparent from Hx & CXR; ? ✓ acute and convalescent serologies
- r/o noninfectious etiologies: BUN, Cr, ANA, RF, screen for common malignancies
- Pericardiocentesis if suspect infxn or malignancy or if effusion large (>2 cm)
  ✓ cell counts, TP, LDH, glc, gram stain & Cx, AFB, cytology
  ADA, PCR for MTb, and specific tumor markers as indicated by clinical suspicion
  "exudate" criteria: TP >3 g/dl, TP$_{eff}$/TP$_{serum}$ >0.5, LDH$_{eff}$/LDH$_{serum}$ >0.6, or glc <60 mg/dl
  high Se (~90%) but *very low* Sp (~20%); overall low utility *(Chest 1997;111:1213)*
- Pericardial bx if suspicion remains for malignancy or tuberculosis

Treatment of pericarditis

- NSAIDs (eg, ibuprofen 600-800 mg tid) ± colchicine 0.5 mg bid *(Circ 2005;112:2012)*
  sx usually subside in 1-3 d, continue Rx for 7-14 d *(JAMA 2003;289:1150)*
- Steroids (usually systemic; occasionally intrapericardial) for systemic autoimmune disorder, uremic, or refractory idiopathic disease
- Avoid anticoagulants
- Infectious effusion → pericardial drainage (preferably surgically) + systemic antibiotics
- Acute idiopathic effusion self-limited in 70-90% of cases
- Recurrent effusion → consider pericardial window (percutaneous vs. surgical)

PERICARDIAL TAMPONADE

Etiology

- Any cause of pericarditis but especially **malignancy, uremia, idiopathic,** proximal aortic dissection with rupture, myocardial rupture
- Rapidly accumulating effusions most likely to cause tamponade as no time for pericardium to stretch (↑ compliance) and accommodate fluid

Pathophysiology *(NEJM 2003;349:684)*

- ↑ intrapericardial pressure, compression of heart chambers, ↓ venous return → ↓ CO
- Diastolic pressures ↑ & equalize in all cardiac chambers → minimal flow of blood from RA to RV when TV opens → blunted y descent
- Pulsus paradoxus (pathologic exaggeration of normal physiology)
  Inspiration → ↓ intrapericardial & RA pressures → ↑ venous return → ↑ RV size → septal shift to left. Also, ↑ pulmonary vascular compliance → ↓ pulm venous return.
  Result is ↓ LV filling → ↓ LV stroke volume & blood pressure
  Defined by respirophasic Δ SBP ≥10 mmHg due to ↑ ventricular interdependence

Clinical manifestations

- **Cardiogenic shock** (hypotension, fatigue) **without pulmonary edema**
- Dyspnea may be due to ↑ respiratory drive to augment venous return

Physical exam

- **Beck's triad: distant heart sounds, ↑ JVP, hypotension**
- Hypotension (50%; occasionally hypertensive), reflex tachycardia, cool extremities
- **Pulsus paradoxus** (>75%) = ↓ SBP ≥10 mmHg during inspiration
  Ddx = PE, hypovolemia, severe obstructive lung disease, constriction (~1/3)
- ↑ JVP with blunted y descent
- Distant heart sounds, ± pericardial friction rub (30%)
- Tachypnea but clear lungs

Diagnostic studies

- ECG: low voltage, electrical alternans, ± signs of pericarditis
- Echocardiogram: ⊕ **effusion,** IVC plethora, **septal shift** with inspiration, **diastolic collapse** of RA (Se 85%, Sp 80%) and/or RV (Se <80%, Sp 90%) **respirophasic Δ's in transvalvular velocities** (↑ across TV & ↓ across MV w/ inspir.)
  postsurgical tamponade may be localized and not easily visible
- Cardiac cath (right heart and pericardial): elevation (15-30) and equalization of intrapericardial and diastolic pressures (RA, RV, PCWP), blunted y descent in RA
  ↑ in stroke volume postpericardiocentesis ultimate proof of tamponade
  if RA pressure remains elevated after drainage, Pt may have effuso-constrictive disease *(NEJM 2004;350:469)* or myocardial dysfxn (eg, from concomitant myocarditis)

Treatment

- Volume (but be careful as overfilling can worsen tamponade) and ⊕ inotropes
- Pericardiocentesis (except if due to aortic or myocardial rupture, in which cases consider removing just enough fluid to reverse PEA while awaiting surgery)

CONSTRICTIVE PERICARDITIS

Etiology
- Any cause of pericarditis but especially **postviral**, **radiation**, **uremia**, **TB**, **postcardiac surgery**, and **idiopathic**

Pathophysiology
- Rigid pericardium limits diastolic filling → ↑ systemic venous pressures
- Venous return is limited only after early rapid filling phase; ∴ rapid ↓ in RA pressure with atrial relaxation and opening of tricuspid valve and *prominent x and y descents*
- Kussmaul's sign: ↑ JVP with inspiration (↑ venous return with inspiration but negative intrathoracic pressure not transmitted to heart because of rigid pericardium)

Clinical manifestations
- Right-sided > left-sided heart failure

Physical exam
- ↑ **JVP** with **prominent y descent**, ⊕ **Kussmaul's sign** (Ddx: TS, acute cor pulmonale, RV infarct, RCMP)
- Hepatomegaly, ascites, peripheral edema
- PMI usually not palpable, **pericardial knock**, usually no pulsus paradoxus

Diagnostic studies
- ECG: nonspecific
- CXR: calcification (MTb most common cause), especially in lateral view (although does not *necessarily* = constriction)
- Echocardiogram: ± thickened pericardium, **"septal bounce"** = abrupt displacement of septum during rapid filling in early diastole
- Cardiac catheterization
  atria: **Ms** or **Ws** (prominent x and y descents)
  ventricles: **dip-and-plateau** or **square-root sign** (rapid ↓ pressure at onset of diastole, rapid ↑ to early plateau)
  discordance between LV & RV pressure peaks during respiratory cycle (*Circ* 1996;93:2007)
- CT or MRI: thickened pericardium with tethering

Treatment
- Diuresis for intravascular volume overload, surgical pericardiectomy

Constrictive Pericarditis vs. Restrictive Cardiomyopathy		
Evaluation	**Constrictive pericarditis**	**Restrictive cardiomyopathy**
Physical exam	⊕ Kussmaul's sign Absent PMI ⊕ pericardial knock	± Kussmaul's sign Powerful PMI, ± S_3 and S_4 ± **Regurgitant murmurs of MR, TR**
ECG	± Low voltage	Low voltage ± **Conduction abnormalities**
Echocardiogram	Normal wall thickness **Septal bounce during early diastole** Inspiration → ↑ flow across TV and MV	± ↑ **wall thickness** **Biatrial enlargement** Inspiration → ↓ flow across TV & MV Slower peak filling rate Longer time to peak filling rate
CT/MRI	**Thickened pericardium with tethering**	Normal pericardium
Cardiac catheterization	Prominent x and y descents Dip-and-plateau sign	
	LVEDP = RVEDP RVSP <50 mmHg RVEDP >1/3 RVSP **Discordance** of LV and RV pressure peaks during respiratory cycle	± **LVEDP > RVEDP** (espec. with vol.) RVSP >60 mmHg RVEDP <1/3 RVSP Concordance of LV and RV pressure peaks during respiratory cycle
Endomyocardial biopsy	Usually normal	± **Specific etiology of RCMP**

JNC VII Classification		
Category	Systolic (mmHg)	Diastolic (mmHg)
Normal	<120	<80
Pre-HTN	120-139	80-89
Stage 1 HTN	140-159	90-99
Stage 2 HTN	≥160	≥100

(JAMA 2003;289:2560)

Epidemiology (JAMA 2003;290:199)
- Prevalence 30% in U.S. adults = 60 million affected (29% in whites, 33.5% in blacks)
- 60% of those w/ HTN are on Rx, only half of whom are adequately controlled

Etiologies
- **Essential** (95%): onset 25-55 y; ⊕ FHx. Unclear mechanism but ? additive microvasc renal injury over time w/ contribution of hyperactive sympathetics (NEJM 2002;346:913)
- **Secondary:** Consider if Pt <20 or >50 y or if sudden onset, severe, refractory or ↑ HTN

Secondary Causes of Hypertension			
Diseases		Suggestive Findings	Initial Workup
RENAL	Renal parenchymal (2-3%)	h/o DM, polycystic kidney disease, glomerulonephritis	CrCl See "Renal Failure"
	Renovascular (1-2%) Athero (90%) FMD (10%, young women) PAN, scleroderma	ARF induced by ACEI/ARB Recurrent flash pulm edema Renal bruit; hypokalemia (NEJM 2001;344:431)	MRA (>90% Se & Sp) Duplex U/S; Angio Plasma aldo:renin <10:1
ENDO	Hyperaldo or Cushing's (1-5%)	Hypokalemia Metabolic alkalosis	See "Adrenal Disorders"
	Pheochromocytoma (<1%)	Paroxysmal HTN, H/A, palp.	
	Myxedema (<1%)	See "Thyroid Disorders"	TFTs
	Hypercalcemia (<1%)	Polyuria, dehydration, Δ MS	ICa
OTHER	Obstructive sleep apnea: morning H/A; PHT; abnl polysomnography		
	Medications: OCP, steroids, licorice; NSAIDs (espec. COX-2); Epo; cyclosporine		
	Coarctation of aorta: ↓ LE pulses, systolic murmur, radiofemoral delay; abnl TTE		
	Polycythemia vera: ↑ Hct		

Standard workup
- Goals: (1) identify CV risk factors or other diseases that would modify prognosis or Rx
  (2) reveal 2° causes of hypertension
  (3) assess for target-organ damage
- History: CAD, CHF, TIA/CVA, PAD, DM, renal insufficiency, sleep apnea; ⊕ FHx for HTN diet, Na intake, smoking, alcohol, prescription and OTC medications, OCP
- Physical exam: ≥2 BP measurements separated by >2 mins; verify in contralateral arm funduscopic, cardiac (LVH, murmurs), vascular, abdominal (masses or bruits), neurologic
- Laboratory tests: electrolytes, BUN, Cr, glc, Hct, U/A, lipids, TSH, ECG (for LVH), CXR

Complications of HTN
- Each ↑ 20 mmHg SBP or 10 mmHg DBP → 2× ↑ CV complications (Lancet 2002;360:1903)
- Neurologic: TIA/CVA, ruptured aneurysms
- Retinopathy: I = arteriolar narrowing, II = copper-wiring, AV nicking, III = hemorrhages and exudates, IV = papilledema
- Cardiac: CAD, LVH, CHF
- Vascular: aortic dissection, aortic aneurysm
- Renal: proteinuria, renal failure

Treatment (NEJM 2003;348:610)
- Goal: <140/90 mmHg; if DM or renal disease goal is <130/80 mmHg, consider <120/80
- Treatment results in 50% ↓ CHF, 40% ↓ stroke, 20-25% ↓ MI (Lancet 2000;356:1955)

- **Lifestyle modifications** (each ↓ SBP ~5 mmHg)
  weight loss: achieve BMI 18.5-24.9; exercise: ≥30 min exercise/d, ≥5d/wk
  diet: rich in fruits & vegetables, low in saturated & total fat (DASH, NEJM 2001;344:3)
  sodium restriction: ≤2.6 g/d or lower
  limit alcohol consumption: ≤2 drinks/d in men; ≤1 drink/d in women & lighter-wt Pts
- **Pharmacologic options** (if HTN or pre-HTN + diabetes or renal disease)
  Pre-HTN: ARB prevents onset of HTN, no ↓ in clinical events (NEJM 2006;354:1685)
  Stage I HTN: thiazide better than ACEI or CCB in preventing CVD (ALLHAT, JAMA 2002;288:2981). β-blockers no longer first choice (Lancet 2005;366:1545)
  Stage 2 HTN: concom. disease may lead to compelling indication for specific drug class
  + **high-risk CAD**: ACEI (HOPE, NEJM 2000;342:145); thiazide (ALLHAT); CCB + ACEI ↓'d mort. by 11% & CV events by 16% c/w βB + diuretic (ASCOT-BPLA, Lancet 2005;366:895)
  + **angina**: β-blockers
  + **post-MI**: β-blockers, ACEI (BHAT, JAMA 1982;247:1707; SAVE, NEJM 1992;327:669)
  + **HF**: ACEI/ARB, β-blockers, diuretics, aldosterone antagonist (see "Heart Failure")
  + **CVA prevention**: ACEI (PROGRESS, Lancet 2001;358:1033) or ARB (LIFE, Lancet 2002;359:995)
  + **diabetes mellitus**: ACEI (UKPDS 39, BMJ 1998;317:713)
  + **chronic kidney disease**: ACEI/ARB (NEJM 1993;329:1456 & 2001;345:851, 861)
  most will require ≥2 antihypertensive drugs to reach goal; if not at goal → optimize doses or add additional drug (if on 2, one should be thiazide)
- **Secondary causes**
  Renovasc: control BP w/ diuretic + ACEI/ARB (watch for ↑ Cr w/ bilat. RAS) or CCB
  Atherosclerosis risk factor modification: quit smoking, ↓ chol.
  If refractory HTN, recurrent HF, UA, or worse CRI, revasc. indicated (JACC 2006;47:1)
  For atherosclerosis: stenting (↑'d restenosis rates w/ PTA alone): 20 mmHg ↓ in SBP, no Δ in Cr, 17% restenosis rate at 9 mos (ASPIRE-2, JACC 2005;46:776)
  For FMD (usually more distal lesions): PTA ± bailout stenting
  Surgery for complex lesions or aortic involvement
  Renal parenchymal: salt and fluid restriction, ± diuretics
  Endocrine etiologies: see "Adrenal Disorders"

HYPERTENSIVE CRISIS

Definitions
- **Hypertensive emergency**: ↑ BP → acute target-organ damage
  neurologic damage: encephalopathy, hemorrhagic or ischemic stroke, papilledema
  cardiac damage: ACS, HF, aortic dissection
  renal damage: proteinuria, hematuria, acute renal failure; scleroderma renal crisis
  microangiopathic hemolytic anemia
  preeclampsia-eclampsia
- **Hypertensive urgency**: SBP >180 or DBP >120 w/ minimal or no target-organ damage

Precipitants
- Progression of essential HTN ± medical noncompliance (espec. clonidine)
- Progression of renovascular disease; acute glomerulonephritis; scleroderma; preeclampsia
- Endocrine: pheochromocytoma, Cushing's
- Sympathomimetics: cocaine, amphetamines, MAO inhibitors + foods rich in tyramine
- Cerebral injury (do not treat HTN in acute ischemic stroke unless Pt getting lysed, extreme, BP, ie, >220/120, or Ao dissection, active ischemia, or CHF; Stroke 2003;34:1056)

Treatment
- Hypertensive emergency: ↓ MAP by 25% in mins to 2 h using IV agents
- Hypertensive urgency: ↓ BP in h using PO agents

Drugs for Hypertensive Crises			
Intravenous agents		**Oral agents**	
Agent	Dose	Agent	Dose
Nitroprusside*	0.25-10 μg/kg/min	Captopril	12.5-50 mg
Nitroglycerin	17-1000 μg/min	Labetalol	200-1200 mg
Labetalol	20-80 mg bolus q10 min or 0.5-2 mg/min	Clonidine	0.2 mg load → 0.1 mg qh
Hydralazine	10-20 mg q 20-30 min	Hydralazine	10-25 mg
Phentolamine	5-15 mg bolus q5-15 min		

* Metabolized to cyanide → Δ MS, lactic acidosis, death. Limit use of very high doses (8-10 μg/kg/min) to <10 min. Monitor thiocyanate levels. Sodium thiosulfate infusion for cyanide toxicity.

Definitions
- **True** aneurysm (involves all 3 layers of aorta) vs. **false** (rupture contained in adventitia)
- **Location**: root (annuloaortic ectasia), thoracic (TAA), thoracoabdominal, abdominal (AAA)
- **Type**: fusiform (circumferential dilation) vs. saccular (localized dilation)

Epidemiology (Circ 2005;111:816; Lancet 2005;365:1577)
- **TAA**: usually involves root/ascending Ao or descending Ao (arch & thoracoabd rare)
  Risk factors: **connective tissue diseases** (Marfan, Ehler's-Danlos type IV), congenital disorders (bicuspid AoV, Turner's); **HTN atherosclerosis; aortitis** (Takayasu's, GCA, spondyloarthropathies, syphilis); familial; chronic Ao dissection; trauma
- **Abdominal aortic aneurysm** (AAA): prev. 5% among individuals >65 y
  5-10× more common in men than women; most infrarenal
  Risk factors = risk factors for atherosclerosis: **smoking**, HTN, hyperlipidemia, age, FHx

Pathophysiology
- **TAA**: cystic medial necrosis
- **AAA**: atherosclerosis & inflammation → matrix degeneration → medial weakening
- Inflammatory and infectious/mycotic aneurysms rare

Screening
- **TAA**: no established guidelines
- **AAA**: ✓ for pulsatile abdominal mass in all Pts; U/S for all men >60 y w/ FHx of AAA and all men 65-75 y w/ prior tobacco use (Lancet 2002;360:1531; Annals 2005;142:203)

Diagnostic studies (Circ 2005;111:816)
- **CXR**: often abnormal, but not definitive in TAA
- **Ultrasound**: screening and surveillance test of choice for AAA
- **Contrast CT**: quick, noninvasive, good Se & Sp for all aortic aneurysms
- **MRI**: preferred for aortic root imaging for TAA, but also useful in AAA
- **TTE/TEE**: useful for root and rest of TAA

Treatment (JACC 2006;47:1)
- **Risk factor modification**: **smoking cessation**, ↓ cholesterol
- **BP control**
  β-blockers (↓ dP/dt) ↓ aneurysm growth (NEJM 1994;330:1335; J Vasc Surg 2002;35:72)
  ACEI assoc. w/ ↓ risk of rupture (Lancet 2006;368:659)
  no burst activity/exercise requiring Valsalva maneuvers
- **Surgery**
  TAA: growing >1 cm/y; ascending ≥5.5 cm; descending >6 cm; Marfan Pt ≥4.5-5 cm, aneurysm ≥4 cm and planned AoV surgery
  AAA: rapidly growing; infrarenal/juxtarenal ≥5.5 cm (NEJM 2002;346:1437, 1445)
- **Endovascular repair** (Circ 2005;112:1663): guidelines evolving; consider for high-risk Pts ↓ AAA mort., but ↑ complic. and no Δ in overall mort. c/w surgery (EVAR 1, Lancet 2005;365:2179; DREAM, NEJM 2005;352:2398); no advantage over medical Rx in Pts unfit for surgery (EVAR 2, Lancet 2005;365:2187)

Complications
- **Pain**: gnawing chest, back, or abdominal
- **Rupture**: risk ↑ w/ diameter, female sex, current smoking, HTN
  TAA: ~2.5%/y if <6 cm vs. 7% if >6 cm; **AAA**: ~1%/y if <5 cm vs. 6.5% if 5-5.9 cm
  may be heralded by ↑ pain; once occurs, usually fatal or Pt may p/w severe constant pain and in hemorrhagic shock; 90% mortality
- **Aortic Dissection** (see following)
- **Thromboembolic ischemic events**
- **Compression of adjacent structures** (eg, SVC, trachea, esophagus)

Follow-up
- Expansion rate ~0.1 cm/y for TAA, ~0.4 cm/y for AAA
- Serial imaging first 3, 6, 9, & 12 mos, then annually
- Screening for CAD, PAD, and aneurysms elsewhere, espec. popliteal. 25% of Pts w/ TAA will also have AAA.

AORTIC DISSECTION

Definitions (*Circ* 2003;108:628)
- **Classic dissection**: intimal tear → extravasation of blood into and along aortic media
- **Intramural hematoma** (IMH): vasa vasorum rupture → medial hemorrhage.
- **Penetrating ulcer**: ulceration of plaque penetrating intima → medial hemorrhage

Classification
- **Proximal**: involves ascending Ao, regardless of origin (= Stanford A, DeBakey I & II)
- **Distal**: involves descending Ao only, distal to subclavian art. (= Stanford B, DeBakey III)

Risk factors (predispose to medial micro apoplexy or "cystic medial necrosis")
- **Hypertension** (h/o HTN in >70% of dissections)
- **Connective tissue disease**

  Marfan (*fibrillin-1* gene): arachnodactyly, joint disloc., pectus, ectopia lentis, MVP
  Ehlers-Danlos type IV (type III procollagen): translucent skin; bowel or uterine rupture
  Annuloaortic ectasia, familial aortic dissection, adult PCKD
- **Congenital aortic anomaly**: bicuspid aortic valve or coarctation (eg, in Turner's)
- **Aortitis**: Takayasu's, giant cell arteritis, Behçet's, syphilis
- **Pregnancy**: typically in 3rd trimester; can also see spont. coronary artery dissections
- **Trauma**: blunt, IABP, cardiac or aortic surgery, cardiac catheterization

Clinical Manifestations and Physical Examination		
Feature	Proximal	Distal
Pain (often abrupt, severe, persistent, tearing)	94% (chest, back)	98% (back, chest, abd)
Syncope (often tamponade)	13%	4%
CHF (usually AI)	9%	3%
CVA	6%	2%
Hypertension	35%	70%
Hypotension/shock (tamp., AI, rupt.)	25%	4%
Pulse deficit	19%	9%
AI murmur	44%	12%

(IRAD *JAMA* 2000;283:897)

Diagnostic studies (*Circ* 2005;112:3802)
- **CXR**: abnormal in 60-90% (↑ mediastinum, effusion), but *cannot* be used to r/o dissection
- **CT**: quick, noninvasive, good Se (80% for proximal; 90-95% for distal); multidetector CT may improve Se; *however*, if ⊖ & *high clin. suspicion → additional studies*
- **TEE**: Se >95% for proximal, 80% for distal; can assess coronaries, pericardium, AI
- **MRI**: Se & Sp >98%, but time-consuming & not readily available
- **Aortography**: Se ~90%, time-consuming, cannot detect IMH; can assess coronaries

Treatment (*Circ* 2003;108:772)
- **Medical**: ↓ **dP/dt** targeting SBP ~110 and HR ~60

  first with IV β-blockers (eg, propranolol, esmolol, labetalol) to blunt reflex ↑ HR & inotropy that will occur in response to vasodilators

  then ↓ **SBP** with IV vasodilators (eg, nitroprusside)

  control pain with MSO$_4$ prn
- **Surgery**

  proximal (root replacement): all acute; chronic if c/b progression, AI or aneurysm
  distal: if c/b progression, signif. branch artery involvement, uncontrolled HTN, aneurysm
- **Endovascular stenting ± fenestration** is an evolving treatment (*NEJM* 1999;340:1539, 1546)

Complications
- **Rupture**: pericardial sac → tamponade; pleural space; mediastinum; retroperitoneum
- **Obstruction of branch artery**

  coronary → AMI (usually RCA → IMI)
  innominate/carotid → CVA, Horner; intercostal/lumbar → spinal cord ischemia/paraplegia
  innominate/subclavian → upper extremity ischemia; iliac → lower extremity ischemia
  celiac/mesenteric → bowel ischemia; renal → acute renal failure
- **AI**: due to annular dilatation or disruption or displacement of leaflet by false lumen

Prognosis
- Acute proximal dissection: mortality 1-2%/h × 48 h
- Acute distal dissection: mortality 10% at 30 d

BRADYCARDIAS, AV BLOCK, AND AV DISSOCIATION

Sinus bradycardia (SB) (NEJM 2000;342:703)
- Etiologies: **medications** (βB, CCB, amiodarone, Li, dig), ↑ vagal tone (incl. IMI), **metabolic** (severe hypoxia, sepsis, myxedema, hypothermia), ↑ **ICP**
- Treatment: usually none required; atropine or pacing if symptomatic

Sick sinus syndrome (SSS)
- Features may include: periods of unprovoked SB, SA arrest, paroxysms of SB and atrial tachyarrhythmias ("tachy-brady" syndrome)
- Treatment: meds alone (? βB w/ intrinsic sympathomimetic activity) usually fail (adeq. control tachy → unacceptable brady); usually need **combination** of meds (βB, CCB, dig) for tachy & **PPM** for brady

	AV Block	
Type	**Features**	
1°	Prolonged PR (>200 ms), all impulses conducted.	
2° Mobitz I (Wenckebach)	Progressive ↑ PR until impulse not conducted (→ "grouped beating"). Abnl AV node due to ischemia (IMI), inflammation (myocarditis), high vagal tone (athletes), MV surgery, drug-induced. Classically (~50%), absolute ↑ in PR decreases over time (→ ↓ RR intervals, duration of pause <2 × preceding RR interval). AVB usually worsens w/ carotid sinus massage, improves w/ atropine. Often paroxysmal / asymptomatic, no Rx required.	
2° Mobitz II	Occasional or repetitive blocked impulses w/ consistent PR interval. Abnl His-Purkinje system due to ischemia (AMI), degeneration of conduction system, infiltrative disease, inflammation, AV surgery. AVB usually improves w/ carotid sinus massage, worsens w/ atropine. Often progresses to 3° AVB. Pacing wire or PPM often required.	
3° (complete)	No AV conduction. Must disting. from other forms of AV dissociation.	

"High-grade" AVB usually refers to block of 2 or more successive impulses.

AV dissociation (not a primary diagnosis, rather a manifestation of 1 of 3 processes)
- *Default*: slowing of SA node allows subsidiary pacemaker (eg, AV junction) to take over
- *Usurpation*: acceleration of subsidiary pacemaker (eg, AV jxnal tachycardia, VT)
- *AV block*: normal pacemaker unable to capture ventricles, subsidiary pacemaker emerges

SUPRAVENTRICULAR TACHYCARDIAS (SVTs)

Arise above the ventricles, ∴ narrow QRS unless aberrant conduction or preexcitation.

	Etiologies of SVT	
	SVT	**Comments**
Atrial	Sinus tachycardia (ST)	Caused by pain, fever, hypovolemia, hypoxia, anemia, anxiety, β-agonists, etc.
	SA node reentrant tachycardia (SANRT)	Rare. Reentrant loop w/in SA node, discern from ST by rapid onset & termination.
	Atrial tachycardia (ATAC)	Originate at site in atria other than SA node Seen w/ CAD, COPD, ↑ catechols, EtOH, dig
	Multifocal atrial tachycardia (MAT)	↑ automaticity at multiple sites in the atria
	Atrial flutter (AFL)	Macroreentry usually within the right atrium
	Atrial fibrillation (AF)	Wavelets irregularly passing down AVN, often originate from the pulmonary veins
AV Jxn	AV nodal reentrant tachycardia (AVNRT)	Reentrant circuit using dual pathways w/in AVN
	Atrioventricular reciprocating tachycardia (AVRT)	Reentrant circuit using AVN and accessory pathway
	Nonparoxysmal junctional tachycardia (NPJT)	↑ automaticity at AV junction May see retrograde P waves or AV dissociation Seen in myo/endocarditis, card. surg, IMI, dig

(NEJM 1995;332:162; NEJM 2006; 354:1039)

Diagnosis of SVT	
Onset	Abrupt onset/offset suggests reentrant (AVNRT, AVRT, SANRT) "Warm up" period suggests ST or ATAC
Rate	Not diagnostic as most SVTs can range from 140-250 bpm, *but*: ST usually <150 bpm AFL often conducts with 2:1 AVB to yield ventricular rate of 150 bpm AVNRT & AVRT are usually >150 bpm
Rhythm	Irregular → AF, AFL w/ variable block, or MAT
P wave morphology	*Upright before QRS* → ST, ATAC (P different from sinus), MAT (≥3 different P waves morphologies) *Retrograde after QRS & inverted in inf. leads* → atrial activation via jxn AVNRT: buried in or distort terminal portion of QRS (pseudo RSR' in V$_1$) AVRT: slightly after but usually distinct from QRS Usually short RP interval (c/w short PR), but can be long RP *Fibrillation or no P waves* → AF *Saw-toothed "F" waves* (best seen in inferior leads & V$_1$) → AFL
Response to vagal stim. or adenosine	↑ automaticity rhythms (ST, ATAC, MAT) → slow rate or ↑ AV block AVN reentry (AVNRT, AVRT) → abruptly terminate (classically with a P wave after last QRS) or no response AFL → ↑ AV block → unmasking of "F" waves

(*NEJM* 2006;354:1039)

Figure 1-4 Approach to SVT

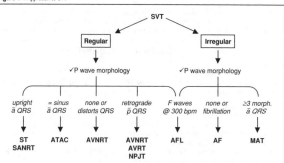

Treatment of SVT		
Rhythm	Acute treatment	Long-term treatment
Unstable	**Cardioversion** per ACLS	n/a
ST	Treat underlying stressor(s)	n/a
ATAC	β-blockers or CCB	β-blockers or CCB, ± antiarrhythmics ? Radiofrequency ablation
AVNRT or AVRT	**Vagal maneuvers** **Adenosine** (caution in AVRT) **CCB** or **β-blockers**	*For AVNRT* (see next section for AVRT): **Radiofrequency ablation** CCB or β-blockers (chronic or prn) ± Class IC AAD (if nl heart)
NPJT	**CCB, β-blockers, amiodarone**	Rx underlying disease (eg, ischemia, dig)
AF	**β-blockers, CCB, digoxin, AAD**	See "Atrial Fibrillation"
AFL	**β-blockers, CCB, digoxin, AAD**	Radiofrequency ablation β-blockers or CCB ± antiarrhythmics
MAT	CCB or β-blockers if tolerated	Treat underlying disease process ? AVN ablation + PPM

Avoid adenosine & nodal agents in AVRT w/ pre-excited tachycardia (i.e., wide-complex tachycardia due to anterograde conduction down accessory pathway). (*JACC* 2003;42:1493)

- *Radiofrequency ablation* has high overall success rate (AFL/AVNRT ~95%, AF ~80%). Complications include stroke, MI, bleeding, cardiac perforation, and conduction block.

ACCESSORY PATHWAYS (WOLFF-PARKINSON-WHITE)

Definitions
- **Accessory pathway** (bypass tract) of conducting myocardium connecting atria to ventricles, allowing impulses to bypass normal AVN conduction delay
- **Preexcitation (WPW) pattern**: ↓ PR interval, ↑ QRS width w/ δ wave (slurred onset, *can be subtle*), ST & Tw abnormalities (can mimic old IMI); only seen w/ pathways that conduct antegrade (if pathway only conducts retrograde then ECG normal during SR → "concealed" bypass tract)
- **WPW syndrome**: accessory pathway + paroxysmal tachycardia

Tachycardias
- **Orthodromic AVRT**: narrow-complex SVT, conducting ↓ AVN & ↑ accessory pathway; requires retrograde conduction and ∴ can occur w/ concealed bypass tracts
- **Antidromic AVRT**: wide-complex SVT, conducting ↓ accessory pathway & ↑ AVN; requires antegrade conduction and ∴ should see WPW pattern during SR
- **AF with rapid conduction** down accessory pathway, ∴ wide-complex irregular SVT; requires antegrade conduction and ∴ should see WPW pattern during SR

Treatment
- **AVRT**: vagal maneuvers, β-blockers, ? CCB; caution w/ adenosine as can precip. AF (see below); *always have defibrillator ready*
- **AF/AFL** w/ conduction down accessory pathway: need to Rx arrhythmia *and* ↑ pathway refractoriness; use ibutilide, flecainide, procainamide *or* cardiovert; avoid CCB & βB (ineffect.) and dig/adenosine (can ↓ refractoriness of pathway → ↑ vent. rate → VF)
- **Long term**: Rx tachycardias w/ radiofrequency ablation *or* antiarrhythmics (IA, IC) consider prophylactic ablation if asx but AVRT or AF inducible on EPS (NEJM 2003;349:1803) risk of SCD related to how short R-R interval is in AF and if SVT inducible w/ exercise

WIDE-COMPLEX TACHYCARDIAS (WCTs)

Etiologies
- **Ventricular tachycardia (VT)**
- **SVT conducted with aberrancy** (either fixed BBB, rate-dependent BBB, or an accessory pathway). Rate-dependent aberrancy usually p/w RBBB morphology.

Ventricular tachycardia
- **Monomorphic** (predominantly upward in V_1 = RBBB-type vs. downward = LBBB-type)
  Structurally *abnormal* heart: **prior MI, CMP**, arrhythmogenic RV dysplasia (ARVD, incomplete RBBB, R-sided TWI, ε wave = terminal notch in QRS in right precordial leads on resting ECG, LBBB-type VT, dx w/ MRI)
  Structurally *normal* heart: RVOT VT (normal resting ECG, LBBB-type VT w/ inf. axis), idiopathic LV VT (responds to verapamil)
- **Polymorphic**: ischemia, **CMP, torsades de pointes** (= polymorphic VT + ↑ QT), Brugada syndrome: pseudo-RBBB w/ STE in V_{1-3} (provoked w/ IA or IC) on resting ECG

Diagnostic clues that favor VT
- Assume all WCT is VT until proven otherwise
- **Prior MI, CHF**, or **LV dysfunction** best predictors that WCT is VT (Am J Med 1998;84:53)
- Hemodynamics and rate do *not* reliably distinguish VT from SVT
- Monomorphic VT is regular, but initially it may be slightly irregular, mimicking AF with aberrancy; grossly irregularly irregular rhythm suggests AF with aberrancy
- ECG features that favor VT (Circ 1991;83:1649)
  AV dissociation (independent P waves, capture or fusion beats) proves VT
  very wide QRS (>140 msec in RBBB-type or >160 msec in LBBB-type)
  extreme axis deviation
  QRS morphology atypical for BBB
    RBBB-type: absence of tall R' (or presence of monophasic R) in V_1, r/S ratio <1 in V_6
    LBBB-type: onset to nadir >60-100 msec in V_1, q wave in V_6
  concordance (QRS in all precordial leads w/ same pattern/direction)

Long-term management (JACC 2006;48:1064)
- Workup: **echo** to √ LV fxn, **cath** or **stress test** to r/o ischemia, ? MRI and/or RV bx to look for infiltrative CMP or ARVD, ? **EP study** to assess for inducibility
- **ICD**: 2° prevention after documented VT/VF (unless due to acute ischemia)
  1° prevention if EF <30-35% (see "Heart Failure"), ? ARVD, ? Brugada, ? certain long QT
- **Medications**: β-blockers, antiarrhythmics (eg, amiodarone) to suppress recurrent VT triggering ICD firing or if not ICD candidate
- **Radiofrequency ablation** if isolated VT focus or if recurrent VT triggering ICD firing

ATRIAL FIBRILLATION

Classification (JACC 2006;48:e149)
- **1st detected** vs. **recurrent** (≥2 episodes)
- **Paroxysmal** (self-terminating) vs. **persistent** (sustained >7 d) vs. **permanent** (typically >1 y and when cardioversion has failed or is foregone)
- **Valvular** (rheumatic MV disease, prosthetic valve, or valve repair) vs. **nonvalvular**
- **Lone AF** = age <60 and w/o clinical or echo evidence of cardiac disease (including HTN)

Epidemiology and etiologies
- ~1% of population has recurrent AF (8% of elderly); mean age at presentation ~75 y
- Acute (up to 50% w/o identifiable cause)
  Cardiac: CHF, myo/pericarditis, ischemia/MI, hypertensive crisis, cardiac surgery
  Pulmonary: acute pulmonary disease or hypoxia (eg, COPD flare, pneumonia), PE
  Metabolic: high catecholamine states (stress, infection, postop, pheo), thyrotoxicosis
  Drugs: alcohol ("holiday heart"), cocaine, amphetamines, theophylline, caffeine
- Chronic: ↑ age, HTN, ischemia, valve dis. (MV, TV, AoV), CMP, hyperthyroidism, obesity

Pathophysiology (NEJM 1998;339:659; Circ 1995;92:1954)
- Commonly originates from ectopic foci in atrial "sleeves" in the pulmonary veins
- Loss of atrial contraction → HF; LA stasis → thromboemboli; ? tachycardia → CMP

Evaluation
- H&P, ECG, CXR, echo (LA size, presence of thrombus, valves, LV fxn, pericardium), TFTs, ? r/o ischemia (AF unlikely due to ischemia *in absence of other sxs*)

Figure 1-5 Approach to acute AF

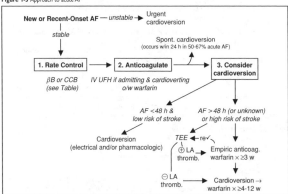

(Adapted from NEJM 2004;351:2408; JACC 2006:48:e149)

Rate Control for AF (Goal HR 60-80, 90-115 with exertion)				
Agent		Acute (IV)	Maint. (PO)	Comments
CCB	Verapamil	5-10 mg over 2′ may repeat in 30′	120-360 mg/d in divided doses	↓ BP (Rx w/ Ca gluc) Watch for CHF
CCB	Diltiazem	0.25 mg/kg over 2′ may repeat after 15′ 5-15 mg/h infusion	120-360 mg/d in divided doses	Preferred if COPD Can ↑ dig levels
βB	Metoprolol	5 mg over 2′ may repeat q 5′ × 3	25-100 mg bid or tid	↓ BP (Rx w/ glucagon) Watch for CHF & bronchospasm Preferred if CAD
βB	Propranolol	1 mg q 2′	80-240 mg/d in divided doses	
Digoxin (takes h)		0.25 mg q2h up to 1.5 mg	0.125-0.375 mg qd (adj for CrCl)	Consider in HF or low BP Poor exertional HR ctrl
Amiodarone		150 mg over 10′ → 0.5-1 mg/min		

IV βB, CCB, and digoxin **contraindicated** if evidence of WPW (ie, pre-excitation or WCT)

Strategies for recurrent AF
- **Rate control**: goal HR 60-80, 90-115 w/ exertion (see above table for options)
  AV node ablation + PPM as a last resort (NEJM 2001;344:1043; NEJM 2002;346:2062)
- **Rhythm control**: no clear survival benefit vs. rate ctrl; perhaps b/c of premature d/c of anticoag & antiarrhythmic drugs can be proarrhythmic (AFFIRM, NEJM 2002;347:1825, 1834)
- **Anticoagulation** (if indicated, see below) to prevent thromboemboli, whether rate or rhythm strategy

Antiarrhythmic Drugs (AAD) for AF				
Agent		**Conversion**	**Maintenance**	**Comments**
III	Amiodarone	5-7 mg/kg IV over 30-60′ → 1 mg/min to achieve 10 g load	200-400 mg qd (most effective drug)	↑ QT but TdP rare Pulm, liver, thyroid toxicity ✓ PFTs, LFTs, TFTs
	Ibutilide	1 mg IV over 10′ may repeat × 1	n/a	Contraindic. if ↓ K or ↑ QT ↑ QT, 3-8% risk of TdP Mg 1-2 g IV to ↓ risk TdP
	Dofetilide	0.5 mg PO bid	0.5 mg bid	↑ QT, ↑ risk of TdP ↓ dose if CrCl < 60
	Sotalol	n/a	90-160 mg bid	✓ for ↓ HR, ↑ QT Need to renally adjust
IC	Flecainide	300 mg PO × 1	100-150 mg bid	PreRx w/ AVN blocker
	Propafenone	600 mg PO × 1	150-300 mg tid	Contraindic. if structural or ischemic heart disease
IA	Procainamide	10-15 mg/kg IV over 1 h	1-2 g bid of slow release	↓ BP; ↑ QT ± PreRx w/ AVN blocker

(Adapted from NEJM 2001;344:1067; Annals 2003;139:1018; JACC 2006;48:e149)

Cardioversion
- Consider pharm or DC cardioversion in Pts w/ 1st episode of AF or in those w/ sx
  if AF >48 h, 2-5% risk stroke w/ cardioversion (pharm. or electric)
  ∴ either TEE to r/o thrombus or therapeutic anticoagulation for ≥3 wks prior
- Likelihood of success dependent on AF duration (better <7d) and atrial size
- Consider preRx w/ antiarrhythmic drugs (especially if 1st attempt fails)
- For pharmacologic cardioversion, class III and IC drugs have best proven efficacy
- Even if SR returns, atria *mechanically stunned*. Also, greatest likelihood of recurrent AF in first 3 mos after return to SR, ∴ must anticoagulate postcardioversion ≥4-12 wks
- "Pill-in-pocket": if IC drugs have been safely tolerated in Pts w/o ischemic or structural heart disease, can take as outPt prn if recurrent sx AF (NEJM 2004;351:2384)

Maintenance of SR (as necessary)
- Lone AF → class IC drugs or sotalol
- CAD → class III drugs
- CHF → dofetilide or amiodarone (NEJM 2007;356:935)

Nonpharmacologic therapy
- Radiofrequency ablation (circumferential pulm. vein isolation): ~80% success (although often requires repeat procedures); consider if ↓ EF or failed antiarrhythmic Rx (NEJM 2004;351:2373 & 2006;354:934; JAMA 2005;293:2634)
- Surgical "maze" procedure (70-95% success rate) option if undergoing cardiac surgery
- Left atrial appendage obliteration in Pts w/ AF undergoing cardiac surgery ↓ risk of stroke

Anticoagulation (JACC 2006;48:e149; Chest 2004;126:429S)
- Risk of stroke ↑↑ in valvular AF, ∴ anticoagulate all
- Risk of stroke ~ 4.5% per year in nonvalvular AF; risk factors include:
  prior stroke/TIA, DM, HTN, older age (≥65 y), HF, ? CAD
  echo: EF ≤35%, dense spontaneous echo contrast in LAA, ? ↑ LA size, ? Ao athero
- Risk of stroke in recurrent paroxysmal AF ≈ persistent AF ≈ permanent AF; AFL ≈ AF
- Treatment options
  warfarin (INR goal 2-3, NEJM 1996;335:540 & 2003;349:1019) → 61% ↓ stroke aspirin (81-325 mg qd): better than placebo (19% ↓ stroke) but inferior to warfarin aspirin + clopidogrel inferior to warfarin (ACTIVE-W, Lancet 2006;367:1903)
- Whom to treat:
  valvular AF, prior stroke/TIA, or ≥ 2 other risk factors → warfarin
  1 risk factor → warfarin or ASA (if age 60-74 and no other risk factors → ? ASA)
  if Pt not good candidate for warfarin (↑ risk of bleeding/falling) → ASA + ? clopidogrel
  lone AF → aspirin or no Rx

SYNCOPE

Definition
- Sudden transient loss of consciousness due to cerebral hypoperfusion

Etiologies (NEJM 2002;347:878; JACC 2006;47:473)
- **Neurocardiogenic** (a.k.a. vasovagal, ~20%; NEJM 2005;352:1004): ↑ sympathetic tone → vigorous contraction of LV → mechanoreceptors in LV trigger ↑ vagal tone (hyperactive Bezold-Jarisch reflex) → ↓ HR (cardioinhibitory) and/or ↓ BP (vasodepressor)
  related disorders: carotid sinus hypersens. (in 39% of elderly, Archives 2006;166:515); cough, deglutition, defecation & micturition syncope
- **Orthostatic hypotension** (10%)
  hypovolemia, diuretics, deconditioning
  vasodilators (especially if combined with ⊖ chronotropes)
  autonomic neuropathy (diabetes, EtOH, amyloid, renal failure, POTS, Shy-Drager)
- **Cardiovascular**
  Arrhythmia (15%)
    Bradyarrhythmias: SSS, high-grade AV block, ⊖ chronotropes, PPM malfunction
    Tachyarrhythmias: VT, SVT (syncope rare unless structural heart disease or WPW)
  Mechanical (5%)
    Endocardial: AS, MS, PS, prosthetic valve thrombosis, myxoma
    Myocardial: pump dysfxn from MI or outflow obstruction from HCMP (but usually VT)
    Pericardial: tamponade
    Vascular: PE, PHT, aortic dissection, subclavian steal
- **Neurologic** (10%): seizure (technically not syncope), TIA/CVA, vertebrobasilar insufficiency, migraine
- **Miscellaneous** (technically not syncope): hypoglycemia, hypoxia, anemia, psychogenic

Workup (etiology cannot be determined in ~35% of cases)
- **History** (from Pt and *witnesses* if available)
  activity and posture before the incident
  precipitating factors: exertion (AS, HCMP, PHT), positional Δ (orthostatic hypotension), stressors such as sight of blood, pain, emotional distress, fatigue, prolonged standing, warm environment, N/V, cough/micturition/defecation/swallowing (neurocardiogenic), head turning or shaving (carotid sinus hypersens.); arm exercise (subclavian steal)
  prodrome (eg, diaphoresis, nausea, blurry vision): cardiac <5 sec, vasovagal >5 sec
  associated sx: chest pain, palp., neurologic, post-ictal, bowel or bladder incontinence (convulsive activity for <10 sec may occur with transient cerebral hypoperfusion)
- **PMH**: prior syncope, previous cardiac or neurologic dis.; no CV disease at baseline → 5% cardiac, 25% vasovagal; CV disease → 20% cardiac, 10% vasovagal (NEJM 2002;347:878)
- **Medications**
  vasodilators: α-blockers, nitrates, ACEI/ARB, CCB, hydralazine, phenothiazines, antidep.
  diuretics; ⊖ chronotropes (eg, β-blockers and CCB)
  proarrhythmic or QT prolonging: class IA, IC or III antiarrhythmics, et al. (see "ECG")
  psychoactive drugs: antipsychotics, TCA, barbiturates, benzodiazepines, EtOH
- **Family history**: CMP, SCD
- **Physical exam**
  VS including *orthostatics* (supine → standing results in >20 mmHg ↓ SBP, >10 mmHg ↓ DBP, or >10-20 bpm ↑ HR), BP in both arms
  cardiac: HF (↑ JVP, displ. PMI, S₃), murmurs, LVH (S₄, LV heave), PHT (RV heave, ↑ P₂)
  vascular exam: ✓ for asymmetric pulses, carotid bruits, carotid sinus massage
  neurologic exam: focal findings, evidence of tongue biting, fecal occult blood test
- **ECG** (abnormal in ~50%, definitively identifies cause of syncope in ~10%)
  sinus bradycardia, sinus pauses, AVB, BBB, SVT, VT
  ischemic changes (new or old); atrial or ventricular hypertrophy
  markers of arrhythmia: ectopy, ↑ QT, preexcitation, Brugada pattern, ε wave (ARVD)

Other diagnostic studies (consider ordering based on results of H&P and ECG)
- Ambulatory ECG monitoring: if suspect arrhythmogenic syncope
  Holter monitoring (continuous ECG 24-48 h): useful if *frequent* events
    arrhythmia + sx (4%); asx but signif. arrhythmia (13%); sx but no arrhythmia (17%)
  Event recorder (activated by Pt to record rhythm strip): useful for infrequent events, but problematic if no prodrome; yield 20-50% over 30-60 d of monitoring
  Loop recorders (continuously save rhythm strip and ∴ can be activated *after* an event): useful for infrequent events including those w/o prodrome

Implantable loop recorders (inserted SC; can record for up to 14 mos): useful for *very infrequent* events; yield 90% after 1 y (AJC 2003;92:1231)
- Echocardiogram: r/o structural heart disease
- ETT: esp. w/ exertional syncope; r/o ischemia- or catecholamine-induced arrhythmias
- Cardiac catheterization: consider if noninvasive tests suggest ischemia
- Electrophysiologic studies (EPS)
   consider if arrhythmia detected, if structural heart disease, or if CAD (esp. with low EF)
   50% abnl (inducible VT, conduction abnormalities) if heart disease, but ? significance
   3-20% abnl if abnl ECG; <1% abnl if normal heart and normal ECG (Annals 1997;127:76)
- Tilt table testing (provocative test for vasovagal syncope): r/o other causes first
   ⊕ in 50% w/ recurrent unexplained syncope; Se 26-80%, Sp ≤90%; reprod. ≤80%
- Cardiac MRI: helpful to dx ARVD if suggestive ECG, echo (RV dysfxn), or ⊕ FH of SCD
- Neurologic studies (cerebrovascular studies, CT, MRI, EEG): if H&P suggestive; low yield

Figure 1-6 Approach to syncope

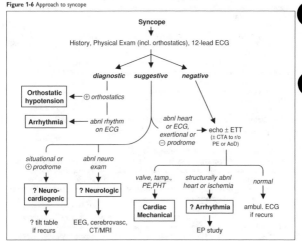

(Adapted from JACC 2006;47:473)

High-risk features (usually warrant admission with telemetry & further testing)
- Age >60 y, h/o CAD, CMP, valvular disease, congenital heart disease, arrhythmias
- Syncope c/w cardiac cause (lack of prodrome, exertional, resultant trauma)
- Abnormal cardiac exam or ECG

Treatment
- Arrhythmia, cardiac mechanical, or neurologic syncope: treat underlying disorder
- Vasovagal syncope: ? midodrine, fludrocortisone, disopyramide, antichlin., theophylline;
   ? 16 oz of H_2O before at-risk situations (Circ 2003;108:2660)
   no proven benefit w/ β-blockers (Circ 2006;113:1164) or PPM (JAMA 2003;289:2224)
- Orthostatic syncope: volume replete; if chronic → rise from supine to standing *slowly*,
   compressive stockings, midodrine, fludrocortisone, high Na diet

Prognosis (Ann Emerg Med 1997;29:459; NEJM 2002;347:878)
- 22% overall recurrence rate
- Cardiac syncope: 2-fold ↑ in mort., 20-40% 1-year SCD rate, median survival ~6 y
- Unexplained syncope w/ 1.3-fold ↑ in mort., but noncardiac or unexplained syncope w/ nl
   ECG, no h/o VT, no HF, age <45 → low recurrence rate and <5% 1-year SCD rate
- Vasovagal syncope: ∅ ↑ in mort., MI, or stroke

Pacemaker Code			
A = atrial, V = vent.	1st letter	2nd letter	3rd letter	4th letter
I = inhibition, D = dual	Chamber	Chamber	Response to	Program
R = rate-adaptive	paced	sensed	sensed beat	features

Common Pacing Modes	
VVI	Ventricular pacing on demand w/ single lead in RV. Sensed ventricular beat inhibits V pacing. Used in chronic AF and symptomatic bradycardia.
DDD	A & V sensing & pacing w/ leads in RA & RV. Sensed A beat inhibits A pacing & *triggers* V pacing → tracking of intrinsic atrial activity; sensed V beat inhibits V pacing. Used if require A & V pacing or to maintain AV synchrony.
Magnet	Placed over generator → Δ setting to DOO/VOO = pacing at fixed rate regardless of intrinsic activity. Use to ✓ ability to capture when output inhibited by intrinsic rhythm. Use when Pt hemodynamically unstable due to bradycardia from inappropriate PPM inhibition or tachycardia that is pacemaker induced.

Indications for Pacing (Circ 2002;106:2145)	
AV block	Symptomatic 3° or 2° AVB; ? Asymptomatic 3° or type II 2° AVB HR <40; pauses ≥3 sec while awake; alternating L and R BBB
Sinus node dysfxn	SB or pauses clearly assoc. w/ sxs or ? in sx Pt w/o clear association Chronotropic incompetence
Acute MI	See "STEMI"
Tachy-arrhythmia	Sx recurrent SVT that can be term. by pacing after failing drugs & ablation Sustained pause-dependent VT; ? high-risk Pts w/ congenital long QT
Syncope	Carotid sinus hypersensitivity with asystole >3 secs ? Neurocardiogenic syncope w/ prominent cardioinhib. response ? Syncope w/ bi- or trifascicular block and not likely 2° to other causes
CMP	Sx DCMP (BiV pacing); ? Sx HCMP w/ significant outflow obstruction

PPM Complications		
Issue	Manifestation	Description
Failure to pace	Bradycardia	Battery depletion, lead fracture/dislodgment, ↑ pacing threshold due to local tissue rxn/injury, or myopotential sensing → inappropriate inhibition.
Failure to sense	Inappropriate pacing	Lead dislodgment or sensing threshold set too high.
PM-mediated tachycardia	Tachycardia	Seen w/ DDD. V depol. → retrograde A activation → sensed by A lead → triggers V pacing → etc.
PM syndrome	Palp., HF	Seen w/ VVI. Due to loss of AV synchrony.

Cardiac Resynchronization Therapy (CRT)/Bivent. (BiV) Pacing (JACC 2005;46:e1)
- 3 lead pacemaker (RA, RV, coronary sinus); R > S in V_1 suggests appropriate LV capture
- **Goal**: enhance "synchronized" RV & LV function (↑ CO, ↓ remodeling)
- **Patient selection**: sx HF despite optimal med Rx, LVEF <35%, ventricular dyssynchrony (QRS ≥120 ms ± imaging evidence of dyssynchrony), ? sinus rhythm
- **Benefits**: ↓ HF sx, ↓ HF hosp., ↑ survival (NEJM 2004;350:2140 & 2005;352:1539)

Implantable Cardiac Defibrillators (ICDs) (NEJM 2003;349:1836; JACC 2006;48:1064)
- RV lead capable of defibrillation & pacing (± antitachycardia pacing, ATP); ± RA lead
- **Goal**: terminate VT/VF w/ shock or pacing, prevent sudden cardiac death (SCD)
- **Patient selection** (Circ 2007;115:1170)
  2° prevention: survivors of VF arrest, unstable VT (AVID, NEJM 1997;337:1576)
  1° prevention: LVEF <30-35% (for ≥1 mo if post-MI or ≥9 mos for nonischemic CMP) HCMP, ARVD, Brugada, LQTS, congenital heart or NM disease: if risk factors for SCD
- **Benefits**: ↓ mortality from SCD c/w antiarrhythmics or placebo
- ICD discharge: ✓ device to see if appropriate; r/o ischemia; 6 mos driving prohibition; if recurrent VT, consider drug Rx (eg, amio + βB; OPTIC, JAMA 2006;295:165) or VT focus ablation. Dual-chamber device may distinguish SVT vs. VT.

Device infection (Circ 2001;104:1029; 2003;108:2015)
- Presents as **pocket infection** (warmth, erythema, tenderness) and/or **sepsis w/ bacteremia**
- Infection in ~1/2 of Pts w/ S. aureus bacteremia (even w/o s/s and w/ ⊖ TTE/TEE)
- Treatment consists of abx and removal of system

Goldman Criteria for General Surgery		
Risk factor		**Points**
History Age >70 y		5
MI within 6 mo		10
Physical exam S_3 or JVD on physical exam		11
Significant aortic stenosis		3
ECG Rhythm other than sinus rhythm on preop ECG		7
>5 PVCs/min at any time preop		7
General status (any of the following)		3
PO_2 <60 mmHg, PCO_2 >50 mmHg,		
K <3 mEq/L, HCO_3 < 20 mEq/L, BUN > 50 mg/dl, Cr >3 mg/dl,		
↑ AST, chronic liver disease, or bedridden due to noncardiac cause		
Operation Intra-abdominal, intrathoracic, or aortic surgery		3
Emergency surgery		4

Class	Points	MI, CHF, VT	Cardiac Death
I	0-5	0.6%	0.2%
II	6-12	3%	1%
III	13-25	11%	2%
IV	>25	12%	39%

(NEJM 1977;297:845, Med Clin North Am 1987;71:416)

Revised Cardiac Risk Index for General Surgery (RCRI)	
Risk factor	**Points**
High risk surgery (intraperitoneal, intrathoracic, aortic)	1
Ischemic heart disease (prior MI, ⊕ ETT, angina, nitrate use, Qw)	1
History of HF	1
History of cerebrovascular disease	1
Insulin therapy for diabetes	1
Preoperative serum Cr >2 mg/dl	1

Class	# Factors	MI, CHF, VF, 3° AVB	
		Derivation Set	Validation Set
I	0	0.5%	0.4%
II	1	1.3%	0.9%
III	2	3.6%	6.6%
IV	3-6	9.1%	11.0%

(Circ 1999;100:1043)

Eagle Criteria for Vascular Surgery			
Clinical variables	**Stress testing**		
Age >70 y	Pts undergoing vasc. surgery have high		
Angina; Q waves on ECG	incidence of CAD. Claudication often limits		
Significant ventricular ectopy	angina. Consider pharmacologic stress test		
Diabetes requiring Rx	(adeno-MIBI or DSE) in Pts w/ 1-2 variables.		
# Variables	**0**	**1-2**	**≥3**
Stress test	n/a	⊖ ⊕	n/a
Event rate	3.1%	3.2% 29.6%	50%

(Annals 1989;110:863)

ACC/AHA Guidelines (Circ 2002;105:1257)

Clinical Markers		
Major	**Intermediate**	**Minor**
• ACS (within 30 d)	• Mild angina	• Age >70
• Decompensated HF	• Prior MI	• Abnormal ECG (eg, LVH,
• Significant arrhythmia (eg,	• Compensated/prior HF	LBBB, ST-T abnl)
high-grade AVB, VT, SVT w/	• Diabetes mellitus	• Rhythm other than sinus
uncontrolled HR)	• Renal insufficiency (Cr	• Low functional capacity
• Severe valvular disease	>2 mg/dl)	• Prior CVA
		• Uncontrolled HTN

Surgery-Specific Risk		
High	**Intermediate**	**Low**
• Emergent operation • Aortic or other major vascular • Peripheral vascular • Prolonged w/ lg fluid shifts or blood loss	• CEA; head & neck • Intraperitoneal/prostate • Intrathoracic • Orthopedic	• Endoscopic • Superficial • Cataract • Breast

Noninvasive Testing Result		
High risk	**Intermediate risk**	**Low risk**
Ischemia at < 4 METs and • ST ↓ ≥1 mm or ST ↑ ≥1 mm • ≥5 abnormal leads • Isch. >3 min after exert • Typical angina	*Ischemia at 4-6 METs and* • ST ↓ ≥1 mm • Typical angina • 3-4 abnormal leads • Isch. 1-3 min after exertion	*No ischemia or at >7 METs and* • ST ↓ ≥1 mm • Typical angina • 1-2 abnormal leads

Figure 1-7 Approach to non-emergent preoperative cardiovascular evaluation

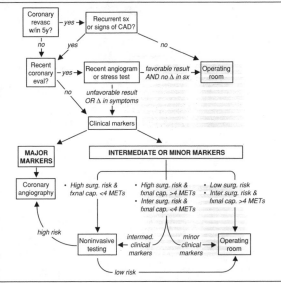

Fxnal capacity: 1-4 METS (ADLs), 4-10 METS (flight of stairs → heavy housework → light exercise), >10 METS (sports) (*Circ* 2002;105:1257).

Preoperative and perioperative monitoring and therapy
• If possible, wait >4-6 wks after MI (even if ⊖ ETT or ⊕ ETT & revascularized). If no revasc, wait 6 mos before elective surgery.
• Optimize BP, treat s/s HF & any SVT. Critical AS w/ sx needs pre-op AVR or valvuloplasty.
• β-blockers (*JACC* 2006;47:2343): use if ischemia, CAD, or major/intermed. clinical markers and undergoing intermed./high-risk surgery; start >1 wk before (titrate to HR ~55) and continue for ≥30 d postop (titrate to HR <80); 65-90% ↓ cardiac death & MI (*NEJM* 1996;335:1713 & 1999;341:1789).
• **Coronary revascularization** should be based on standard indications (ACS, refractory angina, lg territory at risk). No Δ in mort. or postop MI w/ coronary revasc. prior to elective vasc. surgery based on perceived cardiac risk (*NEJM* 2004;351:2795).
• Given need for dual antiplatelet Rx after stenting, wait 4-6 wks after bare metal stent and >12 mos after drug-eluting stent before discontinuing antiplatelet Rx
• ✓ ECG and troponin after surgery to assess for myocardial injury

DYSPNEA

Pathophysiology	Etiologies
Airway obstruction (↑ resistance to airflow)	**Asthma, COPD,** bronchiectasis (permanent dilation of airways with obliteration by secretions, infections, fibrosis), tumor or foreign body
Parenchymal disease (↑ resistance to expansion)	**Pulmonary edema** cardiogenic: LV systolic or diastolic dysfxn noncardiogenic: ALI/ARDS **ILD**
Vascular (V/Q mismatch)	Large vessel: **PE,** tumor emboli Small vessel: **PHT,** vasculitis, emphysema
Bellows (↑ resistance to CW/diaphragm expansion; weakness of respiratory muscles)	**Pleural disease:** effusion, fibrosis **Chest wall/diaphragm:** kyphoscoliosis, ↑ abd girth **Neuromuscular disorders** Hyperinflation (COPD, asthma)
Stimulation of receptors	Chemoreceptors: **hypoxemia,** metabolic acidosis Mechanoreceptors: **ILD, pulmonary edema,** PHT, PE
↓ O₂ carrying cap. (but nl P₄O₂)	**Anemia,** methemoglobinemia, CO poisoning
Psychological	Anxiety, panic attack, depression, somatization

Evaluation
- Cardiopulmonary exam, S_aO_2, CXR, ECG
  predictors of CHF: h/o CHF, PND, S_3, CXR w/ venous congestion, AF (JAMA 2005;294:1944)
  dyspnea w/ nl CXR → CAD, asthma, PE, PHT, early ILD, anemia, acidosis, NM disease
- Based on results of initial evaluation: PFTs, chest CT, TTE, cardiopulmonary testing
- **BNP & NT-proBNP** ↑ in CHF (but also ↑ in AF, RV strain from PE, COPD flare, PHT)
  BNP >100: 90% Se, 76% Sp for CHF causing dyspnea (NEJM 2002: 347:161)
  NT-proBNP: >300 pg/mL → 99% Se, 60% Sp for CHF (∴ use <300 to rule out)
    to rule in use age-related cutpoints: >450 pg/mL if <50 y, >900 if 50-75 y,
    >1800 if >75 y → 90% Se, 84% Sp (EHJ 2006;27:330)
  ↑ in chronic heart failure, ∴ need to compare to known "dry BNP"

PULMONARY FUNCTION TESTS (PFTs)

- **Spirometry:** evaluate for obstructive disease
  Flow-volume loops: diagnose and/or localize obstruction
  Bronchodilator: indicated if obstruction at baseline or asthma clinically suspected
  Methacholine challenge: helps dx asthma if spirometry nl, >20% ↓ FEV_1 → asthma
- **Lung volumes:** evaluate for restrictive disease including NM causes
- **D_LCO:** evaluates functional surface area for gas exchange; helps differentiate causes of obstructive and restrictive diseases and screens for vascular disease & early ILD

Figure 2-1 Approach to abnormal PFTs

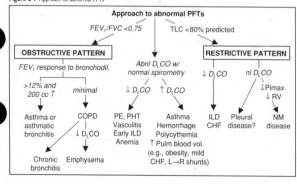

Definition and epidemiology
- Chronic inflamm. disorder w/ **airway hyperrespons.** + var. airflow obstruction
- Affects ~5% population; ~85% of cases by age 40; ? link to ADAM-33 (NEJM 2002;947:936)

Clinical manifestations (NEJM 2001;344:350)
- Classic triad = **wheezing, cough, and dyspnea**; others include chest tightness, sputum; symptoms typically chronic with episodic exacerbation
- Precipitants (**"triggers"**)
  respiratory irritants (smoke, perfume, etc.) & allergens (pets, dust mites, pollen, etc.)
  infections (URI, bronchitis, sinusitis)
  drugs (eg, ASA via leukotrienes, βB via bronchospasm, morphine via histamine release)
  emotional stress, cold air, exercise
- Exacerbations: important to note frequency, severity, duration, and required treatment including need for steroids, ED visits, hospitalizations, and intubations

Physical examination
- Wheezing and prolonged expiratory phase
- Presence of nasal polyps, rhinitis, rash → allergic component
- Exacerbation → ↑ RR, use of accessory muscles of respiration, pulsus paradoxus

Diagnostic studies
- **PFTs**: ↓ peak expiratory flow rate (PEFR)
  spirometry: ↓ FEV_1, ↓ FEV_1/FVC, coved flow-volume loop; lung volumes: ± ↑ RV + TLC
  ⊕ bronchodilator response (↑ FEV_1 ≥12%) strongly suggestive of asthma
  methacholine challenge (↓ FEV_1 ≥20%) if PFTs nl: Se >90% (AJRCCM 2000;161:309)
- Allergy suspected → consider ✓ serum IgE, eosinophils, skin testing/RAST
- Sputum: eos >3% → 86% Se, 88% Sp; can also see Curschmann's spirals (mucus casts of distal airways) and Charcot-Leyden crystals (eosinophil lysophospholipase); normalization of sputum eos count may help guide outPt Rx (Lancet 2002;360:1715)
- Fractional excretion of NO (FeNO) proportional to airway inflammation and sputum eosinophilia: >20 ppb → Se 88%, Sp 79% (AJRCCM 2004;169:473)

Ddx ("all that wheezes is not asthma...")
- Mechanical airway obstruction or structural airway abnormalities (eg, tumor)
- Laryngeal or vocal cord dysfunction (eg, due to GERD or postnasal drip)
- COPD, CHF, vasculitis: consider in older Pts with new dx of "asthma"
- Other pulmonary causes: bronchiectasis, PE, aspiration, sarcoidosis, ILD
- "Asthma + " syndromes (Lancet 2002;360:1313)
  Atopy = asthma + allergic rhinitis + atopic dermatitis
  ASA-sensitive asthma (Samter's syndrome) = asthma + ASA sensitivity + nasal polyps
  ABPA = asthma + pulmonary infiltrates + allergic rxn to Aspergillus
  Churg-Strauss = asthma + eosinophilia + granulomatous vasculitis

Classification of severity
- Intermittent: sx <1/wk, nocturnal sx ≤2/mo, brief exacerb., PEF or FEV_1 ≥80%
- Mild persistent: sx >1/wk but <1/d, nocturnal sx >2/mo; exacerb. may affect activity & sleep, PEF or FEV_1 ≥80%
- Mod. persistent: sx qd, nocturnal sx >1/wk; exacerb. may affect activity & sleep, daily use of short-acting β_2-agonist, PEF or FEV_1 60-80%
- Sev. persistent: sx qd, freq. noct. sx & exacerb., limited physical activity, PEF or FEV_1 ≤60%

"Quick-relief" medications
- Short-acting inhaled β_2-**agonists** (eg, albuterol): treatment of choice
  levoalbuterol (R-isomer) 2x potency with similar side effect profile, no outcome benefit
- Inhaled **anticholinergics** (ipratropium) improve β_2-agonist delivery
- Systemic **corticosteroids**

"Long-term-control" medications
- Inhaled or systemic **corticosteroids**: treatment of choice (SOCS, JAMA 2001;285:2583)
  FeNO can predict responsiveness (AJRCCM 2005;172:453) and guide Rx (NEJM 2005;352:2163)
- Long-acting inhaled β_2-agonists (salmeterol): use w/ caution given concern for ↑ mortality
  (SMART, Chest 2006;129:15; Annals 2006;144:904) possibly due to desensitization of β-receptors
  Pts w/ β_2 receptor genetic polymorphism Arg/Arg (1/6th of asthmatics) do not appear
  to derive long-term benefit and may be harmed by LABA (Lancet 2004;364:1505)
- **Nedocromil/cromolyn**: useful in young Pts, exercise-induced bronchospasm; ineffective unless used before trigger or exercise exposure

- **Theophylline**: useful in hard to control Pts, PO convenience, but high side effect profile
- **Leukotriene modifiers**: some patients very responsive, especially aspirin-sensitive asthma (AJRCCM 2002;165:9); may consider trial in all patients

Other
- Behavior modification: identify and avoid triggers
- Immunotherapy (eg, desensitization): may be useful if significant allergic component
- Anti-IgE (omalizumab): allergic asthma uncontrolled on inhaled steroids (NEJM 2006;354:2689)
- TNF antagonists may be helpful in Pts w/ refractory asthma (NEJM 2006;354:697)
- Bronchial thermoplasty (exp'tal): radiofrequency destruction of airway smooth muscle no Δ in FEV$_1$, but ↓ in sx and # of exacerbations (NEJM 2007;356:1327)

Principles of treatment
- Education and avoidance of environmental triggers for all Pts
- Use quick-relief rescue medication as needed for all Pts
- Rather than fixed Rx based on severity, new goal is to achieve **complete control** = daily sx ≤2/wk, ∅ nocturnal sx or limitation of activity, reliever med ≤2/wk, nl PEFR or FEV$_1$
- Step up treatment as needed to gain control, step down as tolerated

Asthma Stepwise Therapy				
Step 1	Step 2	Step 3	Step 4	Step 5
		Rapid-acting β$_2$-agonists prn		
Controller options	Select one	Select one	Do one or more	Add one or both
	Low-dose ICS	**Low-dose ICS + LABA**	**Δ low-dose ICS to med/high dose (w/LABA)**	Oral steroids (lowest dose)
	LTA	Med/high-dose ICS	Add LTA	Anti-IgE Rx
		Low-dose ICS + LTA	Add Theo	
		Low-dose ICS + Theo		

ICS = inhaled corticosteroid; LABA = long-acting β$_2$-agonist; LTA = leukotriene antag.; Theo = sustained-rel. theophylline
Boldfaced treatments are preferred options.
(Adapted from Global Initiative for Asthma (GINA)–Global Strategy for Asthma Management and Prevention 2006)

EXACERBATION

Direct evaluation
- History
  Previous asthma: baseline PEFR, steroid requirement, ED visits, hospital admissions; **previous need for intubation** a good predictor of risk of death (Thorax 1986;41:833)
  Current exacerbation: duration, severity, potential precipitants, medications used
- Physical exam
  Signs of severity: tachypnea, tachycardia, diaphoresis, cyanosis, fragmented speech, absent breath sounds, accessory muscle use, pulsus paradoxus, abdominal paradox
  Assess for barotrauma: asymmetric breath sounds, tracheal deviation, subcutaneous air → pneumothorax, precordial (Hamman's) crunch → pneumomediastinum
- Diagnostic studies
  ABG: not always considered essential because exam and S$_a$O$_2$ provide equivalent info; low P$_a$CO$_2$ initially; nl or high P$_a$CO$_2$ may signify tiring; may respond to bronchodilator
  PEFR: used to follow clinical course; CXR: not essential unless suspicion for PNA or PTX

Acute Pharmacologic Treatment		
Agent	Dose	Comments
Oxygen	Titrate to achieve S$_a$O$_2$ >90%	
Albuterol	MDI 4-8 puffs q20min or nebulizer 2.5-5 mg q20min continuous nebulizer if severe	First-line therapy (Chest 2002;121:1036)
Corticosteroids	prednisone 60 mg PO or methylprednisolone 80 mg IV	IV not superior to PO (JAMA 1988;260:527)
Ipratropium	MDI 4-8 puffs q30min, or nebulizer 0.5 mg q30min ×3	↑ bronchodilation when combined w/ albuterol (Chest 2002;121:1977)
Magnesium	2g IV over 20 min (Lancet 2003; 361:2114)	↑ PEFR & FEV$_1$

Other treatments
- Epinephrine (0.3-0.5 mL SC of 1:1000 dilution): no advantage over inhaled β_2-agonists
- Antibiotics: not needed unless evidence of bacterial infection, although evidence of improved symptoms/ FEV_1 may be related to anti-inflammatory effect (NEJM 2006;354:1589)
- IV montelukast/zafirlukast: improves FEV_1 acutely (AJRCCM 2003;167:488); ↓ relapse after d/c from emergency department (Chest 2004;126:1480)

Classification of asthma exacerbation severity
- **Mild**: PEFR >80%, dyspnea on exertion, end-expiratory wheezes
- **Moderate**: PEFR 50-80%, dyspnea w/ talking, expiratory wheezes, accessory muscle use
- **Severe**: PEFR <50%, S_aO_2 <91%, P_aCO_2 >42, dyspnea at rest, inspiratory and expiratory wheezes, accessory muscle use, pulsus paradoxus >25 mmHg

Figure 2-2 Initial assessment of asthma exacerbation

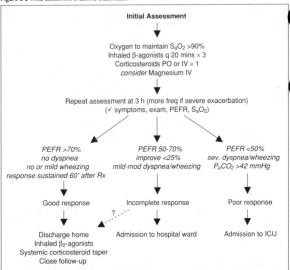

Hospital ward-level care
- ✓ PEFR q8h, S_aO_2 q8h (continuous if <90%), provide supplemental O_2
- **Bronchodilators and steroids usually sufficient**
  continue inhaled β_2-agonist as needed for sx, watch for *tachycardia* and *hypokalemia*
  start steroids at prednisone 60 mg qd or equivalent, begin taper when PEFR >50%

ICU-level care
- **High-dose steroids**: methylprednisolone 125 mg IV q6h (Archives 1983;143:1324)
- **Noninvasive ventilation**: may ↓ need for intubation (Int Care Med 2001;27:486)
- **Heliox**: ? helpful in first hour, especially in more severe Pts (Chest 2003;123:882)
- **Invasive ventilation**
  large ET tube, keep P_{plat} <30 (predicts barotrauma better than PIP), watch for auto-PEEP
  paralysis, inhalational anesthetics, bronchoalveolar lavage w/ mucolytic, and ECMO have been used with success

CHRONIC OBSTRUCTIVE PULMONARY DISEASE

Definition and epidemiology (NEJM 2004;350:26)
- Progressive airflow limitation caused by airway and parenchymal inflammation

Emphysema vs. Chronic Bronchitis		
	Emphysema	**Chronic Bronchitis**
Definition	Dilation/destruction of airspaces (pathologic definition)	Productive cough >3 mo/yr × ≥2 yrs (clinical definition)
Pathophysiology	Parenchyma affected Matched V/Q defects Mild hypoxemia	Small airways affected V/Q mismatch Severe hypoxemia, hypercapnia PHT, cor pulmonale
Clinical manifestations	Severe, constant dyspnea Mild cough	Intermittent dyspnea Copious sputum production
Physical exam	"Pink puffer" Tachypneic, noncyanotic, thin Diminished breath sounds	"Blue bloater" Cyanotic, obese, edematous Rhonchi & wheezes

Pathogenesis (Lancet 2003;362:1053)
- Caused by: **cigarette smoke** (centrilobular emphysema, affects 15-20% of smokers), α_1-antitrypsin deficiency (panacinar emphysema), recurrent airway infections

Clinical manifestations
- Chronic cough, sputum production, dyspnea; later stages → freq exac., a.m. HA, wt loss
- Exacerbation triggers: infxn, other cardiopulmonary disease, incl. PE (Annals 2006;144:390)
  - Infxn: overt tracheobronchitis/pneumonia from viruses, S. pneumoniae, H. influenzae, M. catarrhalis, or triggered by changes in strain of colonizers (NEJM 2002;347:465)
- Physical exam: ↑ AP diameter of chest ("barrel-chest"), hyperresonance, ↓ diaphragmatic excursion, ↓ breath sounds, ↑ expiratory phase, rhonchi, wheezes
  - during exacerbation: tachypnea, accessory muscle use, pulsus paradoxus, cyanosis

Diagnostic studies
- CXR: hyperinflation, flattened diaphragms, ± interstitial markings and bullae
- PFTs:
  - **Obstruction:** ↓↓ FEV_1, ↓ FVC, ↓ FEV_1/FVC, expiratory scooping of flow-volume loop
  - **Hyperinflation:** ↑↑ RV, ↑ TLC, ↑ RV/TLC
  - **Abnormal gas exchange:** ↓ D_LCO (in emphysema)
- ABG: ↓ P_aO_2, ± ↑ P_aCO_2 (in chronic bronchitis, usually only if FEV_1 <1.5 L) and ↓ pH
- ECG: PRWP, S1S2S3, R-sided strain, RVH, ↑ P waves in lead II ("P pulmonale")

Chronic treatment ("COPDer") (JAMA 2003;290:2301, 2313; NEJM 2004;350:2689)
- **C**orticosteroids: (inhaled)
  ~20% ↓ in exacerbations if FEV_1 <2.0 L (Lancet 1998;351:773; BMJ 2000;320:1297)
  may slow FEV_1 loss (NEJM 2000;343:1902 & 2007;356:775)
  ↑ in pneumonia; no Δ in mortality with inh steroids alone (NEJM 2007;356:775)
- **O**xygen: if P_aO_2 ≤55 mmHg or S_aO_2 ≤89% (during rest, exercise, or sleep) to prevent cor pulmonale and ↓ mortality (Annals 1980;93:391 & Lancet 1981;i:681)
- **P**revention: Flu/Pneumovax; smoking cessation → 50% ↓ in lung function decline (AJRCCM 2002;166:675) and ↓ long-term mortality (Annals 2005;142:223)
- **D**ilators: anticholinergics, β_2-agonists, theophylline
  anticholinergic > β_2-agonist; combination *may* be more effective (Chest 1999;115:635)
  LA anticholinergic (tiotropium): ↓ exac., ↑ QoL, ↓ FEV_1 decline in mod/severe disease vs. ipratropium (Cochrane 2005;CD002876), superior to LA β_2-agonist as monotherapy (Chest 2004;125:249), and combination ↑ FEV_1 (Chest 2006;129:509)
  LABA: ~15% ↓ in exacerbations, ↓ FEV_1 decline, trend towards ↓ mort. (NEJM 2007;356:775)
  LABA + inhaled steroid may ↓ mort. (TORCH, NEJM 2007;356:775)
- **E**xperimental
  Lung volume reduction surgery (LVRS): ↑ exer. capacity, ↓ mort. if FEV_1 >20%, upper-lobe emphysema, ↓ baseline exer. capacity (NEJM 2000;343:239; NETT, 2003;348:2059)
  Bronchoscopic LVRS safe and effective (Chest 2006;129:518), await outcome data
  Roflumilast (PDE III inhibitor): ↑ FEV_1 (Lancet 2005;366:563)
- **R**ehabilitation: ↓ dyspnea and fatigue, ↑ exercise tolerance, ↑ QoL (Cochrane 2002;CD003793)

COPD Staging and Recommended Therapies by GOLD Criteria				
Stage	**PFTs (of predicted)**		**Therapies**	
0: ↑ risk	Normal but ± sx		**P**revention	n/a
I: Mild	FEV_1/FVC <70%	FEV_1 ≥80%		**D**ilator prn
IIA: Mod		FEV_1 50-80%		Standing **D**ilator (tiotropium >β ag) **C**orticosteroid if response **R**ehabilitation
IIB: Mod		FEV_1 30-50%		Above + **C**orticosteroid if ↑ exacerbations
III: Severe		FEV_1 <30% *or* respiratory failure *or* right heart failure		Above + **O**xygen if respiratory failure **E**xperimental as indicated

(Adapted from Global Initiative for Chronic Obstructive Pulmonary Disease, WHO/NHLBI 1998)

EXACERBATION

COPD Exacerbation Treatment		
Agent	**Dose**	**Comments**
Ipratropium	MDI 4-8 puffs q1-2h *or* Nebulizer 0.5 mg q1-2h	First-line therapy
Albuterol	MDI 4-8 puffs q1-2h *or* Nebulizer 2.5-5 mg q1-2h	Benefit if component of reversible bronchoconstriction
Corticosteroids	Methylprednisolone 125 mg IV q6h × 72 h *then* Prednisolone 60 mg PO qd × 4 d *then* taper by 20 mg q3-4d *or* Prednisone 30 mg qd × 2 wks if pH >7.26 (*Lancet* 1999;354:456)	↑ FEV_1 (*Lancet* 1999;354:456) & ~30% ↓ in death, intubation, readmit for COPD or need for ↑ Rx (*NEJM* 1999;340:1941; *Archives* 2002;162:2527) OutPt Rx after ED visit ↓ relapse (*NEJM* 2003;348:2618)
Antibiotics	Amoxicillin, TMP-SMX, doxycycline, clarithromycin, anti-pneumococcal FQ, etc., all reasonable (no single abx proven superior)	*H. influenzae, M. catarrhalis, S. pneumonia* freq. precip. ↑ PEFR & chance of clinical resolution (*JAMA* 1995;273:957)
Oxygenation	↑ F_iO_2 to achieve P_aO_2 ≥55-60 *or* S_aO_2 90-93%	**Watch for CO_2 retention** (due to ↑V/Q mismatch, loss of hypoxic resp. drive, Haldane effect) *but must maintain oxygenation!*
Noninvasive positive-pressure ventilation	Initiate *early* if mod/severe dyspnea, ↓ pH / ↑ P_aCO_2, RR >25 Results in 58% ↓ intubation, ↓ LOS by 3.2 d, 59% ↓ mortality Contraindications: Δ MS, inability to cooperate or clear secretions, hemodynamic instability, UGIB (*Cochrane* 2004;CD004104; *Annals* 2003;138:861; *NEJM* 1995;333:817; *ERJ* 2005;25:348)	
Endotracheal intubation	Consider if P_aO_2 <55-60, ↑'ing P_aCO_2, ↓'ing pH, ↑ RR, respiratory fatigue, Δ MS, or hemodynamic instability	
Other measures	Chest physiotherapy, mucolytics *not* supported by data Monitor for cardiac arrhythmias	

(*NEJM* 2002;346:988)

Prognosis

- **FEV_1**: <60% predicted → 5-y mort ~10%; <40% → ~50%; <20% → ~90%
- **BODE** 10-point scale; HR 1.62 for resp. mort for each 1-point ↑
  BMI: ≤21 (+1)
  Obstruction (FEV_1): 50-64% (+1), 36-49 (+2), ≤35 (+3)
  Dyspnea (MMRC scale): walking level (+1), after 100 yds (+2), with ADL (+3)
  Exs capacity (6 min walk): 250-349 m (+1), 150-249 (+2), ≤149 (+3)
  superior to FEV_1 (*NEJM* 2004;350:1005); can predict survival from LVRS (*Chest* 2006;129:873)
- **Continued smoking,** frequent exacerbations also associated w/ poorer prognosis
- Lung transplant: ∅ Δ survival (*Lancet* 1998;351:24), but may improve QoL and symptoms

HEMOPTYSIS

Definition & Pathophysiology
- Expectoration of blood or blood-streaked sputum
- **Massive hemoptysis**: >600cc/24-48 h (though no absolute definition); gas exchange far more important than absolute blood loss
- Massive hemoptysis usually from tortuous or invaded **bronchial arteries**

Etiologies	
Infection/ Inflammation	**Bronchitis** (most common cause of trivial hemoptysis) **Bronchiectasis** incl. **CF** (most common cause of major hemoptysis) Tuberculosis, aspergilloma, pneumonia/lung abscess
Neoplasm	Usually primary lung cancer, sometimes metastasis
Cardiovascular	PE, pulmonary artery rupture (2° to instrumentation), CHF, mitral stenosis, trauma/foreign body, bronchovascular fistula
Other	Vasculitis (Wegener's granulomatosis, Goodpasture's syndrome), AVM, excessive anticoagulation (w/ underlying lung disease), idiopathic pulmonary hemosiderosis, catamenial (lung endometriosis)

Diagnostic workup
- Localize bleeding site
  - **Rule out GI or ENT source** by exam, history; may require endoscopy
  - Pulmonary source: determine whether **unilateral or bilateral, localized or diffuse, parenchymal or airway** by CXR or chest CT, bronchoscopy if necessary
- PT, PTT, CBC to rule out **coagulopathy**
- Sputum culture/stain for bacteria, fungi, and AFB; cytology to **r/o malignancy**
- ANCA, anti-GBM, urinalysis to ✓ for **vasculitis** or **pulmonary-renal syndrome**

Treatment
- Mechanism of death is asphyxiation not exsanguination; maintain gas exchange, reverse coagulation and treat underlying condition; cough supp. may ↑ risk of asphyxiation
- Massive hemoptysis: put bleeding side dependent; selectively intubate nl lung if needed
  - *Angiography:* used for Dx & Rx (vascular occlusion balloons or **selective embolization of bronchial circulation**)
  - *Rigid bronchoscopy:* allows more interventional options (electrocautery, laser) than flex.
  - Surgical resection

SOLITARY PULMONARY NODULE

Principles
- Definition: single, <3 cm, surrounded by normal lung, no LAN or pleural effusion
- Often "incidentalomas," but may represent early potentially curable localized malignancy

Etiologies	
Benign (70%)	**Malignant (30%)**
Granuloma (80%): TB, histo, cocci **Hamartoma** (10%) Bronchogenic cyst, AVM, pulm infarct Echinococcosis, ascariasis, aspergilloma Wegener's, Rheumatoid nodule Lipoma, fibroma, amyloidoma, pneumonitis	**Bronchogenic carcinoma** (75%): adeno & large cell (peripheral) squamous & small cell (central) **Metastatic** (20%): breast, head & neck, colon, testicular, renal, sarcoma, melanoma Carcinoid, primary sarcoma

Risk of Cancer			
Feature	Low	Intermediate	High
Diameter (cm)	<1.5	1.5-2.2	≥2.3
Nodule shape	smooth	scalloped	spiculated
Age (y)	<45	45-60	>60
Smoking	never	current (≤1 ppd)	current (>1 ppd)
Smoking cessation	none, quit ≥7 y	quit <7 y ago	never quit

(NEJM 2003;348:2535)

Initial evaluation
- **History**: h/o cancer, smoking, age (<30 y = 2% malignant; +15% ea. decade >30)
- **CT**: size/shape, Ca, LAN, effusions, bony destruction, **c/w old studies**
  $\varnothing$ Ca → ↑ likelihood malignant; laminated → granuloma; "popcorn" → hamartoma

Diagnostic studies
- **PET**: detects metab. activity of tumors, 97% Se & 78% Sp for malig. (espec if >8 mm) also useful for surgical staging b/c may detect unsuspected mets (*Lancet* 2001;2:659) useful in deciding which lesions to bx vs. follow w/ serial CT (*J Thor Oncol* 2006;1:71)
- **Transthoracic needle biopsy**: if tech. feasible, 97% will obtain definitive tissue dx (*AJR* 2005;185:1294); if non-informative or malignant → resect
- **Video-assisted thoracoscopic surgery** (VATS): for percutaneously inaccessible lesions; highly sensitive and allows resection; has replaced thoracotomy
- Transbronchial bx: most lesions too small to reliably sample w/o endobronchial U/S (*Chest* 2003;123:604); bronch w/ brushings low-yield unless invading bronchus
- PPD, fungal serologies, ANCA

Management
- **Low-risk**: serial CT (q3mos × 4, then q6mos × 2); shared decision w/ Pt regarding bx
- **Intermediate-risk**: PET, transthoracic needle bx or transbronchial bx depending on location, co-morbidities and Pt preference; if non-informative → VATS
- **High-risk** (and surgical candidate): VATS → lobectomy if malignant

CXR/CHEST CT

Distribution, morphology, & clinical correlation help narrow Ddx

Pattern	Pathophysiology	Ddx
Consolidation	Radiopaque material in air space & interstitium patent airway → "air bronchograms"	*Acute:* water (**pulm edema**), pus (**PNA**), **blood** *Chronic:* neoplasm (BAC, lymphoma), aspiration, inflammatory (BOOP, eosinophilic PNA), PAP, granuloma (TB/fungal, alveolar sarcoid)
Ground glass (CT easier than CXR)	Interstitial thickening or partial filling of alveoli (but vessels visible)	*Acute:* pulm edema, infxn (PCP, viral, resolving bact. PNA) *Chronic:* ILD w/o fibrosis: acute hypersens., DIP/RB, PAP w/ fibrosis: IPF
Septal lines Kerley A & B	Radiopaque material in septae	**Cardiogenic pulm edema**, interstitial PNA (viral, mycoplasma), lymphangitic tumor
Reticular	Lace-like net (ILD)	**ILD** (espec. IPF, CVD, bleomycin, asbestos)
Nodules	Tumor Granulomas Abscess	*Cavitary:* **Primary or metastatic cancer**, **TB** (react. or miliary), fungus, Wegener's, RA septic emboli, PNA *Noncavitary:* any of above + **sarcoid**, hypersens. pneum., HIV, Kaposi's sarcoma
Wedge opac.	Peripheral infarct	**PE**, cocaine, angioinv. aspergillus, Wegener's
Tree-in-bud (best on CT)	Inflammation of small airways	**Bronchopneumonia**, endobronchial TB/MAI, viral PNA, aspiration, ABPA, CF, asthma, BOOP
Hilar fullness	↑ LN or pulm arteries	**Neoplasm** (lung, mets, lymphoma) **Infxn** (AIDS); **Granuloma** (sarcoid/TB/ fungal) Pulmonary hypertension
Upper lobe	n/a	**TB**, fungal, sarcoid, hypersens. pneum., CF, XRT
Lower lobe	n/a	**Aspiration**, bronchiect., IPF, RA, SLE, asbestos
Peripheral	n/a	BOOP, IPF & DIP, eos PNA, asbestosis

CXR in heart failure
- ↑ cardiac silhouette (in systolic dysfxn, not in diastolic)
- Pulmonary venous hypertension: cephalization of vessels (vessels size > bronchi in upper lobes), peribronchial cuffing (fluid around bronchi seen on end → small circles), Kerley B lines (horizontal 1-2 cm lines at bases), ↑ vascular pedicle width, loss of sharp vascular margins, pleural effusions (~75% bilateral)
- Pulmonary edema: ranges from ground glass to consolidation; often dependent and central, sparing outer third ("bat wing" appearance)

INTERSTITIAL LUNG DISEASE

WORKUP OF ILD

Rule-out mimickers of ILD
- **Congestive heart failure**
- **Infection**
  viral (influenza, parainfluenza, adenovirus, coronavirus, RSV, CMV)
  bacterial (especially atypicals such as *Mycoplasma*, *Chlamydia*, and *Legionella*)
  fungal (PCP, histoplasmosis, coccidioidomycosis); mycobacterial (MTb and MAI)
  parasitic (see Löffler's syndrome below)
- **Malignancy**
  lymphangitic carcinomatosis: adenoCa (breast, pancreas, stomach, lung) > squamous
  bronchoalveolar cell carcinoma (although usually appears as air-space disease)
  lymphoproliferative disorders (leukemia and lymphoma)

History and physical exam
- Occupational, travel, exposure, medications, precipitating event
- Tempo (acute → infection, CHF, hypersensitivity pneumonitis, eos PNA, AIP, COP)
- Extrapulmonary s/s (skin Δs, arthralgias/arthritis, neuropathies, etc.)

Diagnostic studies
- CXR and **high-resolution chest CT**: reticular, nodular, or ground glass pattern
  upper → coal, silicosis, hypersens., sarcoid, TB, RA, LCG; lower → IPF, asbestosis
  adenopathy → sarcoidosis, berylliosis, silicosis, malignancy, fungal infections
  pleural disease → collagen-vascular diseases, asbestosis, infections, XRT
- PFTs: restrictive pattern ($\downarrow$ volumes), $\downarrow D_LCO$, $\downarrow P_aO_2$ (especially w/ exercise)
- Serologies: ✓ ACE, ANA, RF, ANCA, anti-GBM, HIV
- Bronchoalveolar lavage: dx in infections, hemorrhage, PIE syndromes, PAP
- Biopsy (transbronchial, CT-guided, VATS, open): dx in granulomatous diseases (sarcoid, hypersens., Wegener's, Churg-Strauss, LCG), pneumoconioses, IIPs, infection, malig
  ∴ consider if no clear precipitant and noninvasive workup unrevealing

ETIOLOGIES OF ILD

Sarcoidosis *(Lancet 2003;361:1111; JAMA 2003;289:330)*
- Prevalence: African Americans, northern Europeans, and females; onset in 3rd–4th decade
- Pathophysiology: depression of cellular immune system peripherally, activation centrally
- Clinical manifestations: **asx hilar LAN ± ILD** or fever, malaise, dyspnea, arthralgias, rash
  Stages: I = bilateral hilar LAN; II = LAN + ILD; III = ILD only; IV = diffuse fibrosis
  Extrathoracic: erythema nodosum and/or skin plaques (~25%); uveitis (~25%);
  hepatomegaly ± granulomatous hepatitis (~25%); BM & splenic granulomas (~50%);
  CNS/ peripheral neuropathy (~5%); cardiac conduction dis. (~5%); ↑ parotid (<10%)
  Löfgren's syndrome: erythema nodosum + hilar adenopathy + arthritis
  Ddx erythema nodosum: idiopathic (34%), infection (33%, Strep, TB), sarcoid (22%), drugs (OCP, PCNs), vasculitis (Behçet's), IBD, lymphoma *(Arthritis Rheum 2000;43:584)*
- Diagnostic studies: **LN bx → noncaseating granulomas** + multinucleated giant cells
  ↑ **ACE** (Se 60%, 90% w/ active dis.; Sp 80%, false ⊕ in granulomatous diseases)
  hypercalciuria and hypercalcemia (10%, due to vitamin D hydroxylation by Mφ);
  lymphopenia, eosinophilia, ↑ ESR, polyclonal ↑ IgG, cutaneous anergy (70%)
- Treatment: steroids if sx, or extrathoracic organ dysfxn, but controversial
  (JAMA 2002;287:1301; ERJ 2006;28:627); anti-TNF, MTX, AZA, cyclophosphamide also used
- Prognosis: some spontaneously remit (60-80% of stage I, 50-60% stage II, 30% stage III), 40% improve on Rx, 20% go on to irreversible lung injury

Iatrogenic
- Chemo: bleomycin (triggered by hyperoxia), busulfan, cyclophosphamide, MTX, nitrosourea
- Other drugs: nitrofurantoin, sulfonamides, thiazides, amiodarone, INH, hydralazine, gold
  amio (~10%; dose & duration depend.): chronic interstitial pneumonia ↔ ARDS;
  bx → vacuolized Mφ w/ lamellar inclusions on EM; Rx: d/c amio, steroids
- Radiation (→ BOOP): oftentimes with sharply linear, non-anatomic boundaries

Idiopathic interstitial pneumonias (IIPs) (AJRCCM 2005;172:268)
- Definition: **ILD of unknown cause**; dx by clinical, radiographic and histologic features
- Idiopathic pulmonary fibrosis (**IPF** = usual interstitial pneumonia (UIP); (AJRCCM 2000;161:646): sx >12 mos; HRCT: peripheral, subpleural, basal reticular opacities, traction bronchiectasis & honeycombing, Rx: ? IFN-γ ↓ mort. (NEJM 2004;350:125; Chest 2005;128:203) NAC 600 tid slowed ↓ lung fxn (NEJM 2005;353:2229); 5-y mort. 80%
- Acute interstitial pneumonia (**AIP**, "Hamman-Rich syndrome"): sx 1-2 wks; HRCT: ground glass w/ lobar sparing; Rx: ? steroids; 6-month mort. 60%
- Cryptogenic organizing pneumonia (**COP**, also called bronchiolitis obliterans w/ organizing pneumonia, **BOOP**, if cause known): prolif. granulation tissue in small bronchioles and inflammation of surrounding alveoli. Causes of **BOOP**: post-infxn, drugs (amiodarone, bleomycin), rheum. diseases, post-HSCT or XRT (Archives 2001;161:158); sx <3 mos; HRCT: subpleural, peribronchial nodules or patchy consolidation; Rx: steroids; 5-y mort. <5%
- Desquamative interstitial pneumonia (**DIP**) & respiratory bronchiolitis-associated ILD (**RBILD**): Mφ in alveoli in smokers age 30-50; RBILD milder form; sx wks-mos; HRCT: DIP w/ diffuse ground glass mid/lower lobes; RBILD w/ nodules, bronchial thickening, patchy ground glass; Rx: quit smoking, ? steroids; death rare
- Nonspecific interstitial pneumonia (**NSIP**): histologic mimic of CTDs & hypersens.; cellular & fibrotic types; sx for mos-y; HRCT: symmetric basal subpleural homogenous ground glass or consolidation; Rx: steroids; 5-y mort. 10% (fibrotic ↑)
- Lymphocytic interstitial pneumonia (**LIP**): polyclonal B-cell infiltration of lung; sx >1 yr; HRCT: diffuse ground glass, nodules, thin-walled cysts; Rx: steroids; prog unknown

Environmental & occupational exposures (NEJM 2000;342:406)
- **Pneumoconioses** (inorganic dusts)
  Coal worker's: upper lobe coal macules; may progress to massive fibrosis
  Silicosis: upper lobe opacities ± "eggshell calcification" of lymph nodes; ↑ risk of TB
  Asbestosis: lower lobe fibrosis, calcified pleural plaques; ↑ risk of mesothelioma
  Berylliosis: multisystemic granulomatous disease that mimics sarcoidosis
- **Hypersensitivity pneumonitides** (organic dusts): loose, noncaseating granulomas
  Antigens: "farmer's lung" (spores of thermophilic actinomyces); "pigeon fancier's lung" (proteins from feathers and excreta of birds); "humidifier lung" (thermophilic bacteria)
  Pathophysiology: immunologic rxn; either acute (6 h after exposure) or chronic

Collagen vascular diseases (ERJ 2001;18:69S; NEJM 2006;355:2655)
- **Rheumatologic disease**
  Scleroderma: fibrosis in ~67%; PHT seen in ~10% of CREST Pts
  PM-DM: ILD & weakness of respiratory muscles; MCTD: PHT & fibrosis
  SLE & RA: pleuritis and pleural effusions more often than ILD
- **Vasculitis** (can p/w diffuse alveolar hemorrhage)
  Wegener's granulomatosis (⊕ c-ANCA) w/ necrotizing granulomas
  Churg-Strauss syndrome (⊕ c- or p-ANCA) w/ eosinophilia & necrotizing granulomas
  Microscopic polyangiitis (⊕ p-ANCA) w/o granulomas

Diffuse alveolar hemorrhage (DAH)
- CHF-like CXR appearance, but does not resolve w/ diuresis; ± hemoptysis, ↓ Hct, ↑ D$_L$CO
- Goodpasture's syndrome = DAH + RPGN; typically in smokers; ⊕ anti-GBM in 90%
- Idiopathic pulmonary hemosiderosis (IPH): a rare disease and dx of exclusion
- Other: ANCA ⊕ vasculitis, SLE, PM, APLA, crack cocaine, HSCT, XRT

Pulmonary infiltrates w/ eosinophilia (PIE) = eos on BAL ± periph. blood
- **Allergic bronchopulmonary aspergillosis (ABPA)**: allergic reaction to Aspergillus
  Criteria: asthma, pulm infiltrates (transient or fixed), skin rxn & serum precipitins to Aspergillus, ↑ IgE to Aspergillus & total (>1000), ↑ eos, central bronchiectasis
  Rx: steroids ± itraconazole for refractory cases (NEJM 2000;342:756)
- Löffler's syndrome: transient pulmonary infiltrates + cough, dyspnea, eos due to parasites (Ascariasis, hookworm, Strongyloides) or drugs (nitrofurantoin, crack)
- Acute eosinophilic pneumonia (AEP): acute hypoxic febrile illness; Rx: steroids
- Chronic eosinophilic pneumonia (CEP): "photonegative" of CHF, typically in women
- Other: Churg-Strauss syndrome; hypereosinophilic syndrome

Miscellaenous
- Pulmonary alveolar proteinosis (PAP): accumulation of surfactant-like phospholipids; male smokers; cough w/ white & gummy sputum; BAL milky fluid (NEJM 2003;349:2527)
- Langerhans cell granulomatosis (LCG): affects young male smokers; cysts; PTX in ~25%

PLEURAL EFFUSION

Pathophysiology
- **Systemic factors** (eg, ↑ PCWP, ↓ oncotic pressure) → *transudative* effusion
- **Local factors** (ie, Δ pleural surface permeability) → *exudative* effusion

Transudates
- **Congestive heart failure (40%)**: 80% bilateral, usually cardiomegaly on CXR occasionally exudative (especially after aggressive diuresis or if chronic), but ~75% of exudative effusions in CHF Pts found to have non-CHF cause (*Chest* 2002;122:1518)
- Constrictive pericarditis
- **Cirrhosis** ("hepatic hydrothorax"): diaphragmatic defect w/ passage of ascitic fluid often right-sided (2/3) & massive (even w/o marked ascites)
- Nephrotic syndrome: usually small, bilateral, asymptomatic (r/o PE b/c hypercoag)
- Other: PE (usually exudate), malignancy (lymphatic obstruction), myxedema, CAPD

Exudates
- **Lung parenchymal infection (25%)**
  bacterial (parapneumonic): can evolve along spectrum of *exudative* (but sterile) → *fibropurulent* (infected fluid) → *organization* (fibrosis & formation of rigid pleural peel)
  mycobacterial: >50% lymphs 80% of the time, ADA >40, pleural bx ~70% Se
  fungal, viral (usually small), parasitic (eg, amebiasis, echinococcosis, paragonimiasis)
- **Malignancy (15%)**: primary lung cancer most common, metastases (especially breast, lymphoma, etc.), mesothelioma (✓ serum osteopontin levels; *NEJM* 2005;353:15)
- **Pulmonary embolism (10%)**: effusions in ~40% of PEs; exudate (75%) > transudate (25%); hemorrhagic—must have high suspicion b/c presentation highly variable
- **Collagen vascular disease**: RA (large), SLE (small), Wegener's, Churg-Strauss
- **Gastrointestinal diseases**: pancreatitis, esophageal rupture, abdominal abscess
- Hemothorax (Hct_{eff}/Hct_{blood} >50%): trauma, PE, malignancy, coagulopathy, leaking aortic aneurysm, aortic dissection, pulmonary vascular malformation
- Chylothorax (triglycerides >110): thoracic duct damage due to trauma, malignancy, LAM
- Other
  Post-CABG: left-sided; initially bloody, clears after several wks
  Dressler's syndrome (pericarditis & pleuritis post-MI), uremia, post-radiation therapy
  Asbestos exposure: benign; ⊕ eosinophils
  Drug-induced (eg, nitrofurantoin, methysergide, bromocriptine, amiodarone): ⊕ eos.
  Meigs' syndrome = benign ovarian tumor → ascites & pleural effusion
  Yellow-nail syndrome: yellow nails, lymphedema, pleural effusion, bronchiectasis

Diagnostic studies
- **Thoracentesis**
  Indications: all effusions >1 cm in decubitus view
    if suspect due to CHF, can diurese and see if effusions resolve (75% do so in 48 h)
    asymmetry, fever, chest pain, or failure to resolve → thoracentesis
    parapneumonics should be tapped ASAP (cannot exclude infxn clinically)
  Diagnostic studies: ✓ total protein, LDH, glucose, cell count w/ differential, gram stain & culture, pH; remaining fluid for additional studies as dictated by clinical scenario
  Complications: PTX (5-10%), hemothorax (~1%), re-expansion pulm. edema (if >1.5 L removed), spleen/liver lac.; post-tap CXR not routinely needed (*Annals* 1996;124:816)
- **Transudate vs. exudate** (*Annals* 1972;77:507)
  Light's criteria: exudate = TP_{eff}/TP_{serum} >0.5 or LDH_{eff}/LDH_{serum} >0.6 or LDH_{eff} >2/3 ULN of LDH_{serum}; 98% Se, 83% Sp; best Se of all methods (*Chest* 1995;107:1604); however will misidentify 25% of transudates as "exudates"; ∴ if clinically suspect transudate but meets criterion for exudate, confirm w/ test w/ higher Sp
  exudative criteria w/ better Sp: serum-effusion alb gradient ≤1.2; Se 87%, Sp 92% chol$_{eff}$ >45 mg/dl and LDH$_{eff}$ >200; 90% Se, 98% Sp (no serum required)
  CHF effusions: TP may ↑ with diuresis or chronicity → "pseudoexudate"; use albumin gradient ≤1.2, chol$_{eff}$ >60 md/dl (Se 54%, Sp 92%), or clinical judgment to help distinguish (*Chest* 2002;122:1524)
- **Complicated vs. uncomplicated parapneumonic** (*Chest* 1995;108:299)
  complicated = ⊕ gram stain or culture or pH <7.2 or glucose <60
  complicated parapneumonic effusions usually require **drainage** to achieve resolution
  empyema = frank pus, also needs drainage to achieve resolution

- Additional pleural fluid studies (NEJM 2002;346:1971)
  WBC & diff. exudates tend to have ↑ WBC vs. transudates but nonspecific
    neutrophils → parapneumonic, PE, pancreatitis
    lymphocytes (>50%) → cancer, TB, rheumatologic
    eos (>10%) → blood, air, drug rxn, asbestos, paragonimiasis, Churg-Strauss, PE
  RBC: Hct_{eff} 1–20% → cancer, PE, trauma; Hct_{eff}/Hct_{blood} >50% → hemothorax
  AFB: yield in TB 0-10% w/ stain, 11–50% w/ culture, ~70% w/ pleural bx
  adenosine deaminase (ADA): seen w/ granulomas, >70 suggests TB, <40 excludes TB
  cytology: yield is 55% w/ 1 sample, 70% w/ 3 samples; ↑ sample volume → no Δ Se
  glucose: <60 mg/dl → malignancy, infection, RA
  amylase: seen in pancreatic disease and esophageal rupture (salivary amylase)
  rheumatoid factor, C_H50, ANA: limited utility in dx collagen vascular disease
  triglycerides: >110 → chylothorax, 50-110 → ✓ lipoprotein analysis for chylomicrons
  cholesterol: >60; seen in chronic effusions (eg, CHF, RA)
  creatinine: effusion/serum ratio >1 → urinothorax
- Chest CT; pleural biopsy; VATS

Characteristics of Pleural Fluid (not diagnostic criteria)						
Etiology	Appear	WBC diff	RBC	pH	Glc	Comments
CHF	clear, straw	<1,000 lymphs	<5,000	normal	≈serum	bilateral, cardiomegaly
Cirrhosis	clear, straw	<1,000	<5,000	normal	≈serum	right-sided
Uncomplicated parapneumonic	turbid	5-40,000 polys	<5,000	normal to ↓	≈ serum (>40)	
Complicated parapneumonic	turbid to purulent	5-40,000 polys	<5,000	↓↓	↓ (<40)	need drainage
Empyema	purulent	25-100,000 polys	<5,000	↓↓↓	↓↓	need drainage
Tuberculosis	serosang.	5-10,000 lymphs	<10,000	normal to ↓	normal to ↓	⊕ AFB ⊕ ADA
Malignancy	turbid to bloody	1-100,000 lymphs	<100,000	normal to ↓	normal to ↓	⊕ cytology
Pulmonary embolism	sometimes bloody	1-50,000 polys	<100,000	normal	≈serum	no infarct → transudate
Rheumatoid Arthritis/SLE	turbid	1-20,000 variable	<1,000	↓	RA ↓↓↓ SLE nl	↑ RF, ↓ C_H50 ↑ imm. complex
Pancreatitis	serosang. to turbid	1-50,000 polys	<10,000	normal	≈serum	left-sided, ↑ amylase
Esophageal rupture	turbid to purulent	<5,000 >50,000	<10,000	↓↓↓	↓↓	left-sided, ↑ amylase

Treatment
- Symptomatic effusion: therapeutic thoracentesis, treat underlying disease process
- Parapneumonic effusion (Chest 2000;118:1158)
  uncomplicated → antibiotics for pneumonia
  >½ hemithorax or complicated or empyema → tube thoracostomy
    (o/w risk of organization and subsequent need for surgical decortication)
  loculated → tube thoracostomy or VATS; intrapleural lytics w/o clear benefit
    (although largest trial used lytics late and w/ small-bore chest tubes, NEJM 2005;352:865)
- Malignant effusion: serial thoracenteses vs. tube thoracostomy + pleurodesis (success
  rate ~80-90%) (Cochrane database 2004; CD002916); pleurodesing agent (talc, bleo, doxy)
  controversial; systemic steroids and pH <7.2 assoc. w/ ↑ likelihood to fail pleurodesis
- TB effusions: effusion will often resolve spontaneously; however, treat Pt for active TB
- Hepatic hydrothorax
  Rx: Δ pressure gradient (ie, ↓ ascitic fluid volume, NIPPV)
  avoid chest tubes; prn thoracenteses, pleurodesis, TIPS or VATS closure of diaphragmatic
    defects if medical Rx fails; NIPPV for acute short-term management
  spontaneous bacterial empyema (SBEM) can occur (even w/o SBP being present),
    ∴ thoracentesis if suspect infection
  transplant is definitive treatment and workup should begin immediately

VENOUS THROMBOEMBOLISM (VTE)

Definitions
- Calf-vein thrombosis: less likely to cause significant thromboembolism, 80% resolve spont.
- Proximal deep venous thrombosis (DVT): thrombosis of popliteal, femoral, or iliac veins (nb, "superficial" femoral vein is part of the deep venous system)
- Pulmonary embolism (PE): thrombosis that originates in the venous system and embolizes to the pulmonary arterial circulation; ~600,000 cases per yr

Risk factors (JAMA 1990;263:2735)
- Virchow's triad for thrombogenesis
  - **alterations in blood flow** (ie, stasis): bed rest, inactivity, CHF, CVA w/in 3 mos, air travel >8 h (NEJM 2001;345:779)
  - **injury to endothelium**: trauma, surgery, prior DVT
  - **thrombophilia** (50% ⊕): APC resistance, protein C or S deficiency, APS, prothrombin gene mutation, hyperhomocysteinemia OCP, HRT, tamofixen, raloxifene
- Malignancy (12% of "idiopathic" DVT/PE)
- History of thrombosis

Clinical manifestations (Chest 1991;100:598 & Am J Card 1991;68:1723)
- DVT: calf pain, edema, venous distention, pain on dorsiflexion, asx
  - *phlegmasia cerulea dolens:* stagnant blood → edema, cyanosis, pain
- PE: dyspnea (73%), pleuritic chest pain (66%), cough (37%), hemoptysis (13%), asx massive PE with acute cor pulmonale → syncope, hypotension, PEA
- 50% of Pts with symptomatic DVT have asx PE; 60% of patients with PE have DVT

Physical exam (Chest 1991;100:598 & 2000;117:39; Am J Card 1991;68:1723)
- DVT (Se 60-88%, Sp 30-72%, JAMA 1998;279:1094): lower extremity swelling (>3 cm c/w unaffected leg), edema, erythema, warmth, tenderness, palpable cord, ⊕ Homan's sign (calf pain on dorsiflexion, seen in <5% of patients)
- PE: tachypnea (>70%), crackles (51%), tachycardia (30%), fever, cyanosis, pleural friction rub, loud P₂; submassive/massive: ↑ JVP, R-sided S₃, Graham Steell's (PR) murmur

Pretest Probability of DVT	
Major points	**Minor points**
• Active cancer	• Trauma to symptomatic leg w/in 60 d
• Paralysis, paresis, immobilization of foot	• Pitting edema in symptomatic leg
• Bed rest × >3d or major surg. w/in 4 wks	• Dilated superficial veins (nonvaricose) in symptomatic leg only
• Localized tenderness along veins	• Hospitalization w/in previous 6 mos
• Swelling of thigh *and* calf	• Erythema
• Swelling of calf >3 cm c/w asx side	
• ⊕ FHx of DVT (≥2 1° relatives)	
High probability (~85% ⊕ DVT)	**Low probability** (~5% ⊕ DVT)
≥3 major + *no* alternative dx	1 major + ≥2 minor + alternative dx
≥2 major + ≥2 minor + *no* alternative dx	1 major + ≥1 minor + *no* alternative dx
Intermediate prob (~33% ⊕ DVT)	0 major + ≥3 minor + alternative dx
neither high nor low probability	0 major + ≥2 minor + *no* alternative dx

(Lancet 1995;345:1326; NEJM 1996;335:1816)

Diagnostic studies (DVT)
- Compression ultrasonography >95% Se & Sp (BMJ 1998;316:17); U/S ⊕ in 60% Pts w/ PE

Figure 2-3 Approach to suspected DVT

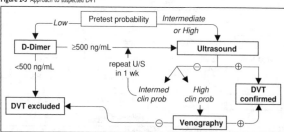

(Based on data from Lancet 1995;345:1326 & 1997;350:1795; NEJM 1996;335:1816 & 2003;349:13.)

"Modified Wells" Pretest Probability Scoring of PE	
Variable	**Point Score**
• PE as likely or more likely than alternate dx; clin. s/s of DVT	3 each
• HR >100 bpm; prior DVT or PE	1.5 each
• Immobilization (bed rest ≥3 d) or surgery w/in 4 wks	1.5
• Hemoptysis; malignancy	1 each

"Modified Wells" Pretest Probability Assessment (Use for V/Q)		
Score <2	Score 2-6	Score >6
Low probability	Intermediate probability	High probability

"Dichotomized Wells" Pretest Probability Assessment* (Use for CTA)	
Score ≤4: PE "Unlikely"	Score >4: PE "Likely"

(*Ann Int Med* 2001;135:98) (**JAMA* 2006;295:172)

Diagnostic studies (PE)
- CXR (limited Se & Sp): 12% nl, atelectasis, effusion, ↑ hemidiaphragm, Hampton hump, (wedge-shaped density abutting pleura); Westermark sign (avascularity distal to PE)
- ECG (limited Se & Sp): sinus tachycardia, AF; signs of RV strain → RAD, P pulmonale, RBBB, TWI V_1-V_4 (McGinn-White pattern; *Chest* 1997;111:537), $S_IQ_{III}T_{III}$
- ABG: hypoxemia, hypocapnia, respiratory alkalosis, ↑ A-a gradient (*Chest* 1996;109:78) 18% w/ room air P_aO_2 85-105 mmHg, 6% w/ nl A-a gradient (*Chest* 1991;100:598)
- D-dimer: high Se, poor Sp (~25%); ⊖ ELISA has >99% NPV and can be used to r/o PE in Pts w/ "unlikely" pretest prob. (see below) (*JAMA* 2006;295:172)
- Echocardiography: useful for risk stratification (RV dysfxn), but not dx (Se <50%)
- V/Q scan: use at CTA-inexperienced institutions or if contraindication to CTA
- **CT angiography (CTA):** Se. ~90% & Sp ~95% w/ MDCT, + CTV, and experienced readers (PIOPED II, *NEJM* 2006:354:2317); PPV & NPV >95% if imaging concordant w/ clinical suspicion, ≤80% if discordant (∴ need to consider both); CT may also provide other dx
- Pulmonary angiography: ? gold-standard (morbidity 5%, mortality <0.5%)
- MR angiography: Se 84% (segmental) to 100% (lobar) (*Lancet* 2002;359:1643)
- **Diagnostic algorithms:** CTA-experienced institutions use CTA algorithm (fig. 2-4); CTA inexperience, contraindic., *or* inconclusive CTA use V/Q algorithm (fig. 2-5)

Figure 2-4 Approach to suspected PE using CTA

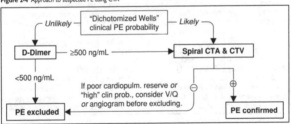

Based on data from *NEJM* 2005;352:1760 & 2006;354:22; *JAMA* 2005;293:2012 & 2006;295:172

Figure 2-5 Approach to suspected PE using V/Q scan

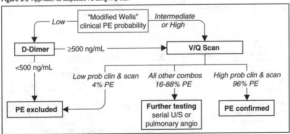

Based on data from *JAMA* 1990:263:2753; *Annals* 2001;135:98

Workup for Idiopathic VTE
- **Thrombophilia workup:** recurrent or idiopathic DVT/PE + (age <50, ⊕ FHx, unusual location, massive); *may not predict recurrence*, ? utility of w/u (*JAMA 2005;293:2352*)
- **Malignancy workup:** 12% pts w/ "idiopathic" DVT/PE will have a malignancy; initial screening is adequate: H&P (breast, abd, FOBT, pelvic, rectal), basic labs (CMP, CBC, U/A); CXR, up-to-date mammo., colonoscopy; avoid extensive w/u (*NEJM 1998;338:1169*)

Risk stratification for Pts with PE
- **Clinical:** hypotension and/or tachycardia (~30% mortality), hypoxemia
- **CTA:** RV / LV dimension ratio >0.9 (*Circ 2004;110:3276*)
- **Biomarkers:** ↑ troponin (*Circ 2002;106:1263*),↑ BNP (*Circ 2003;107:1576*)
- **Echocardiogram:** RV dysfxn (2× ↑ mort)

Treatment of VTE (*Chest 2004;126:401-S*)
- **Calf-vein DVT:** sx, extending to proximal veins or associated PE → anticoagulate
- **UE DVT:** *spontaneous* → anticoagulate (? catheter-lysis, angioplasty, surgery)
  catheter-associated: if sx → anticoagulate & ? catheter removal; asx → observe
- **Acute anticoagulation** (*initiate immediately if high clinical suspicion!*)
  IV UFH: 80 U/kg bolus → 18 U/kg/h → titrate to goal PTT 60-85 sec (1.5-2.3 × cntl), *or*
  SC UFH: 333 U/kg ×1 → 250 U/kg bid (*JAMA 2006;296:935*), *or*
  LWMH: enoxaparin 1 mg/kg SC bid *or* dalteparin 200 IU/kg SC qd (*Annals 1999;130:800*)
    LWMH preferred over UFH except: renal failure (CrCl <25), ? extreme obesity, hemodynamic instability or bleed risk (*Chest 2004;126:401S & Cochrane 2004;CD001100*)
    attractive option as outPt bridge to long-term oral anticoagulation
  Fondaparinux: 5-10 mg SC qd ≈ UFH (*MATISSE, NEJM 2003;349:1695*), used in HIT ⊕ Pts
  Direct thrombin inhibitors (eg, argatroban, lepirudin) used in HIT ⊕ Pts
- **Thrombolysis** (TPA 100 mg over 2 h *or* 0.6 mg/kg over 3-15 min)
  extensive DVT or massive PE causing *hemodynamic compromise*
  controversial for *RV dysfunction alone* no mort. benefit (*NEJM 2002;347:1143*)
- **Thrombectomy:** if large, proximal PE + hemodynamic compromise + contra. to lysis; also consider in experienced ctr if lg prox. PE + RV dysfxn (*J Thorac CV Surg 2005;129:1018*)
- **IVC filter:** if anticoagulation contraindication, failure, bleed or ↓ CP reserve; temp. filter if risk time-limited; PE ↓ 1/2, DVT ↑ 2 ×, no mort. diff. (*NEJM 1998;338:409; Circ 2005;112:416*)
- **Long-term anticoagulation**
  Warfarin: start when PTT therapeutic or after 1st dose of LMWH; overlap × 5 d w/ heparin; goal INR 2-3 (superior to 1.5-2; *ELATE, NEJM 2003;349:631*)
  Reversible or time-limited risk factor: 3-6 mos of warfarin
  Idiopathic PE/DVT: long-term (~5 y) superior to 6 mos (*PREVENT, NEJM 2003;348:1425*)
  2nd event, cancer, nonmodifiable risk factor: 12 mos – lifelong (*DURAC II, NEJM 1997;336:393*)
  Pts w/ cancer: long-term Rx w/ LMWH superior to warfarin (*CLOT, NEJM 2003;349:146*)
  ✓ head CT if melanoma, renal cell, thyroid, or chorioCA as brain mets tend to bleed

Complications & Prognosis
- Post-thrombotic syndrome (25%): pain, swelling; ↓ with compression stockings × 3 mos
- Recurrent VTE: 1%/y (after 1st VTE) to 5%/y (after recurrent VTE)
  after only 6 mos of Rx: 5%/y & >10%/y, respectively
  predictors: D-dimer ≥250 after d/c anticoag (*JAMA 2003;290:1071*); ⊕ U/S after 3 mos of anticoag (*Annals 2002;137:955*); thrombin generation >400 nM (*JAMA 2006;296:397*)
- Chronic thromboembolic PHT after acute PE ~3.8% (*NEJM 2004;350:2257*)
- Mortality: 17% at 3 mos (PE, cancer, resp. failure); 75% of those die during initial hosp.

Thromboprophylaxis

Risk	Patient & situation	Prophylaxis
Low VTE << 1%	• minor surgery, age <40, no RF	early ambulation
Moderate DVT 2-4% PE 1-2%	• minor surgery + age 40-60 *or* RF • major surgery + age <40, no RF	**LDUH** 5,000 U q12h **LMWH** dalt 2,500 qd *or* enox 20 mg qd IPC + ES
High DVT 4-8% PE 2-4%	• minor surgery + age >60 *or* RF • major surgery + age >40 *or* RF • MI, CVA, bed rest, chronic illness	**LDUH** 5,000 U q8h **LMWH** dalt 5,000 U qd *or* enox 40 mg qd IPC + ES
Highest DVT 10-20% PE 4-10%	• orthopedic surgery, trauma • major surgery + age >40 *and* RF • acute spinal cord injury	**LMWH** dalteparin 5,000 U qd *or* enoxaparin 30 mg bid **fondaparinux** 2.5 mg qd

RF = risk factor; includes: immobility, varicose veins, CHF, malignancy, thrombophilia, prior VTE; ES = elastic stockings; IPC = intermittent pneumatic compression; LDUH = low-dose SC UFH (*Chest 2004;126:388-S*)

PULMONARY HYPERTENSION (PHT)

PA mean pressure >25 mmHg at rest or >30 mmHg with exertion

Pathobiology *(NEJM 2004;351:1655)*
- Imbalance between vasoconstrictors and vasodilators
  - ↑ vasoconstrictors: thromboxane A_2 (TXA_2), serotonin (5-HT), endothelin-1 (ET-1)
  - ↓ vasodilators: prostacyclin (PGI_2), nitric oxide (NO), vasoactive peptide (VIP)
- Smooth muscle & endothelial cell proliferation: ↑ VEGF, ET-1, 5-HT; ↓ PGI_2, NO, VIP; mutations in bone morphogenic protein receptor 2 (*BMPR2*; gene involved in prolif. & apoptosis) seen in ~50% familial and ~26% sporadic cases of PPH *(NEJM 2001;345:319)*
- *In situ* thrombosis: ↑ TXA_2, 5-HT, PAI-1; ↓ PGI_2, NO, VIP, tissue plasminogen activator

Etiologies of Pulmonary Hypertension (Venice Classification)	

Pulmonary arterial HTN (PAH)	• Idiopathic (IPAH)
	• Familial (FPAH)
	• Associated conditions (APAH)
	  Connective tissue disorders: CREST, SLE, MCTD, RA, PM, Sjögren
	  Congenital L → R shunts: ASD, VSD, PDA
	  Portopulmonary HTN (? 2° vasoactive substances not filtered in ESLD; ≠ hepatopulmonary syndrome)
	  HIV; Drugs & toxins: anorexic agents, rapeseed oil, L-tryptophan
	• Pulmonary veno-occlusive disease: ? 2° chemo, BMT; orthopnea, CHF, pl eff, nl PCWP; art vasodil. worsen CHF *(AJRCCM 2000;162:1964)*

Left heart disease	• Left ventricular systolic or diastolic dysfunction • MS/MR
Respiratory system disorders or chronic hypoxia	• COPD • Alveolar hypoventilation (eg, NM disease) • ILD • Chronic hypoxemia (eg, high altitude) • Sleep apnea • Pneumonia (transient and mild PHT)
Chronic thrombotic or embolic disease	• Acute pulmonary embolism (transient PHT) • Chronic thromboembolic pulmonary HTN (CTEPH) • Nonthrombotic emboli (tumor, foreign body, parasites)
Miscellaneous	• Sarcoidosis, histiocytosis X, lymphangiomatosis, schistosomiasis • Compression of pulmonary vessels (adenopathy, tumor, fibrosis)

(EHJ 2004;25:2243)

Clinical manifestations
- Dyspnea, exertional syncope (hypoxia, ↓ CO), exertional chest pain (RV ischemia)
- Symptoms of R-sided CHF (eg, peripheral edema, RUQ fullness, abdominal distention)
- IPAH: mean age of onset 36 (men older than women); female:male = 1.7-3.5:1

Physical exam
- PHT: prominent P_2, R-sided S_4, RV heave, PA tap & flow murmur, PR (Graham Steell), TR
- ± RV failure: ↑ JVP, hepatomegaly, peripheral edema

Diagnostic studies
- CXR: dilatation and pruning of pulmonary arteries, enlargement of RA and RV
- ECG: RAD, RBBB, RAE ("P pulmonale"), RVH (Se 55%, Sp 70%)
- PFTs: ↓ D_{LCO}, mild restrictive pattern
- ABG: ↓ P_aO_2 and S_aO_2 (especially with exertion), ↓ P_aCO_2, ↑ A-a gradient
- Echocardiogram: ↑ RVSP (estimated from TR jet), flattening ("D") of septum, TR, PR
- Cardiac catheterization: ↑ RA, RV, and PA pressures, ↑ PVR, ↓ CO, normal PCWP

Workup (IPAH yearly incidence 1-2 per million, r/o 2° causes)
- Echocardiogram: r/o LV dysfxn, mitral valve disease, and congenital heart disease
- Cardiac catheterization: definitive evaluation of filling pressures, r/o ↑ PCWP, r/o shunt
- CXR and high resolution chest CT: r/o parenchymal lung disease
- PFTs: r/o obstructive and restrictive lung disease, check D_{LCO}
- ABG & polysomnography: r/o hypoventilation, OSA
- CTA (large/med vessel), V/Q scan (small vessel), ± pulmonary angiogram: r/o PE
- Vasculitis labs: ANA (commonly ⊕ in PPH), RF, anti-Scl-70, anti-centromere, ESR
- LFTs & HIV: r/o portopulmonary and HIV-associated PAH
- 6-min walk test (6MWT) or cardiopulmonary exercise testing to establish fxnl capacity

Treatment *(Archives 2002;162:1925; NEJM 2004;351:1425; JIM 2005;258:199)*
- Principles
  1) prevent and reverse vasoactive substance imbalance and vascular remodeling
  2) prevent RV failure: ↓ wall stress (↓ PVR, PAP, RV diam); ensure adeq. systemic DBP

- **Supportive**
  Oxygen: maintain S_aO_2 >90-92% (reduces vasoconstriction)
  Diuretics: ↓ RV wall stress and relieve RHF sx; *gentle* because RV is preload depend.
  Digoxin: control AF, ? counteract neg. inotropic effects CCB
  Dobutamine and inhaled NO for decompensated PHT
  Anticoagulation: ↓VTE risk of RHF; ? prevention of *in situ* microthrombi; ? mort. benefit (*Circ* 1984;70:580; *Chest* 2006;130:545)

- **Vasodilators**
  acute vasoreactivity test: use inhaled NO, adenosine, or prostacyclin to identify Pts likely to have a long-term response to oral CCB (⊕ vasoreactive response defined as ↓ PAP >10 mmHg to a level <40 mmHg with ↑ or stable CO); ~10% Pts are acute responders; no response → still candidates for other vasodilators (*NEJM* 2004;351:1425)

Vasodilators	Comments
Oral CCB (nifedipine, diltiazem) (*NEJM* 1992;327:76)	Given if ⊕ acute vasoreactive response. Only 1/2 will be long-term responder (= NYHA I or II & near-normal hemodynamics), but they have ↓ **mortality**. Side effects: hypoTN, lower limb edema
IV Prostacyclin (epoprostenol; Flolan) (*NEJM* 1996;334:296)	Vasodilation, ↓ plt agg, ↓ smooth muscle proliferation; benefits ↑ with time (? vascular remodeling) (*NEJM* 1998;338:273) ↑ 6MWT 45 m, ↓ PVR ~50%, ↓ PAP 5 mmHg, ↓ **mortality** H/A, flushing, jaw/leg pain, abd cramps, nausea, diarrhea, central venous catheter dysfxn and infection
Prostacyclin analogues Inhaled (Iloprost) (*NEJM* 2002;347:322) SC (Treprostinil) (*AJRCCM* 2002;165:800) Oral (Beraprost)	Same mechanism as prostacyclin IV, but easier to take and w/o central venous catheter system side effects ↓ sx, ↑ 6MWT 36 m, ↓ PVR 25%; ↓ PAP 5 mmHg; trend to ↓ clinical events; requires 6-12 inhalations daily ↓ sx, ↑ 6MWT 16 m, ↓ PVR 10%; ↓ PAP 3 mmHg; no Δ in clinical events; given via SC microcatheter; infusion site rxn common No sustained Δ in 6MWT, PAP or PVR, or clinical events (n/a in US)
Endothelin-1 antag (bosentan) (*NEJM* 2002;346:896)	↓ smooth muscle remodeling, ↑ vasodilation, ↓ fibrosis ↓ sx, ↑ 6MWT 44 m, ↓ PVR 25%, ↓ PAP 2 mmHg, ↓ clinical events Side effects: ↑ LFTs, headache, anemia, edema
PDE-5 Inhibitor (sildenafil) (*NEJM* 2005;353:2148)	↑ cGMP → ↑ NO → vasodilation, ↓ smooth muscle proliferation ↓ sx, ↑ 6MWT 51 m, ↓ PVR 28%, ↓ PAP 5 mmHg, no Δ clinical Low side effect profile: H/A, vision Δ's, sinus congestion

- Treat underlying causes of 2° PHT; can use vasodilators, although little evidence to support
- Refractory PHT
  balloon atrial septostomy: R → L shunt causes ↑ CO, ↓ S_aO_2, net ↑ tissue O_2 delivery
  lung transplant (single or bilateral); heart-lung needed if Eisenmenger physiology

Figure 2-6 Treatment of PAH

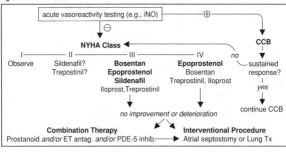

Prognosis
- Median survival after diagnosis ~2.8 y
  PAH (all etiologies): 2-y 66%, 5-y 48% (*Chest* 2004;126:78-S)
- ↑ NT-ProBNP is associated with RV dysfunction and ↑ mortality in PHT (*Chest* 2006;129:1313)
- Lung transplant: 1-y survival 66-75%; 5-y survival 45-55% (*Chest* 2004;126:63-S)

Hypoxemia → $P_AO_2 = F_iO_2 \times (760 - 47) - \dfrac{P_aCO_2}{R}$

- **A-a gradient** = $P_AO_2 - P_aO_2$: normal (*on room air*) = "4 + age/4" or "2.5 + (.21 × age)" hypoxemia + normal A-a gradient → problem is excess P_aCO_2 (ie, hypoventilation)
- **S_vO_2** (mixed venous O_2 sat, nl 60-80%): measure of O_2 consumption vs. delivery low $S_vO_2 \to \downarrow O_2$ delivery ($\downarrow S_aO_2$, nl S_aO_2 but $\downarrow$ CO or anemia) or excessive O_2 consump.
- **V/Q mismatch** and **shunt** represent spectrum w/ both coexisting in alveolar disease 100% O_2 can overcome V/Q mismatch but not lg shunt given sigmoidal Hg-O_2 curve
- $\downarrow P_iO_2$ (high altitude) and diffusion impairment (ILD + exercise) not causes of *acute* $\downarrow P_aO_2$

Figure 2-7 Workup of acute hypoxemia

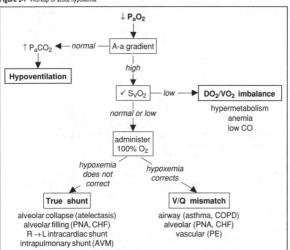

Hypercapnia → $P_aCO_2 = k \times \dfrac{\dot{V}_{CO_2}}{RR \times V_T \times \left(1 - \dfrac{V_D}{V_T}\right)}$

↑P_aCO_2			
"Won't breathe"	"Can't breathe"		
Respiratory Drive	**NM System**	**Lung/Airways**	**CW/Pleura**
↓ RR	↓V_T	↓V_T and/or ↑V_D	↓V_T
↓ P_{100}	↓ PI_{max}	Abnl PFTs	Abnl PEx
Voluntary hypervent.	↓ PE_{max}		Abnl CXR/CT
Nl PI_{max} & A-a gradient			
Chemoreceptors	**Neuropathies**	**Lung parenchyma**	**Chest wall**
metab. alkalosis	cervical spine	emphysema	obesity
1° neurologic	phrenic nerve	ILD/fibrosis	kyphosis
brainstem stroke	GBS, ALS, polio	CHF, PNA	scoliosis
tumor	**NMJ**	**Airways**	**Pleura**
1° alveolar hypovent.	MG, LE	asthma, COPD	fibrosis
2° neurologic	botulism	bronchiectasis	effusion
sedatives	**Myopathies**	CF	
CNS infection	diaphragm	OSA	
hypothyroidism	PM/DM		
	musc dystrophies		
	hypophosphatemia		

↑VCO_2 typically transient cause of ↑ P_aCO_2; Ddx: exercise, fever, hyperthyroidism, ↑ work of breathing, ↑ carbs.

Indications
- Apnea
- Improve gas exchange
  - ↑ oxygenation
  - ↑ alveolar ventilation and/or reverse acute respiratory acidosis
- Relieve respiratory distress
  - ↓ work of breathing (can account for up to 50% of total oxygen consumption)
  - ↓ respiratory muscle fatigue
- Airway protection
- Pulmonary toilet

Choosing settings (NEJM 2001;344:1986)
1) Pick ventilator mode
2) Choose volume-targeted or pressure-targeted
3) Set or ✓ remaining variables

Step 1: Pick Ventilator Mode	
Mode	Description
Assist control (AC)	Vent delivers a minimum number of supported breaths Additional Pt-initiated breaths trigger *fully-assisted* vent breaths ∴ Vent-triggered breaths identical to Pt-triggered breaths Tachypnea → ? respiratory alkalosis, breath-stacking, & auto-PEEP May be pressure-targeted or volume-targeted
Synchronized intermittent mandatory vent (SIMV)	Vent delivers min. no. of supported breaths (synch. to Pt's efforts) Additional Pt-initiated breaths → V_T determined by *Pt's efforts* ∴ Vent-assisted breaths ≠ spontaneous breaths Must overcome resp. circuit during spont. breaths → ↑ fatigue SIMV = AC in patients who are not spontaneously breathing
Pressure support vent (PSV)	Vent supports Pt-initiated breaths with a set inspiratory pressure A mode of *partial* vent support because no set rate Can combine with SIMV to partially assist spontaneous breaths
Continuous positive airway pressure (CPAP)	Pt breathes spont. at their own rate while vent maintains constant positive airway pressure throughout respiratory cycle (7 cm H_2O overcomes 7 Fr ETT)
T-piece	No airway pressure, no rate set; patient breathes through ETT
Other	High-frequency vent (AJRCCM 2002;166:801; CCM 2003;S-31:S-317) ECMO and ECCO₂R (Ann Surg 2004;240:595)

Step 2: Choose Volume-Targeted or Pressure-Targeted	
Volume-targeted	Vent delivers a set V_T Airway pressures depend on airway resist. & lung/chest wall compliance **Benefit:** ↑ control over ventilation (ideal initial ventilator setting); evidence-based benefit in ALI/ARDS; easy to measure mechanical respiratory properties (PIP, P_{plat}, airway resistance, compliance) **Risk:** Patient at risk for ↑ *pressures* → barotrauma (and volutrauma if set volume to high!)
Pressure-targeted	Vent delivers a fixed inspiratory pressure regardless of V_T V_T depends on airway resistance and lung/chest wall compliance **Benefit:** May ↑ patient comfort (PSV) requiring less sedation **Risk:** Pt at risk for ↓ *volumes* → inadequate V_E
General principles	**Institutional/practitioner preference** and **patient comfort** usually dictate ventilator strategy; no strategy has proven superior **Common reasons for changing ventilator strategies include:** dysynchrony, poor gas exchange, Δ mechanical respiratory properties, Δ goals of care (eg, sedation, weaning, lung protection) **Alarms** can be set for ↑ volumes and ↑ airway pressures in pressure-targeted and volume-targeted strategies, respectively

Step 3: Set or ✓ Remaining Variables	
F_iO_2	Fraction of inspired air that is oxygen

Positive end-expiratory pressure (PEEP)	Positive pressure applied during exhalation
	Generated by a resistor in exhalation port
	Benefits: prevents alveoli collapse, ↓ intrapulmonary shunt, ↑ O_2
	Cardiac effects:
	  ↓ preload by ↑ intrathoracic pressure and impeding venous return
	  ↓ afterload by ↓ cardiac transmural pressure
	  may ↑ or ↓ CO and may ↑ or ↓ oxygen delivery based on the above
	"Auto-PEEP" or "intrinsic PEEP": inadequate exhalation time → lungs unable to completely empty before the next breath (ie, "breath stacking"); if flow at end-expiration must be pressure = auto-PEEP
	  Will ↓ preload and may ↓ CO, especially if Pt. hypovolemic
	  Will ↑ work of breathing as must be overcome by Pt to trigger breaths; can prevent Pt from successfully triggering ventilator
	  Can be detected if end-expiratory flow ≠ 0 before next breath
	  Can measure by occluding expiratory port of vent at end-expiration

Inspiratory time	Normally I:E ratio is ~1:2; however, can alter I time (and consequently flow rate, see below); use in pressure control mode
Inspiratory flow rates	↑ flow rate → ↓ I time → ↑ E time and ∴ improved ventilation in obstructive disease; use in volume control mode
Peak inspiratory pressure (PIP)	Dynamic measurement during inspiration Determined by airway resistance and lung/chest wall compliance Set in pressure-targeted ventilation ↑ PIP w/o ↑ P_{plat} → ↑ airway resist (eg, bronchospasm, plugging) ↓ PIP → ↓ airway resistance or air leak in the system
Plateau pressure (P_{plat})	Static measurement at the end of inspiration when there is no flow Determined by resp system compliance (resist. not a factor since ∅ flow) ↑ P_{plat} → ↓ lung or chest wall compliance (eg, PTX, pulmonary edema, pneumonia, atelectasis), ↑ PEEP, or auto-PEEP

Initial Settings				
Mode	Tidal volume	Respiratory rate	F_iO_2	PEEP
Assist control Volume-targeted	~ 8 mL/kg IBW	12-14 breaths/min	1.0 (ie, 100%)	? 5 cm H_2O

Initial V_T ≥9 mL/kg is risk factor for subsequent development of VILI in non-ALI acute respiratory failure (*CCM* 2004;32:1817); ∴ start with ~8 mL/kg and subsequently tailor.

Noninvasive Ventilation	
Continuous positive airway pressure (CPAP)	≈ PEEP No limit on O_2 delivered (ie, can give hi-flow → F_iO_2 ≈ 1.0) Used in Pts whose primary problem is **hypoxemia** (eg, CHF) CHF: ↓ intub. & mortality (*JAMA* 2005;294:3124; *Lancet* 2006;367:1155)
NPPV/Bilevel positive airway pressure (BiPAP) (nb, recent trials w/ ICU-style NIV w/ alarms, new modes, ↑ O_2 delivery, etc.; ? equivalent to basic BiPAP device)	≈ PSV + PEEP Able to set both inspiratory (usually 8-10 cm H_2O) and expiratory pressures (usually <5 cm H_2O); O_2 delivery limited **COPD**: ↓ intub. & mortality (*Lancet* 2000;355:1931) **PNA**: controversial → ↑ secretions, ↓ mort, ↓ intubations in subgroup w/ acute hypoxemic resp. failure (*AJRCCM* 2003;168:1438) **Immunocompromised**: ↓ mort., ↓ intub., ↓ infections **Postextubation**: if high risk (age >65 y, CHF, APACHE-II >12) routine NIV × 24 h → ↓ reintub. and, if P_aCO_2 >45 during SBT, ↓ mortality (*AJRCCM* 2006;173:164) Rescue strategy after failed extubation: ↑ mort. (*NEJM* 2004;350:2452)
Mask ventilation	Tight-fitting mask connecting patient to a standard ventilator Can receive pressure support of up to 20-30 cm H_2O, PEEP of up to 10 cm H_2O, F_iO_2 of up to 1.0 Used for short-term support (<24 h) for a reversible process (asthma, CHF, COPD)
Contraindications: altered MS, vomiting, unable to protect airway, extrapulmonary organ failure, hemodynamic instability, severe UGIB, inability to fit mask (*JAMA* 2002;288:932)	

Tailoring the ventilator settings
- To improve oxygenation: ↑ F_iO_2, ↑ PEEP (optimize based on lung mechanics)
- To improve ventilation: ↑ V_T or inspiratory pressures, ↑ RR (may need to ↓ I time to accomplish Δs)
- Permissive hypercapnia: tolerating ↑ P_aCO_2 to avoid excessive barotrauma or volutrauma may have protective effect in ALI/ARDS (*CCM* 2006;34:1)
  V_T = 4-6 mL/kg IBW (as long as P_aCO_2 <80 and pH >7.15) (*NEJM* 1995;332:345)
  rel. contraindic.: cerebrovascular disease, hemodynamic instability, renal failure, PHT

Acute ventilatory deterioration (usually ↑ PIP)
- Response to ↑ PIP: disconnect Pt from vent., bag, auscultate, suction, ✓ CXR & ABG

Figure 2-8 Approach to acute ventilatory deterioration

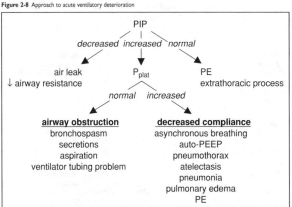

(Adapted from Marino, P.L. *The ICU Book*, 2nd ed., Baltimore: Williams & Wilkins, 1990:430)

Weaning from the ventilator
- Weaning strategy (no single proven approach): spontaneous breathing trial (SBT) ? better than PSV (↓ 2-4 cm H_2O q12h) and SIMV (↓ RR 2-4 breaths/min q12h + backup 5 cm H_2O PSV); IMV not effective (*NEJM* 1995;332:345)
- Identify Pts who can breathe spontaneously (*NEJM* 1991;324:1445 & 1996;335:1864)
  screening criteria: sedation reversed, VS stable, minimal secretions, adequate cough, cause of respiratory failure or previously failed SBT reversed
  vent parameters: P_aO_2/F_iO_2 >200, PEEP ≤5, f/V_T <105, V_E <12 L/min, VC >10 mL/kg
  SBT (CPAP or T-piece × 30-120 min) (*AJRCCM* 1999;159:512)
  failure if: deteriorating ABGs, ↑ RR, ↑ or ↓ HR, ↑ or ↓ BP, diaphoresis, anxiety
  rapid shallow breathing index (f/V_T) >105 predicts failure; NPV 0.95 (*NEJM* 1991;324:1445)
- If tolerate SBT → consider extubation
- If fail SBT → ? cause → work to correct on comfortable vent settings → retry SBT qd

Complications
- Barotrauma and volutrauma (eg, pneumothorax, pneumomediastinum)
  high PIPs are usually not harmful unless ↑ P_{plat} (? >33 cm H_2O, but the lower the better) → alveolar damage
- Oxygen toxicity (theoretical); proportional to duration + degree of ↑ oxygen (F_iO_2 >0.6)
- Alterations in cardiac output
- Ventilator associated pneumonia (1%/day, mortality rate ~30%)
  typical pathogens: MRSA, *Pseudomonas*, *Acinetobacter* and *Enterobacter* species
  preventive strategies (*AJRCCM* 2005;171:388)
    nonpharm: wash hands, semirecumbent position, non-nasal intubation, enteral nutrition rather than TPN, routine suction of subglottic secretions
    pharm: avoid unnecessary abx and transfusions, routine oral antiseptic, daily sedation withdrawal, stress-ulcer prophylaxis w/ ? sucralfate (↓ VAP,↑ GIB) vs. H_2-ant or PPI
- Laryngeal
  edema: for Pts ventilated >36h, ? consider *methylprednisolone* 20 mg IV 12 h before extubation and q4h until tube removed → 86% ↓ in clinically evident laryngeal edema and 50% ↓ in reintubation (*Lancet* 2007;369:1003)
  ulceration: consider *tracheostomy* for patients in whom expect >14 d of mech. vent → ↓ duration mech. vent,↑ # ICU days (*BMJ* 2005;330:1243)

ACUTE RESPIRATORY DISTRESS SYNDROME

Definition (NEJM 2000;342:1334)
- Acute respiratory distress syndrome (ARDS) / Acute lung injury (ALI)
  clinical = acute onset, severe hypoxemia, refractory to O_2 w/ bilateral infiltrates
  pathophys. = noncardiogenic pulmonary edema
  path. = diffuse alveolar damage (DAD)
- American-European Consensus Conference (1994): 4 criteria to define ARDS w/o bx
  1) acute onset
  2) bilateral patchy air-space disease (need not be diffuse)
  3) PCWP <18 mmHg or no clinical evidence of ↑ LA pressure
  4) P_aO_2/F_iO_2 ≤200 → ARDS; P_aO_2/F_iO_2 ≤300 → ALI

Etiologies			
Direct Injury		**Indirect Injury**	
• Pneumonia (~40%)	• Inhalation injury	• Sepsis (~25%)	• Pancreatitis
• Aspiration (~15%)	• Lung contusion	• Shock	• Trauma/multiple fractures
• Near drowning		• DIC	• Hypertransfusion (TRALI)

Pathophysiology
- ↑ intrapulmonary shunt (∴ refractory to ↑ FiO_2); can develop 2° PHT
- ↓ compliance (V_T/P_{plat} - PEEP) <50 cc/cm H_2O

Diagnostic studies
- CXR: bilateral infiltrates developing w/in 24 h of appearance of air-space disease
- Chest CT: patchy infiltrate mixed w/ normal lung, densities greater in dependent areas
- Lung biopsy: not required, but often provides useful dx information (Chest 2004;125:197)

Treatment (primarily supportive) (Lancet 2007;369:1553)
- Mech. vent.: maintain systemic O_2 deliv. while min. ventilator-induced lung injury (VILI)

Mechanisms of VILI	Ventilator Strategies
Barotrauma/volutrauma: alveolar overdistention → mech. damage; biotrauma → SIRS	V_T ≤6 mL/kg, P_{plat} ≤30 cm H_2O, tolerate ↑ P_aCO_2 (but keep pH >7.15), sedation/paralysis as needed (but try to minimize); ↓ mortality (NEJM 2000;342:1301)
Atelectrauma: repetitive alveoli recruitment & decruitment	**Titrate PEEP to prevent tidal alveolar collapse** may ↓ mortality (NEJM 1997;338:347), but no mortality diff. in high v. low PEEP strategy at a given V_T (ALVEOLI, NEJM 2004;351:327).
Hyperoxia: O_2 rad. → ? injury	↑ **PEEP** rather than F_iO_2 (keep <0.60)

- **Fluid balance:** target CVP 4-6 cm H_2O (if nonoliguric & normotensive) → ↑ ventilator/ICU free days, but no mortality difference (FACTT, NEJM 2006;354:2564)
- Routine PA catheter use to guide fluid management in ARDS offers no advantage over central venous catheter (FACTT, NEJM 2006;354:2213)
- **Steroids:** early ARDS → no benefit (NEJM 1987;317:1505). However,
  ARDS onset 7-13 d: ? benefit → ↑ ventilator/ICU free days, no mort. difference
  ARDS onset ≥14 d: clear harm → ↑ mortality (LaSRS, NEJM 2006;354:1671)
- **Experimental:**
  Inhaled nitric oxide: transient ↓ PAP, ↑ P_aO_2/F_iO_2, no ↓ mort. (JAMA 2004;291:1603)
  Prone ventilation: ↑ P_aO_2, no ↓ mortality (JAMA 2004;292:2379)
    ? ↓ mortality if initiated early and for longer (17 h/d) (AJRCCM 2006;173:1233)
  IV B_2 agonist: ↓ lung H_2O, ↓ P_{plat} (AJRCCM 2005;173:281); await results of large RCT
  Lung recruitment: insp. hold to recruit lung and then ↑ PEEP to maintain (NEJM 2006;354:1775 & 1839)
  ECMO: selected Pts. (young, immunocompetent w/o MODS) (Arch Surg 1999;134:375)

Prognosis
- Mortality: ~40% overall; 9-15% resp. causes, 85-91% extrapulmonary (MODS)
- Higher dead-space fraction [($(P_aCO_2-P_ECO_2)/P_aCO_2$)] predicts ↑ mort. (NEJM 2002;346:1281)
- Sequelae: PFTs ~normal, ↓ D_LCO, muscle wasting, weakness persists (NEJM 2003;348:683)

ESOPHAGEAL AND GASTRIC DISORDERS

DYSPHAGIA

Definition
- Difficulty swallowing and passing food from the esophagus to the stomach

Etiologies (*BMJ* 2003;326:433)

Figure 3-1 Etiologies of and approach to dysphagia

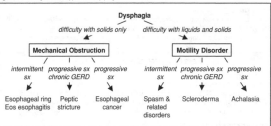

Diagnostic studies
- Barium swallow 1st-line test for both mechanical and motility disorders
- EGD: ideal for structural/mechanical lesions; provides limited motility information
- Manometry: if motility disorder suspected following completion of above studies

Achalasia
- Etiology: idiopathic (most common), pseudoachalasia (due to GE junction tumor), Chagas
- Diagnosis: barium swallow → dilated esophagus with distal "bird's beak" narrowing; manometry → low-amplitude contractions, incomplete relaxation of lower esophageal sphincter (± LES hypertension)
- Treatment: Heller myotomy; pneumatic balloon dilatation (2% risk of esophageal perforation); botulinum toxin injection (primarily used for high-risk surgical candidates)

DYSPEPSIA ("INDIGESTION")

Definition
- Discomfort centered in the upper abdomen

Etiologies
- **Functional causes** ("nonulcer dyspepsia" or NUD, ~60%): some combination of visceral afferent hypersensitivity and abnormal gastric motility
- **Organic causes**: peptic ulcer disease (15-20%), gastric cancer (<2%), other (lactose intolerance, biliary pain, chronic pancreatitis, mesenteric ischemia)
- *Alarm factors* that suggest organic cause and warrant EGD: dysphagia, ⊕ FOBT or anemia, persistent anorexia or vomiting, weight loss, palpable mass or adenopathy, age >55 y

Treatment
- *H. pylori* eradication useful for PUD → empiric Rx if ⊕ serology (*NEJM* 1998;339:1869)
- Functional dyspepsia: acid suppression w/ PPI, H_2-blocker; trials of prokinetic agents, TCAs

GASTROESOPHAGEAL REFLUX DISEASE (GERD)

Pathophysiology
- Excessive transient relaxations of lower esophageal sphincter (LES) or incompetent LES
- Esophageal mucosal damage (esophagitis) due to prolonged contact with acid, etc.
- Hiatal hernia: contributes to ↓ LES tone; acts as reservoir for refluxed gastric contents

Clinical manifestations
- **Heartburn**, atypical chest pain; regurgitation of stomach contents, water brash, dysphagia
- Cough (chronic nocturnal aspiration), asthma, hoarseness (vocal cord inflammation)
- **Precipitants**: large meals, supine position, fatty foods, caffeine, alcohol, cigarettes, CCB

Diagnosis
- Often based on Hx, trial of PPI (although Se & Sp of improved sx after empiric PPI for dx of GERD are surprisingly low: 78% & 54% respectively) (*Annals* 2004;140:518)
- EGD to detect esophagitis, ulcer, Barrett's esophagus, or stricture (*JAMA* 2002;287:1972)
- 24-h ambulatory esophageal pH monitoring if diagnosis is uncertain

Treatment
- Lifestyle measures: avoid precipitants, small meals, avoid late meals, elevate head of bed
- Medical: antacids, H_2-blockers, PPI, prokinetic agents
- Surgical: fundoplication (often laparoscopic), success rate >90% (*NEJM* 1992;326:786)

Complications
- Esophagitis, *Barrett's esophagus* (specialized intestinal metaplasia with ~30-60 × ↑ risk of adenocarcinoma, ~0.8% per y, *NEJM* 1999;340:825 & 2002;346:846), stricture
- If Barrett's found, endoscopic surveillance (eg, q 3 y) for *dysplasia* is warranted

---

PEPTIC ULCER DISEASE (PUD)

Epidemiology
- Lifetime prevalence ~10%
- **Duodenal ulcer (DU)** and **gastric ulcer (GU)** prevalence ↓ over last decade (↓ DU > ↓ GU), due in part to ↓ incidence *H. pylori*; incidence of hospitalization for complications unΔ'd (in fact ↑ in elderly; likely 2° to ↑ NSAID use in this group)

Principal etiologies (*Lancet* 2002;360:933)
- ***H. pylori* infection:** 90% of DU and 70% GU
  ~30% of population colonized with *H. pylori*, but only 15% will develop an ulcer
- **NSAIDs** (15-30% GU, 0.1-4% UGIB) and **ASA**
- Gastrinoma (Zollinger-Ellison) & other hypersecretory states (consider if mult. recur. ulcers)
- Malignancy (5-10% of GU)
- Other: smoking, stress ulcers (if CNS process = "Cushing's"; if burn = "Curling's"), XRT, chemo, CMV (immunocompromised Pts), bisphosphonates; steroids alone not risk factor, however, may exacerbate NSAID-induced ulceration

Clinical manifestations
- **Epigastric abdominal pain**, relieved with food (duodenal) or worsened by food (gastric)
- **Complications** include UGIB, perforation & penetration, gastric outlet obstruction

Diagnostic studies
- Tests for *H. pylori*
  serology (90% Se, 70-80% Sp, not useful in confirming erad. as can stay ⊕ wks to y)
  urea breath test (UBT, Se & Sp >90%)
  stool antigen (HpSA, 89-98% Se, >90% Sp, useful in confirming eradication)
  EGD + rapid urease testing (eg, CLOtest, Se & Sp >95%) or bx and histology
- EGD more sensitive (>95%) than UGI series to detect PUD
  biopsies should be taken of all GU; DU rarely malignant, ∴ routine biopsy not rec.

Treatment (*NEJM* 2002;347:1175)
- ***H. pylori* eradication: clarithromycin** 500 mg bid + **amoxicillin** 1 g bid + **PPI** bid × 10-14 d is 1st line Rx, but recent ↓ in eradication rates to ~70% b/c ↑ clarithro resist.
  metronidazole 500 mg bid can be substituted for amoxicillin in penicillin-allergic Pts
  quadruple therapy (MNZ + tetracycline + bismuth subsalicylate + PPI) can be given in cases of *H. pylori* resistance to clarithromycin or MNZ
  eradication should be documented via UBT or HpSA in Pts w/ hx GIB or perforated ulcer
- If *H. pylori* negative, **acid suppression with PPI**
- **Discontinue NSAIDs**; if must continue, consider:
  adding PPI (*NEJM* 1998;338:719 & 727)
  adding misoprostol (*Annals* 1995;123:241); however, causes diarrhea
  Δ to COX-2 selective inhibitor (↓ PUD and UGIB *but* ↑ risk of serious CV events) consider only in Pts w/ low CV risk not on ASA (as no GI benefit if concomitant ASA)
- Lifestyle changes: discontinue smoking and ? EtOH; diet irrelevant
- Endoscopy: acutely to control UGIB (also see "Gastrointestinal Bleeding"); to document resolution of GU after Rx (∴ indicated only if ulcer suspicious for malignancy); if sx do not resolve; or ulcer was large or complicated on previous endoscopy
- Surgery: usually reserved for rare cases refractory to medical management (rule out surreptitious NSAID use) or for complications (see above)

Definition
- Intraluminal blood loss anywhere from the oropharynx to the anus
- Classification: **upper** = above the ligament of Treitz; **lower** = below the ligament of Treitz
- Signs: **hematemesis** = blood in vomitus (UGIB); **hematochezia** = bloody stools (LGIB or rapid UGIB); **melena** = black, tarry stools from digested blood (usually UGIB, but can be anywhere above and including the right colon)

Etiologies of upper GI bleed (UGIB)
- Oropharyngeal bleeding and epistaxis → swallowed blood
- **Erosive esophagitis** (10%): GERD/Barrett's esophagus, XRT
  if immunocompromised also consider CMV, HSV, Candida
- **Varices** (10-30%; *NEJM* 2001;345:669): esophageal ± gastric, 2° to portal HTN;
  present in 40-60% cirrhotics; if isolated gastric need to r/o splenic vein thrombosis
- **Mallory-Weiss tear** (10%; GE junction tear due to retching against closed glottis)
- **Gastritis/gastropathy** (15%; NSAIDs, ASA, alcohol, stress-related mucosal disease)
- **Peptic ulcer disease** (PUD) (50%; *H. pylori*, NSAIDs, gastric hypersecretory states)
- **Vascular malformations** (5%)
  Dieulafoy's lesion: superficial ectatic artery usually in cardia → sudden, massive UGIB
  vascular lesions: AVMs, angioectasias (submucosal, may involve any part of the gut)
  gastric antral vascular ectasia (GAVE): "watermelon stomach," tortuous, dilated vessels
  aorto-enteric fistula: AAA or aortic graft erodes into 3rd portion of duodenum;
    p/w "herald bleed"; if suspected, diagnose by endoscopy or CT
  vasculitis
- Neoplastic disease: esophageal or gastric carcinoma, GIST

Etiologies of lower GI bleed (LGIB)
- **Diverticular hemorrhage** (33%; 60% of diverticular bleeding localized to right colon)
- **Angiodysplasia** (8%; most commonly located in ascending colon and cecum)
- **Neoplastic disease** (19%; usually occult bleeding, rarely severe)
- **Colitis** (18%; infection, ischemic, radiation, inflammatory bowel disease [UC >> CD])
- **Anorectal** (4%; hemorrhoids, anal fissure, rectal ulcer)
- Post-polypectomy

Clinical manifestations
- UGIB > LGIB: nausea, vomiting, hematemesis, coffee-ground emesis, epigastric pain, vasovagal reactions, syncope, melena
- LGIB > UGIB: diarrhea, tenesmus, BRBPR or maroon stools

Workup (performed concurrently with initial stabilization)
- **Goal**: *where* (anatomic location), *why* (etiology), and *how much* (amt of blood loss)
- **History**
  acute or chronic GIB, number of episodes, most recent episode
  hematemesis, vomiting *prior* to hematemesis, melena, hematochezia
  abdominal pain, weight loss, anorexia, Δ in stool caliber
  use of aspirin, NSAIDs, anticoagulants, or known coagulopathy
  alcohol abuse, cirrhosis, known liver disease, risk factors for liver disease
  abdominal/rectal radiation, history of cancer
  prior GI or aortic surgery
- **Physical exam**
  tachycardia at 10% volume loss; orthostatic hypotension at 20% loss; shock at 30% loss
  pallor, telangiectasis (alcoholic liver disease or Osler-Weber-Rendu syndrome)
  signs of liver disease: jaundice, spider angiomata, gynecomastia, testicular atrophy,
    palmar erythema, caput medusae, Dupuytren's contractures, hepatosplenomegaly
  localizable abdominal tenderness or peritoneal signs, masses, LAN, signs of prior surgery
  rectal exam: appearance/color of stools, presence of hemorrhoids or anal fissures
- **Laboratory studies: Hct** (*may be normal* early in acute blood loss before equilibration, which may take 24 h; ↓ 2-3% → loss of 500 cc blood), MCV, **platelet count**, **PT**, **PTT**, BUN/Cr (ratio >36 in UGIB due to GI resorption of blood and/or prerenal azotemia), LFTs
- **Nasogastric tube**: useful for localization. Most helpful if returns fresh blood → active UGIB; coffee grounds → recent UGIB (but can be confused w/ bile); nonbloody bile suggests lower source, but does not exclude active UGIB; ⊕ Hemoccult of no value.
- Dx studies in UGIB: **EGD** (potential Rx as well; consider erythro 250 mg IV ×1 30-60 min prior to promote gastric emptying of blood and ↑ Dx/Rx yield)

- Diagnostic studies in LGIB (r/o UGIB before attempting to localize presumed LGIB)
  bleeding spontaneously stops → **colonoscopy** (identifies cause in >70%, potential Rx)
  stable but continued bleeding → colonoscopy after rapid purge (GoLYTELY 4-6 L)
  unstable → **arteriography** (detects bleeding rates ≥0.5 ml/min; therapeutic potential
  [intraarterial vasopressin or embolization]); **tagged RBC scan** (bleeding rates
  ≥0.1 ml/min, but localization unreliable) often used as screening prior to angio
  exploratory **laparotomy**

Treatment
- **Acute treatment of GIB is hemodynamic resuscitation with IV fluid and blood**
  establish **access** with 2 large-bore (18-gauge or larger) intravenous lines
  volume resuscitation with normal saline or lactated Ringer's solution
  transfusion (blood bank sample for type & cross; use O-neg blood if Pt exsanguinating)
  correct coagulopathies (FFP to normalize PT, platelets to keep count >50,000/mm^3)
  nasogastric tube lavage if hematemesis
  intubation for emergent EGD if shock, poor resp status, ongoing hematemesis, ΔMS

Etiology	Options
Varices	*Pharmacologic* **octreotide** 50 µg IVB → 50 µg/h infusion (84% success; *Lancet* 1993;342:637). Usually × 5 d, but most benefit w/in 24-48 h. Antibiotics in Pts w/ascites for SBP prophylaxis (norfloxacin 400 mg PO bid or Bactrim DS PO bid × 7 d) (*Hepatology* 2004;39:746) *Non-pharmacologic* **endoscopic** band ligation (>90% success) has replaced sclerotherapy (88% success) b/c ↓ compl. (*NEJM* 1992;326:1527) octreotide + endoscopic Rx (>95% success; *NEJM* 1995;333:555) balloon tamponade (Sengstaken-Blakemore) if bleeding severe; mainly used as rescue procedure and bridge to TIPS **TIPS** for esophageal variceal hemorrhage refractory to above, or for gastric varices (main side effect: encephalopathy) surgery (portocaval/splenorenal shunts, Sugiura procedure)
PUD	*Pharmacologic* **PPI** (omeprazole 80 mg IVB → 8 mg/h) before EGD accelerates resolution of bleeding, ↓ need for Rx during EGD, and ↓ LOS (*NEJM* 2007;356:1631) ? octreotide 50 µg IVB → 50 µg/h if unstable and EGD not immediately available (*Annals* 1997;127:1062) *Non-pharmacologic* **endoscopic therapy** (epinephrine inj, bipolar cautery, hemoclip) arteriography with infusion of vasopressin or embolization surgery if endoscopic and pharmacologic therapy fails
Mallory-Weiss	*Usually stops spontaneously; endoscopic therapy if active*
Esophagitis Gastritis	PPI, H$_2$-antagonists
Diverticular disease	*Usually stops spontaneously (~75%)* Endoscopic therapy (eg, epinephrine injection, cautery, banding, or hemoclip), arterial vasopressin or embolization, surgery
Angiodysplasia	*Usually stops spontaneously (~85%)* Endoscopic Rx (cautery), arterial vasopressin/embolization, surgery

Poor prognostic signs in UGIB
- Demographics: age >60, comorbidities, variceal or neoplastic etiology
- Severity: bright red blood in NGT, ↑ transfusion requirement, hemodynamic instability

Obscure GIB
- Etiologies: angiodysplasia, small intestinal tumors, Meckel's diverticulum (congenital ileal abnormality: incomplete obliteration of vitelline duct w/ heterotopic gastric mucosa that can lead to peptic ulceration), Crohn's disease, mesenteric ischemia, vasculitis
- Workup: repeat EGD, push enteroscopy, bleeding scan, angiography (to look for abnormal "vascular blush"), ^{99m}Tc-pertechnetate scan ("Meckel's scan"), video capsule endoscopy, double-balloon enteroscopy

DIARRHEA

Infections (NEJM 2004;350:38)
- **Acute**
  Preformed toxins ("food poisoning," <24 h): *S. aureus, C. perfringens, B. cereus*
  Viruses: rotaviruses, noroviruses, adenovirus, CMV (immunosuppressed Pts)
  Noninvasive bacteria
    enterotoxin-producing (⊖ fecal WBC or blood): enterotoxigenic *E. coli, Vibrio cholera*
    cytotoxin-producing (⊕ fecal WBC and blood): *E. coli* O157:H7, *C. difficile*
  Invasive bacteria (⊕ fecal WBC and blood): enteroinvasive *E. coli* (EIEC), *Salmonella,*
    Shigella, Campylobacter, Yersinia, V. parahaemolyticus
  Parasites: *Giardia* (⊖ fecal WBC and blood); *E. histolytica* (⊖ fecal WBC, ⊕ blood)
  Opportunistic: *Cryptosporidia, Isospora, Microsporidia, Cyclospora,* MAC, CMV
- **Chronic:** *Giardia, E. histolytica, C. difficile,* opportunistic organisms
- Clues as to etiology
  Travel: *E. coli,* parasites (*Giardia* with ingestion of water from streams)
  Shellfish: noroviruses, *Vibrio* sp.; Undercooked hamburger: *E. coli* O157:H7;
  Poultry: *Campylobacter, Salmonella*
  Antibiotic use: *C. difficile* (see below)

Medications (cause ↑ secretion, ↑ motility, Δ flora, ↑ cell death, or inflammation)
- **Antibiotics,** antacids, lactulose, sorbitol, chemoRx, colchicine, gold, ASA, NSAIDs

Malabsorption (↓ diarrhea with fasting, ↑ osmotic gap, ↑ fecal fat)
- **Bile salt deficiency**
  ↓ synthesis: liver disease (cirrhosis) or cholestasis (primary biliary cirrhosis)
  bacterial overgrowth: deconjugation of bile salts or ↓ nutrient absorption
  ileal disease (eg, Crohn's, surgery): interruption of enterohepatic circulation
- **Pancreatic insufficiency:** most commonly from chronic pancreatitis
- **Mucosal abnormalities**
  Celiac sprue: intestinal reaction to α-gliadin in gluten → loss of villi & absorptive area
    other s/s: Fe-defic anemia, dermatitis herpetiformis (pruritic papulovesicular rash)
    Dx: anti-tissue transglutaminase or anti-endomysial IgA; small bowel bx
    treatment: gluten-free diet (Lancet 2003;362:383)
  Tropical sprue: affects residents of the tropics; treatment with antibiotics, folate, B_{12}, iron
  Whipple's disease (NEJM 2007;365:55): infxn w/ *T. whipplei* affects middle-aged white men
    other s/s: fever, LAN, edema, arthritis, CNS Δs, gray-brown skin pigmentation, AI &
    MS, oculomasticatory myorhythmia (eye oscillations + mastication muscle contract.)
    treatment: PCN G + streptomycin, or 3rd-gen ceph × 10-14 d → Bactrim for ≥1 y
- **Lactose intolerance:** 1° or 2° mucosal abnormality, viral/bacterial enteritis, s/p resection
  clinical manifestations: bloating, flatulence, discomfort, diarrhea
  Dx: lactose hydrogen breath test or empiric lactose-free diet
  treatment: lactose-free diet, use of lactaid milk and lactase enzyme tablets
- **Other:** Crohn's disease, eosinophilic gastroenteritis, intestinal lymphoma

Inflammatory (fever, hematochezia, abdominal pain)
- **Inflammatory bowel disease**
- Radiation enteritis, ischemic colitis, diverticulitis, neoplasia (colon cancer, lymphoma)

Secretory (normal osmotic gap, no Δ diarrhea after NPO, nocturnal diarrhea freq described)
- **Hormonal:** VIP (VIPoma, Verner-Morrison), serotonin (carcinoid), calcitonin (medullary
  cancer of the thyroid), gastrin (Zollinger-Ellison), glucagon, substance P, thyroxine
- **Laxative abuse**
- Neoplasm: carcinoma, lymphoma, villous adenoma
- Idiopathic bile salt malabsorption
- Lymphocytic colitis, collagenous colitis (often associated with meds, including NSAIDs)

Motility
- **Irritable bowel syndrome** (10-22% of adults; NEJM 2001;344:1846): Rome III criteria →
  recurrent abd pain ≥3 d/mo over last 3 mos *plus* 2 or more of the following:
  1) improvement w/defecation, 2) onset w/Δ freq of stool, 3) onset w/Δ in form of stool
  treatment (NEJM 2003;349:2136): constipation → fiber; diarrhea → anti-diarrheals; pain
  → anti-spasmodics
- Scleroderma (pseudo-obstruction); diabetic autonomic neuropathy; hyperthyroidism

Diarrhea workup

Figure 3-2 Workup of acute diarrhea (<3 wks duration)

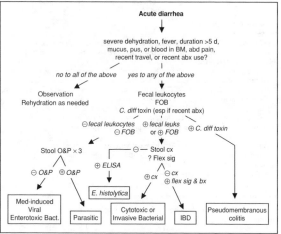

Figure 3-3 Workup of chronic diarrhea (>3 wks duration)

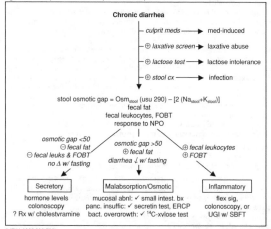

(NEJM 1995;332:725)

Empiric treatment for acute, community-acquired, likely infectious diarrhea
- Mild: bismuth subsalicylate & loperamide prn
- Moderate-severe or fever, blood, or pus: consider empiric fluoroquinolone × 1-5 d (if no suspicion for *E. coli* O157:H7 or fluoroquinolone-resistant *Campylobacter*)

CLOSTRIDIUM DIFFICILE

Pathogenesis
- Infxn when nl colonic flora altered by **abx** (eg, clinda, β-lactams, quinolones) or chemoRx and Pt colonized by *C. difficile* (or its spores) w/ subsequent toxin release
- **Toxin A + B** → colon brush border → necrosis & inflammation → **pseudomembranes**
- New highly toxigenic strains → ↑ mort. & length of hosp. (esp in elderly; *NEJM* 2005;353:2442)

Clinical manifestations (spectrum)
- Asx colonization <3% in healthy adults; 15-21% in inpatients treated w/ abx
- Acute watery diarrhea (occ bloody) ± mucus, often w/ lower abd pain, fever, ↑↑↑ WBC
- Pseudomembranous colitis: above sx + pseudomembranes + bowel wall thickening
- Fulminant colitis (2-3%): **toxic megacolon** (colon dilatation ≥6 cm on KUB, colonic atony, systemic toxicity) and/or bowel perforation
- Ddx: infectious colitis, ischemic colitis, IBD

Diagnosis
- **Stool ELISA**: detects toxin A and/or B; fast (2-6 h); Se ~90% if high clinical suspicion and 1st test ⊖, consider repeating some ELISAs only detect A (∴ miss B-prod. strains)
- Stool cytotoxin assay: gold standard, highly Se & Sp; takes 24-48 h

Treatment (*NEJM* 2002;346:334)
- Discontinue antibiotics as soon as possible; avoid antimotility agents
- **Metronidazole** 500 mg PO tid (1st choice) × 10-14 d; if need to stay on original abx, continue MNZ for ≥7 d post-abx cessation. IV MNZ w/ similar efficacy; should be used if ↓ gut motility or absorption, or inability to tolerate POs; there is ↑'ing rate of MNZ resistance
- **Vancomycin** 125-500 mg PO qid × 10-14 d; efficacy = MNZ, but ↑ cost; can select for VRE indicated if diarrhea/colitis severe, Pt pregnant or <10 y, or no improvement w/ MNZ
- Recurrent *C. difficile* infection (15-30% of Pts) (*Gastro* 2006;130:1311)
  1st relapse: conservative Rx if sx mild; 14 d MNZ or vanco if mod/severe
  2nd relapse: PO vanco taper
  Further relapses: prolonged vanco + *S. boulardii* or cholestyramine; ? IVIG
- Adjunctive Rx: *Saccharomyces boulardii*, lactobacillus, cholestyramine, fecal enemas
- Consider flex sig if dx uncertain and/or evidence of limited improvement w/ standard Rx
- Stool carriage may persist 3-6 wks post-cessation of sx and should not trigger further Rx

---

CONSTIPATION & ADYNAMIC ILEUS

Constipation (*NEJM* 2003;349:1360)
- Definition (Rome III criteria): must include 2 of the following (in at least ¼ of BMs): straining during defecation, lumpy/hard stools, incomplete evacuation, sensation of anorectal obstruction/blockage; stool frequency <3 per wk
- Etiology: fxnal (nl transit, slow transit, pelvic floor disorders, IBS); **obstruction** (cancer, stricture); **metabolic** (DM, hypothyroid, hypoK, preg., panhypopit., hyperCa); **meds** (opioids, anticholinergics incl. TCAs & antipsychotics, iron, CCB); **neurogenic** (Parkinson's, Hirschsprung's, amyloid, MS, Chagas, autonomic neuropathy)
- Treatment (fiber supplementation → osmotic laxative → stimulant laxative)
  bulk laxatives (psyllium, methylcellulose, polycarbophil): ↑ colonic residue, ↑ peristalsis
  osmotic laxatives (Mg, sodium phosphate, lactulose, etc.): draw water into intestines
  stimulant laxatives (senna, castor oil, bisacodyl, docusate sodium): ↑ motility & secretion
  rectal enema/suppository (phosphate, mineral oil, tap-water, soapsuds, bisacodyl)
  tegaserod: ↑ motility, but recently withdrawn from market b/c ? CV toxicity
  lubiprostone: ↑ secretion (useful for severe constipation)

Adynamic ileus
- Definition: loss of intestinal peristalsis in absence of mechanical obstruction
  Ogilvie's = acute colonic adynamic ileus in presence of competent ileocecal valve
- Precipitants: intra-abd. process (surgery, pancreatitis, peritonitis); severe medical illness (eg, PNA, sepsis); intestinal ischemia; meds (opiates, anticholinergics); electrolyte abnl
- Clinical manifestations: abd. discomfort, N/V, hiccups, abd. distention, ↓ or absent bowel sounds, no peritoneal signs; cecum ≥10-12 cm → ↑ rupture
- Dx: supine & upright abdominal films → gas-filled loops of small & large intestine; must exclude mechanical obstruction (absence of gas in rectum); consider abd. CT
- Treatment: NPO, mobilize (walk, roll), d/c drugs that ↓ intestinal motility, enemas; decompression (NGT, rectal tubes, colonoscope); erythromycin, neostigmine

DIVERTICULAR DISEASE

DIVERTICULOSIS

Definition and Pathology (Lancet 2004;363:631)
- Acquired herniations of colonic mucosa and submucosa through the colonic wall
- More common on the **left side** (90%, mostly sigmoid) than the right side of the colon
- May be a consequence of a **low-fiber diet** → colonic musculature contracting against small, hard stools → ↑ intraluminal pressure → herniation of mucosa + submucosa

Epidemiology
- Affects 20-50% of persons over the age of 50; most prevalent in "Westernized" societies

Clinical manifestations
- Usually asx, but can be complicated by **diverticulitis** or **diverticular hemorrhage**

DIVERTICULITIS

Pathophysiology (NEJM 1998;338:1521)
- Retention of undigested food and bacteria in diverticulum → fecalith formation → obstruction → compromise of diverticulum's blood supply, infection, perforation
- Microperforation (localized infection) or macroperforation (abscess, peritonitis, obstruction)

Clinical manifestations
- **LLQ abdominal pain, fever**, nausea, vomiting, constipation

Physical exam
- Mild: LLQ tenderness, ± palpable mass, ± positive FOBT (~25%)
- Severe: peritonitis, septic shock

Diagnostic studies
- **Plain abdominal radiographs** to r/o free air, ileus, or obstruction
- Abdominal CT (I⁺) may show thickening of colon (sigmoid); usually reserved for Pts who fail to respond to therapy or if suspect pericolic abscess
- Sigmoidoscopy/colonoscopy *contraindicated* in acute setting because of ↑ risk of overt perforation; colonoscopy recommended 2-6 wks after resolution to rule out neoplasm

Treatment
- **Mild**: PO antibiotics (FQ + MNZ) and liquid diet × 7-10 d
- **Severe**
  NPO, IV fluids, NGT (if ileus)
  IV antibiotics (GNR & anaerobic coverage): amp/gent/MNZ or piperacillin-tazobactam
- Abscess drainage percutaneously or surgically
- Surgery if medical therapy fails, free perforation, large abscess that cannot be drained percutaneously, recurrent disease (≥2 severe episodes)
- If surgery deferred after 2nd attack, consider prophylactic Rx w/ mesalamine ± rifaximin

DIVERTICULAR HEMORRHAGE (also see "GASTROINTESTINAL BLEEDING")

Pathophysiology
- Erosion of blood vessel feeding diverticulum by a fecalith
- Diverticula more common in left colon; *but bleeding diverticula are often in right colon*

Clinical manifestations
- Usually painless hematochezia, but can have abdominal cramping
- Usually stops spontaneously (~75%) but resolution may occur over hrs-days; ~20% recur

Physical exam
- Usually benign

Diagnostic studies
- Colonoscopy or angiography ± tagged RBC scan if severe bleeding

Treatment (see "Gastrointestinal Bleeding" for persistent bleeding)
- Colonoscopy: epinephrine injection ± electrocautery (NEJM 2000;342:78), hemoclip, banding
- Arteriography: intraarterial vasopressin infusion or embolization
- Surgery

INFLAMMATORY BOWEL DISEASE

Definition (NEJM 2002;347:417)
- **Ulcerative colitis (UC)**: idiopathic inflammation of the colonic *mucosa*
- **Crohn's disease (CD)**: idiopathic *transmural* inflammation of the GI tract, *skip areas*
- In 5-10% of Pts with chronic colitis a clear distinction between UC and CD cannot be made even with mucosal biopsy ("indeterminate colitis")

Differential diagnosis
- Infectious: bacterial (SSCY, *E. coli* O157:H7), pseudomembranous, amebic, CMV, STDs
- Ischemic colitis
- Intestinal lymphoma or carcinoma; collagenous colitis
- Irritable bowel syndrome
- Drugs (NSAIDs, OCP, gold, allopurinol, penicillamine)

ULCERATIVE COLITIS

Epidemiology
- Prevalence 1:1000
- Age of onset 20-25 y; ↑ incidence in Caucasians, especially Jews; familial in ~10%
- Appendectomy prior to age 20 for appendicitis (NEJM 2001;344:808) and tobacco use (NEJM 1987;316:707) have been reported to protect against the development of UC

Pathology
- Extent: involves rectum (95%) and extends proximally and *contiguously*
  50% of Pts have proctosigmoiditis, 30% left-sided colitis, and 20% pan-colitis
- Appearance: granular, friable mucosa with diffuse ulceration; *pseudopolyps*
  barium enema → hazy margins (fine mucosal granularity), loss of haustra ("lead pipe")
- Microscopy: superficial inflammation + micro-ulcerations; crypt abscesses (PMNs)

Clinical manifestations
- **Grossly bloody diarrhea**, lower abdominal cramps, urgency, tenesmus
- **Fulminant colitis** (15%): progresses rapidly over 1-2 wks with ↓ Hct, ↑ ESR, fever, hypotension, >6 bloody BMs per day, distended abdomen with absent bowel sounds
- Extracolonic (25%)
  erythema nodosum, pyoderma gangrenosum, aphthous ulcers, iritis, episcleritis, thromboembolic events, autoimmune hemolytic anemia
  seronegative arthritis, chronic hepatitis, cirrhosis, primary sclerosing cholangitis (PSC; with ↑ risk of cholangiocarcinoma)
- Serologies: p-ANCA in 60-70% (associated with pancolitis and PSC)

Complications
- **Toxic megacolon** (5%): colon dilatation (≥6 cm on KUB), colonic atony, systemic toxicity requires IV steroids and broad-spectrum abx; surgery if fails to improve w/in 48-72 h
- Perforation → pneumoperitoneum, peritonitis
- Stricture (5%): occurs in rectosigmoid after repeated episodes of inflammation
- **Colon cancer**: risk with *pancolitis* is greatest (7-16% cumulative risk at 20 y); Pts w/ left-sided colitis and PSC also at ↑ risk; risk *not* increased with ulcerative proctitis
- Surveillance: yearly *colonoscopy* with random biopsies after 8 y of pancolitis or 15 y of left-sided colitis to look for dysplasia (low grade → ~20% have cancer; high grade or dysplasia associated lesion/mass (DALM) → ≥40% have cancer) → colectomy if present

Prognosis
- Intermittent exacerbations in 80%; continual active disease in 10-15%; severe initial attack requiring urgent colectomy in 5-10%
- Mortality rate for severe attack of ulcerative colitis is <2%
- No difference in life expectancy compared to individuals without ulcerative colitis

CROHN'S DISEASE

Epidemiology (Lancet 2007;369:1627)
- Prevalence 1:3000
- Bimodal with peaks in 20s and 50-70; ↑ incidence in Caucasians, Jews, and smokers
- Mutation of the *NOD2/CARD15* gene found in 20% of Pts (Nature 1996;379:821)
  homozygotes have ~40-fold risk, heterozygotes ~7-fold risk of developing Crohn's

Pathology
- Extent: can affect any portion of GI tract from mouth to anus, with *skip lesions* 30% of Pts have ileitis, 50% ileocolitis, and 20% colitis; isolated upper-tract disease rare
- Appearance: nonfriable mucosa, cobblestoning, aphthous ulcers, deep & long **fissures** barium enema → sharp lesions, cobblestoning, long ulcers & fissures, "string sign"
- Microscopy: **transmural inflammation** with mononuclear cell infiltrate, noncaseating **granulomas** (seen in <25% of mucosal biopsies), fibrosis, ulcers, fissures

Clinical manifestations
- **Smoldering disease with abdominal pain,** fevers, malaise, weight loss
- Mucus-containing, **nongrossly bloody diarrhea**
- ($\downarrow$ albumin, $\uparrow$ ESR, $\downarrow$ Hct (due to Fe, B_{12}, folate deficiency, or chronic disease)
- Extracolonic: same as UC, plus *gallstones* (malabsorption of bile salts, $\downarrow$ bile/cholesterol ratio, $\uparrow$ lithogenicity) and *kidney stones* (Ca oxalate stones due to binding of intraluminal Ca^{++} by unabsorbed free fatty acids allowing $\uparrow$'d oxalate absorption)
- Serologies: anti-*Saccharomyces cerevisiae* antibodies (ASCA) in 60-70%

Complications
- Perianal fissures, perirectal abscesses (up to 33% of Pts)
- **Stricture**: postprandial abdominal pain and bloating; can lead to complete obstruction
- **Fistulas**: perianal, enteroenteric, rectovaginal, enterovesicular, enterocutaneous
- **Abscess**: fever, tender abd mass, $\uparrow$ WBC; steroids mask sx, $\therefore$ need high-level suspicion
- **Cancer**: small intestinal/colorectal; risk of colorectal cancer in CD $\approx$ to that in UC; recs for colonoscopic surveillance in Pts w/ Crohn's pancolitis are same as those for UC

TREATMENT

General measures
- Avoid NSAIDs (both UC and CD) & tobacco (CD)
- Antidiarrheals only in *mild* disease; limited role for TPN, but may be needed in severe dz
- Rule out infection before treating with immunosuppressants and biologics

Acute Flare Treatment	
Severity	**Options**

Mild	**5-ASA compounds (oral)**
	Sulfasalazine (5-ASA + sulfa): bacterial reductases release 5-ASA in *colon*
	Mesalamine (5-ASA in pH-sensitive or time-dependent capsules)
	    Asacol: dissolves at pH 6-7 → 5-ASA released in *terminal SI & colon*
	    Pentasa: 5-ASA released throughout the *small intestine & colon*
	    Olsalazine & Balsalazide (5-ASA dimer): cleaved in the *colon*
	rectal 5-ASA (enemas, suppositories) for distal UC, proctitis
	Antibiotics
	metronidazole: useful in perianal, fistulizing, and active colonic CD
	ciprofloxacin ± metronidazole, or clarithromycin useful for active CD

Moderate	**Oral steroids:** prednisone; budesonide (oral steroid useful in *ileocecal* CD; low systemic absorption)
Severe	**Intravenous steroids** ± infliximab (refractory or fistulizing CD; NEJM 1997;337:1029 & 1999;340:1398; refractory UC; NEJM 2005;353:2462) ± cyclosporine for UC (NEJM 1994;330:1841) Serial abd exams + radiographs/CT to r/o dilatation, perforation, or abscess

(*Lancet* 2007;369:1641)

Maintenance of remission
- 5-ASA compounds (? UC only): appropriate formulation to treat affected areas
- **Azathioprine/6-MP**: mainstay of maintenance treatment for CD and UC. Thiopurine methyltransferase (TPMT) genotype may be checked before initiation to avoid toxicity.
- **Infliximab** for CD (ACCENT 1, *Lancet* 2002;359:1541)
- Other: methotrexate for CD (NEJM 2000;342:1627); ? budesonide; adalimumab

Indications for surgery
- UC (25% of all Pts): failed medical therapy, hemorrhage, perforation, stricture, fulminant colitis, toxic megacolon, growth retardation, high-grade dysplasia, or carcinoma
- CD (75% of all Pts): hemorrhage, failed medical therapy, ? chronic steroid requirement, stricture, fistula, abscess, high-grade dysplasia, or carcinoma

ACUTE MESENTERIC ISCHEMIA

SMALL BOWEL

Etiologies
- **SMA embolism** (50%): from LA (AF), LV (↓ EF), or valves; SMA most prone to embolism
- **Nonocclusive mesenteric ischemia** (25%): transient intestinal hypoperfusion due to ↓ CO, atherosclerosis, sepsis, drugs that ↓ gut perfusion (pressors, cocaine, dig, diuretic)
- **SMA thrombosis** (10%): usually at site of atherosclerosis, often at origin of artery
- **Venous thrombosis** (10%): due to hypercoaguable states, portal hypertension, malignancy, inflammation (pancreatitis, peritonitis), pregnancy, trauma, surgery
- **Focal segmental ischemia of the small bowel** (5%): vascular occlusion to small segments of the small bowel (vasculitis, atheromatous emboli, strangulated hernias, XRT)

Clinical manifestations
- Sudden onset of abdominal pain out of proportion to abdominal tenderness on exam
- Abdominal distension w/o pain (usually with nonocclusive disease); nausea/vomiting
- GI bleed due to mucosal sloughing (right colon is supplied by superior mesenteric artery)
- "Intestinal angina": postprandial abdominal pain & early satiety may occur wks to mos before the onset of acute pain in Pts w/ chronic mesenteric ischemia

Physical exam
- May be unremarkable, or may only show abdominal distention or occult blood in stool
- Bowel infarction suggested by peritoneal signs (diffuse tenderness, rebound, guarding)

Diagnostic studies
- Diagnosis relies on high level of suspicion; rapid diagnosis essential to avoid infarction
- Laboratory evaluation: may be normal; ↑ WBC; ↑ amylase and LDH; metabolic acidosis and ↑ lactate (late)
- Imaging
  plain radiograph: normal prior to infarction, "thumbprinting" & ileus in later stages
  abdominal CT: early signs nonspecific; colonic dilatation, bowel wall thickening, pneumatosis of bowel wall; best test to detect mesenteric vein thrombosis
  CT angiogram: more sensitive than CT alone, less invasive than standard angio
  angiography: gold standard; potentially therapeutic; indicated if suspect occlusion

Treatment
- Volume resuscitation, optimization of hemodynamics, discontinue pressors if possible
- Broad spectrum **antibiotics** (amp/gent/MNZ) for infarction, sepsis
- Intraarterial infusion of **thrombolytic** agent for acute arterial embolism
- **Anticoagulation** for arterial and venous thrombosis and embolic disease
- Intraarterial infusion of **papaverine** (vasodilator) for nonocclusive mesenteric ischemia
- Surgery: **embolectomy** for acute arterial embolism; revascularization for acute superior mesenteric arterial thrombosis; resection of infarcted bowel

Prognosis
- Mortality 20-70%; dx prior to infarction strongest predictor of survival

---

ISCHEMIC COLITIS

Definition and pathophysiology
- Non-occlusive disease 2° to Δs in systemic circulation or anatomic/fxnal Δs in local mesenteric vasculature
- Most common ischemic bowel syndrome
- **"Watershed"** areas (splenic flexure and recto-sigmoid) are most susceptible

Clinical manifestations, diagnosis, and treatment
- Disease spectrum: reversible colopathy (35%), transient colitis (15%), chronic ulcerating colitis (20%), stricture (10%), gangrene (15%), fulminant colitis (<5%)
- Usually p/w **cramping LLQ pain with ⊕ FOBT** or overtly bloody stool; fever and peritoneal signs should raise clinical suspicion for infarction
- Diagnosis: r/o infectious colitis; consider **flexible sigmoidoscopy** or **colonoscopy** if sx persist and no alternative etiology identified (only if peritonitis not present)
- Treatment: bowel rest, IV fluids, **broad spectrum abx**, serial abd. exams; **surgery** for infarction, fulminant colitis, hemorrhage, failure of medical Rx, recurrent sepsis, stricture
- Resolution w/in 48 h with conservative measures occurs in over 50% of cases

ACUTE PANCREATITIS

Etiologies
- Common
  alcohol (30% of cases, typically in men): usually chronic, with acute flares
  gallstones (35% of cases, typically in women): usually small (<5 mm) stones are culprit
- Rare
  Obstructive: ampullary or pancreatic tumors, ? pancreas divisum
  Metabolic: hypertriglyceridemia (TG need to be >1000 and usually ~4500; seen w/ type I and type V familial hypertriglyceridemia), hypercalcemia
  Drugs: furosemide, thiazides, sulfa, didanosine, protease inhibitors, estrogen, 6-MP, azathioprine, ACE-I (occur via hypersensitivity, toxic metabolite, or direct toxicity)
  Infection: echovirus, coxsackievirus, mumps, rubella, EBV, CMV, HIV, HAV, HBV, Ascaris
  Trauma: blunt abdominal trauma, post-ERCP (35-70% with ↑ amylase, ~5% with clinical, overt pancreatitis)
  Familial: autosomal dominant with variable penetrance (PRSS 1, CFTR, SPINK 1 genes)
  Ischemia: vasculitis, cholesterol emboli, hypotension, hemorrhagic shock
  Scorpion sting (in Trinidad): mechanism believed to be hyperstimulation of pancreas
- Idiopathic ~20% (many cases probably due to microlithiasis)

Clinical manifestations
- **Epigastric abdominal pain**, radiating to back, constant, some relief w/ leaning forward
- Nausea and vomiting; fever is common
- Ddx: biliary disease, perforated viscus, intestinal obstruction, mesenteric ischemia, IMI, AAA leak, distal aortic dissection, ruptured ectopic pregnancy

Physical exam
- Abdominal tenderness and guarding, ↓ bowel sounds (adynamic ileus)
  ± palpable abdominal mass; ± jaundice if biliary obstruction
- Signs of retroperitoneal hemorrhage (Cullen's = periumbilical; Grey Turner's = flank) rare
- ± hypotension or shock

Diagnostic studies (JAMA 2004;291:2865)
- Laboratory
  ↑ **amylase**: levels $>3 \times$ ULN very suggestive of pancreatitis, but level ≠ severity
    false ⊖: acute on chronic (eg, alcoholic); hypertriglyceridemia (↓ amylase activity)
    false ⊕: other abd. or salivary gland process, acidemia, renal failure, macroamylasemia (amylase binds to other proteins in serum, cannot be filtered out)
  ↑ **lipase**: may be more specific than amylase
    false ⊕: renal failure, other abd. process, diabetic ketoacidosis, HIV, macrolipasemia
  ALT $>3 \times$ ULN → gallstone pancreatitis (Am J Gastro 1994;89:1863); Aφ, bili not helpful
  other labs depending on severity: ↑ WBC, ↓ Hct, ↑ BUN, ↓ Ca, ↑ glucose
- Imaging studies
  abdominal CT not required in Pts at time of dx. Obtain if needed to exclude other dx, stage severity, r/o complic. Assessment of necrosis req. IV contrast, which may want to avoid for 1st few days b/c theoretical concern of ↑ necrosis (and spont. necrosis may not be radiographically apparent for 48-72 h)
  abdominal ultrasound to evaluate for gallstones, CBD dilatation, ascites, pseudocyst pancreas often obscured by bowel gas; if seen → diffusely enlarged, hypoechoic
  MRCP can be used to assess for gallstones & pancreatic ductal disruption
  endoscopic U/S (EUS) most Se test for gallstones; limited role in acute pancreatitis
- CT-guided abscess drainage or fine-needle aspiration to r/o infection if Pt w/ persistent fevers, ↑ WBC, or organ failure and pancreatic necrosis present on CT (96% Se, 99% Sp); has risk of seeding sterile necrosis

Treatment (Lancet 2003;361:1447; NEJM 2006;354:2142)
- Supportive therapy
  fluid resuscitation (may need up to 10L/d if hemodynamically severe pancreatitis)
  enteral nutrition: ↓ infectious complications and disease severity, and trend toward ↓ mortality c/w TPN (BMJ 2004;328:1407). Ideally via NJ tube, but NG acceptable.
  analgesia with IV meperidine, morphine (theoretical risk of sphincter of Oddi spasm, but has not been shown to adversely affect outcome), or hydromorphone
- Prophylactic systemic antibiotics (eg, imipenem) of unclear benefit and remain controversial (Gastro 2007;132:2019); if used, reserve for severe necrotizing pancreatitis (>30% necrosis by CT) for no more than 14 d

- ERCP + sphincterotomy: may ↓ biliary sepsis in severe gallstone pancreatitis if performed w/in 72 h (NEJM 1993;328:228); no effect on local or systemic pancreatitis complications; most effective if obstructive jaundice (bili ≥5) and/or cholangitis (NEJM 1997;336:237; Ann Surg 2007; 245:10)
- Surgery
  débridement: indicated if infected necrosis (usually after confirmation of infection by FNA); up to 65% mortality if surgery performed w/in first few days (Pancreat 2002;2:565); should be delayed ≥2 wks unless Pt worsening
  cholecystectomy if gallstones (as soon as Pt recovers and inflammatory process ↓)

Complications
- Systemic: shock, ARDS, renal failure, GI hemorrhage, DIC
- Metabolic: hypocalcemia, hyperglycemia, hypertriglyceridemia
- **Acute fluid collection** (30-50%): seen early, no capsule, no Rx required
- **Pseudocyst** (10-20%): fluid collection, persists for 4-6 wks, encapsulated suggested by persistent pain & elevation of amylase or lipase, or mass on exam most resolve spont.; if >6 cm or persists >6 wks + pain → endo/perc/surg drainage
- **Sterile pancreatic necrosis** (20%): area of nonviable pancreatic tissue Rx conservatively with prophylactic antibiotics (eg, imipenem; NEJM 1999;340:1412) if severe necrosis & supportive measures for as long as possible; surgery if Pt unstable
- **Infection** (5% of all cases, 30% of severe): fever and ↑ WBC; usually 2° enteric GNR
  infected pancreatic necrosis (aspiration → ⊕ bacterial culture): antibiotics + surgical débridement (100% mortality w/o débridement; Hepatogastroenterology 1991;38:116)
  pancreatic abscess: circumscribed collection of pus (usually w/o pancreatic tissue) treat with antibiotics + drainage (CT-guided if possible)
- Pancreatic ascites or pleural effusion: indicates disrupted pancreatic duct; consider early ERCP with stent placement across duct
- Scarring of pancreatic duct → stricture → chronic pancreatitis

Prognosis
- Severe pancreatitis = organ failure or local complications (necrosis, abscess, pseudocyst)
- Scoring systems: Apache II, Ranson's criteria, CT Severity Index (CTSI; Balthazar grade score + necrosis score)
  APACHE II: assigns points for age, previous health status, temp, HR, RR, MAP, P_aO_2, pH, K, Na, Cr, Hct, WBC, GCS → severe pancreatitis if ≥8 (>13 = ↑↑↑ mortality) advantage: can be used on admission (before 48 h) and on daily basis
  Ranson's: severe pancreatitis when ≥3 criteria; takes 48 h to compute
  CT Severity Index: most helpful to assess severity; combine with Ranson's

Ranson's Criteria		Prognosis	
At diagnosis	**At 48 hours**	**# of criteria**	**Mortality**
age >55	Hct ↓ >10%	≤2	<5%
WBC >16,000/mm³	BUN ↑ >5 mg/dl	3-4	15-20%
glucose >200 mg/dl	base deficit >4 mEq/L	5-6	40%
AST >250 U/L	Ca <8 mEq/L	≥7	>99%
LDH >350 U/L	P_aO_2 <60 mmHg		
	fluid sequestration >6 L		

(Am J Gastroenterol 1982;77:633)

CT Grade	Description	Points	Necrosis	Points	Total Index	Mortality
A	Normal pancreas c/w mild pancreatitis	0	<33%	2	0-3	3%
B	Enlarged pancreas but w/o inflammation	1	33-50%	4	4-6	6%
C	Pancreatic or peripancreatic inflammation	2	>50%	6	7-10	17%
D	Single peripancreatic fluid collection	3				
E	≥2 Peripancreatic fluid collections or gas in the pancreas or retroperitoneum	4				

(Radiology 1990;174:331)

ABNORMAL LIVER TESTS

Abnormal liver tests in hepatocellular injury or cholestasis
- **Aminotransferases** (AST, ALT): intracellular enzymes released 2° necrosis/inflammation
  ALT more specific for liver than is AST (also in heart, skeletal muscle, kidney, brain)
  ALT > AST → viral hepatitis or fatty liver/nonalcoholic steatohepatitis (pericirrhotic)
  AST:ALT >2:1 → alcoholic hepatitis; ↑↑↑ LDH → ischemic or toxic hepatitis
- **Alkaline phosphatase** (Aφ): enzyme bound in hepatic canicular membrane
  besides liver, also found in bone, intestines, kidney, and placenta
  confirm liver origin with: ↑ 5'-NT, ↑ GGT, or Aφ heat fractionation
  ↑ levels seen with biliary obstruction or intrahepatic cholestasis (eg, hepatic infiltration)

Tests of hepatic function
- **Albumin**: marker for liver protein synthesis, ↓ slowly in liver failure ($t_{1/2}$ ~20 d)
- **Prothrombin time** (PT): depends on synthesis of coag factors; because $t_{1/2}$ of some
  of these factors (eg, V, VII) is short, ↑ PT can occur w/in h of liver dysfxn
- **Bilirubin**: product of heme metab. in liver; unconjugated (indirect) or conjugated (direct)
  ↑ conjugated can be from obstruction (intra/extra-hepatic) or congenital disorder

Patterns in liver injury
- **Hepatocellular**: ↑↑ aminotransferases, ± ↑ bilirubin or Aφ
  ↑↑↑ aminotransferases (>1000): severe viral hepatitis, acetaminophen, ischemia
- **Cholestasis**: ↑↑ Aφ and bilirubin, ± ↑ aminotransferases
- **Isolated hyperbilirubinemia**: ↑↑ bilirubin, normal Aφ and aminotransferases
- *Jaundice* is a clinical sign seen when bilirubin >2.5 mg/dl (especially in sclera or under
  tongue); if hyperbilirubinemia conjugated → ↑ urine bilirubin
- **Infiltrative**: ↑ Aφ, ± ↑ bilirubin or aminotransferases

Figure 3-4 Approach to abnormal liver tests with hepatocellular pattern

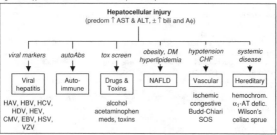

Figure 3-5 Approach to abnormal liver tests with cholestatic pattern

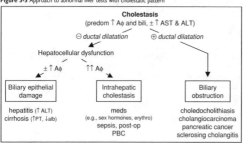

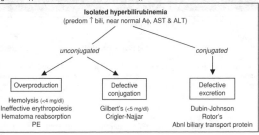

Figure 3-7 Approach to abnormal liver tests with infiltrative pattern

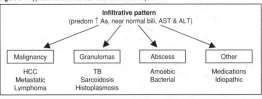

Abnormal liver tests in asymptomatic patients (*NEJM* 2000;342:1266)
- **Hepatocellular**
    evaluate for most common causes: alcohol, NAFLD, HBV/HCV, hemochromatosis, meds
        (NSAIDs, statins, abx)
    if unrevealing → rule out nonhepatic causes (✓ CPK, aldolase, TFTs)
    if hepatic → consider less common causes: autoimmune hepatitis, Wilson's disease,
        celiac disease, α_1-antitrypsin deficiency
    if unrevealing → liver biopsy if ALT or AST >2 × ULN for >6 mos; o/w observe
- **Cholestatic**: ✓ 5'-NT or GGT, if ↑ → ✓ RUQ U/S, AMA
    careful review of med list → eliminate potential cholestatic meds
    if biliary dilatation or obstruction → ERCP/MRCP to eval for choledocholithiasis or
        stricture
    liver biopsy if AMA ⊕ and U/S ⊖, or AMA ⊖ and U/S w/ abnormal parenchyma
    if AMA & U/S ⊖: Aφ >1.5 ULN → consider biopsy; Aφ <1.5 ULN → observe
- **Isolated hyperbilirubinemia**: ✓ conjugated vs. unconjugated
    conjugated → perform abdominal U/S → MRCP and/or ERCP if dilatation or
        obstruction
    unconjugated → ✓ hct, retic count, smear, LDH, haptoglobin

VIRAL

Hepatitis A
- Transmission: fecal-oral route; contaminated food, water, shellfish; day-care ctr outbreaks
- Incubation: 2-6 wks, no chronicity
- Diagnosis: acute hepatitis = ⊕ IgM anti-HAV; past exposure = ⊕ IgG anti-HAV (⊖ IgM)
- Prevention: vaccinate children (>2 y) and those at high risk (2 doses at 0, 6-12 mos)
- Postexposure prophylaxis: IG 0.02 ml/kg IM + start vaccine w/in 2 wks of exposure

Hepatitis B (Lancet 2003;362:2089)
- Transmission: blood, sexual, perinatal
- Incubation: 1-6 mos; mean 2-3 mos
- Extrahepatic syndromes: PAN (<1%), MPGN, arthritis, dermatitis, PMR
- Natural history
  acute infection: 70% subclinical, 30% jaundice, <1% fulminant hepatitis
  chronic: <5% (adult-acquired), >90% (perinatally-acquired)
- Serologic and virologic tests
  HBsAg: appears before symptoms; used to screen blood donors
  HBeAg: evidence of viral replication and ↑ infectivity
  IgM anti-HBc: first Ab to appear; indicates acute infection
   window period = HBsAg become ⊖, anti-HBs not yet ⊕, anti-HBc only clue to infection
  IgG anti-HBc: indicates previous (HBsAg ⊖) or ongoing (HBsAg ⊕) HBV infection
  anti-HBe: indicates waning viral replication, ↓ infectivity
  anti-HBs: indicates resolution of acute disease & immunity (sole marker after vaccination)
  HBV DNA: presence in serum correlates with active viral replication in liver

Figure 3-8 Serologic course of acute HBV infection with resolution

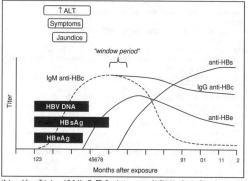

(Adapted from Friedman LS & Keeffe EB. Serologic course of HBV. *Handbook of Liver Disease* 1998;38; Hoofnagle JH & DiBisceglie AM. Serologic diagnosis of acute and chronic viral hepatitis. *Semin Liver Dis* 1991;11:73.)

Diagnosis	HbsAg	anti-HBs	anti-HBc	HBeAg	anti-HBe	HBV DNA
Acute hepatitis	⊕	⊖	IgM	⊕	⊖	⊕
Window period	⊖	⊖	IgM	±	±	⊕
Recovery	⊖	⊕	IgG	⊖	±	⊖
Immunization	⊖	⊕	⊖	⊖	⊖	⊖
Chronic hepatitis *HBeAg ⊕*	⊕	⊖	IgG	⊕	⊖	⊕
Chronic hepatitis *HBeAg ⊖*	⊕	⊖	IgG	⊖	⊕	±*

*Precore mutant: HBeAg not generated, but anti-HBe can develop due to cross-reactivity with HBcAg; high serum HBV DNA levels

- Treatment for acute HBV: supportive
- Treatment for chronic HBV (⊕ HBsAg & DNA) if: HBeAg ⊕ and DNA >10^5 copies/ml; HBeAg ⊖ and DNA >10^4 copies/ml; ALT ≥2 × ULN; or inflammation on bx
  options: IFN-α-2b (NEJM 1990;323:295), peg IFN-α-2a (NEJM 2005;352:2682) for 48 wks, **lamivudine** (NEJM 1999;341:1256) (development of resist. at ↑ rates), **adefovir** (NEJM 2003;348:800&808) (30% resist. at 5 y), **telbivudine** (some X-resist. w/ lamivudine), or **entecavir** (NEJM 2006;354:1001); oral agents preferred b/c ↓ tox.; entecavir most potent
  Rx endpoint: if HBeAg ⊕ → HBeAg ⊖ + anti-HBe; if HBeAg ⊖ → ALT nl + HBV DNA ⊖
  liver transplantation: HBIG and/or nucleoside analog effective in preventing reinfection
- Risk of hepatocellular carcinoma: 10-390 × ↑ risk (highest: perinatal acquired and high HBV DNA level; JAMA 2006;295:65); screen with serum AFP and hepatic U/S q6mos
- Prevention: vaccinate if at high risk (3 doses at 0, 1, and 6 mos)
- Postexposure ppx: HBIG ± vaccine (if unvaccinated or known nonresponder)

Hepatitis C (Lancet 2003;362:2095)
- Transmission: blood >> sexual; ~20% without a clear precipitant
- Incubation: 1-5 mos; mean 2 mos
- Extrahepatic syndromes: cryoglobulinemia, porphyria cutanea tarda, MPGN, lymphoma
- Natural history
  acute infection: 75% subclinical; 25% jaundice; fulminant hepatitis very rare
  chronic: 50-80% → chronic hepatitis, 20-30% of whom develop cirrhosis (after ~20 y), hepatocellular carcinoma develops in 2-5% of cirrhotics/y (usually after 20-30 y)
- Serologic and virologic tests
  anti-HCV (ELISA): ⊕ in 6 wks, does not imply recovery, may become ⊖ after recovery
  HCV RNA: ⊕ within 2 wks, marker of active infection
  HCV RIBA: used to confirm ⊕ anti-HCV ELISA in Pts with undetectable HCV RNA
  HCV genotype: used to guide duration and predict response to Rx (genotype 2,3 >1,4)
- Diagnosis
  acute hepatitis = ⊕ HCV RNA, ± anti-HCV
  resolved hepatitis = ⊖ HCV RNA, ± anti-HCV
  chronic hepatitis = ⊕ HCV RNA, ⊕ anti-HCV
  consider liver biopsy to assess grade of inflammation and stage of fibrosis
- Treatment
  Indications: HCV RNA ⊕, bx w/ fibrosis stage >1, and compensated liver disease (for genotype 2 or 3, may proceed to Rx w/o biopsy due to high response rate ~80%)
  Contraindications: decompensated cirrhosis, pregnancy, psych illness, active substance abuse, severe cardiac/pulm disease, uncontrolled DM, seizure d/o, autoimmune dis.
  PEG-IFNα-2a + ribavirin →55% sustained virologic response rate (NEJM 2006;355:2444)
  genotypes 2 or 3: Rx 24 wks, ? 12 wks total if HCV RNA ⊖ at 4 wks (NEJM 2005;352:2609)
  genotypes 1 or 4: Rx 48 wks if HCV RNA ↓ 2 log by 12 wks
  Predictors of response: low HCV RNA, absence of cirrhosis, female, age <40 y, wt <75 kg, nongenotype 1, white/Hispanic, adherence, absence of HIV coinfection
- Postexposure ppx: none (IG not effective); if HCV RNA → ⊕, consider Rx w/in 3 mo

Hepatitis D
- Transmission: blood or sexual
- Pathogenesis: requires HBV to cause either simultaneous or superimposed infection
- Natural history: more severe hepatitis, faster progression to cirrhosis
- Serologic/virologic tests: anti-HDV; follow HDV RNA during Rx (high relapse rate)

Hepatitis E
- Transmission: fecal-oral; travelers to Pakistan, India, SE Asia, Africa, and Mexico
- Natural history: acute hepatitis with ↑ mortality (10-20%) during pregnancy
- Diagnosis: IgM anti-HEV (through CDC)

Other viruses (CMV, EBV, HSV, VZV)

AUTOIMMUNE HEPATITIS

Hepatitis + ↑ globulins + AutoAbs

- **Classification** (NEJM 2006;354:54; Gastro 2001;120:1502)
  - Type 1: anti-smooth muscle Ab (ASMA), ANA; 3/4 female; ± autoimmune thyroiditis, UC anti-soluble liver antigen (anti-SLA) associated with more severe disease and relapse
  - Type 2: anti-liver/kidney microsome type 1 (anti-LKM1); children (age 2-14)
  - Diagnosis: combination of autoimmune serologies, ↑ globulin, exclusion of other causes of liver disease, and liver biopsy showing plasma cell infiltrate with interface hepatitis

Overlap syndromes
- Autoimmune hepatitis + primary biliary cirrhosis or primary sclerosing cholangitis

Treatment
- Indic.: AST 10× ULN, AST 5× ULN + glob 2× ULN, or bridging/multiacinar necrosis
- **Prednisone** ± azathioprine → 65% remission w/in 3 y; 50% relapse on withdrawal of meds at 6 mos; up to 90% by 3 y; ∴ most will require long-term Rx

OTHER CAUSES OF HEPATITIS OR HEPATOTOXICITY

Alcoholic hepatitis
- Aminotransferases usually <300-500 w/ AST:ALT >2:1, in part b/c concomitant B_6 defic.
- Treatment: discriminant function >32 or encephalopathy (w/o GIB or infection)
  discriminant function = (4.6 × [PT-control]) + total bilirubin (mg/dl)
  prednisolone or prednisone 40 mg PO qd × 1 mo then taper over 4-6 wks ↓↓ mortality
  (NEJM 1992;326:507)
  pentoxifylline 400 mg PO tid × 1 mo ↓ mortality and HRS (Gastro 2000;119:1637)

Acetaminophen hepatotoxicity
- Normal metabolism via glucuronidation and sulfation → nontoxic metabolites
- Overdose (usually >10 g): CYP2E1 hydroxylation → reactive electrophilic species (NAPQI) that are scavenged by glutathione until reserves exhausted → hepatotoxicity
- CYP2E1 *induced* by fasting and alcohol (allowing for "therapeutic misadventure" in malnourished alcoholics taking even low doses (2-6 g) of acetaminophen)
- Liver dysfunction may not be apparent for 2-6 d
- Treatment: NG lavage, activated charcoal if presenting w/in 4 h
  N-acetylcysteine: administer up to 36 h after ingestion if acetaminophen level above "no-risk" zone or if time of ingestion unknown or reliable hx of major poisoning (>10 g) should have low threshold for NAC (even if low or undetectable acetaminophen levels)
  PO NAC (preferred): 140 mg/kg loading dose → 70 mg/kg q4h × 17 additional doses
  IV NAC: 150 mg/kg load over 1h → 50 mg/kg over 4 h → 100 mg/kg over 16 h
  risk of anaphylaxis; use if unable to tolerate PO, GIB, preg., fulminant hepatic failure

Figure 3-9 Acetaminophen toxicity nomogram

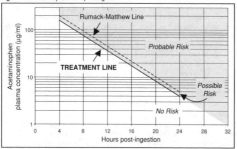

(Adapted Archives 1981;141:382 & Guidelines for Management of Acute Acetaminophen Overdose. McNeil, 1999.)

Other drugs and toxins that may cause hepatitis (NEJM 2006;354:731)
- Amiodarone, azoles, INH, methyldopa, phenytoin, PTU, rifampin, sulfonamides, minocycline, chemotherapy drugs, herbal medications, statins (rare)
- Halothane, CCl_4, solvents, toxic mushrooms (Amanita phalloides)

Ischemic hepatitis: "shock liver" w/ AST & ALT >1000 + ↑↑ LDH; 2° CHF, sepsis, HoTN

Nonalcoholic fatty liver disease (NAFLD) (Annals 1997;126:137; JAMA 2003;289:3000)
- Spectrum of fatty infiltration ± inflammation ± fibrosis in absence of EtOH abuse
- Prevalence 7-9%; metabolic syndrome (associated w/ DM, hyperinsulinemia, obesity, hypertriglyceridemia), HAART, meds (tamoxifen, amiodarone)
- Clinical: usually asx 2-3 × ↑ in ALT; ± RUQ pain, fatigue; may → cirrhosis (~5%)
- Dx: exclusion of other causes of hepatitis or cirrhosis; U/S → hyperechoic liver; ⊕ bx
- Rx: wt loss, glycemic/lipid control; if IGT/DM & bx-confirmed steatohepatitis thiazolidinediones ↓ steatosis & aminotransferases (NEJM 2006;355:2297); ? ursodeoxycholic acid + vitamin E, ? metformin

Definition
- Acute hepatic disease + coagulopathy + encephalopathy
- Fulminant = develops w/in 8 wks; subfulminant = develops between 8 wks and 6 mos

Etiology
- **Viral**
  HAV, HBV, HCV (rare), HDV + HBV, HEV (especially if pregnant)
  HSV (immunocompromised Pt), EBV, CMV, adenovirus, paramyxovirus, parvovirus B19
- **Drugs/Toxins**
  Drugs: acetaminophen (most common cause; ~40% of all cases), phenytoin, INH, rifampin, sulfonamides, tetracycline, telithromycin, amiodarone, PTU
  Toxins: fluorinated hydrocarbons, CCl_4, *Amanita phalloides*
- **Vascular:** ischemic hepatitis, Budd-Chiari syndrome, hepatic SOS, malignant infiltration
- **Autoimmune hepatitis** (usually initial presentation)
- **Misc.:** Wilson's disease, acute fatty liver of pregnancy, HELLP, Reye's syndrome
- Idiopathic (~20%)

Clinical manifestations
- Initial presentation usually nonspecific, w/ nausea, vomiting, malaise, followed by jaundice
- Neurologic
  encephalopathy: stage I = ΔMS; stage II = lethargy, confusion; stage III = stupor; stage IV = coma
  asterixis in stage I/II/III encephalopathy; hyperreflexia, clonus, rigidity in stage III/IV
  cerebral edema → ↑ ICP, ↓ CPP → cerebral hypoxia, uncal herniation, Cushing's reflex (hypertension + bradycardia), pupillary dilatation, decerebrate posturing, apnea
- Cardiovascular: **hypotension** with low SVR
- Pulmonary: **respiratory alkalosis**, impaired peripheral O_2 uptake, pulm edema, ARDS
- Gastrointestinal: GIB (↓ clotting factors, ↓ plts, DIC, fibrinolysis), pancreatitis (? hypoxia)
- Renal: ATN, **hepatorenal syndrome**, hyponatremia, hypokalemia, hypophosphatemia
- Hematology: **coagulopathy** (due to ↓ synthesis of clotting factors ± DIC)
- **Infection** (~90%): especially w/ Staph, Strep, GNRs, and fungi (↓ immune fxn, invasive procedures); SBP in 32% of Pts; *fever and ↑ WBC may be absent*
- Endocrine: **hypoglycemia** (↓ glc synthesis), metabolic acidosis (↑ lactate)

Workup
- Viral serologies
- Toxicology screen (acetaminophen levels q1-2h until peak determined)
- Imaging studies (RUQ U/S or abd CT, Doppler studies of portal and hepatic veins)
- Other tests: autoimmune serologies, ceruloplasmin and urine copper
- Liver biopsy (unless precluded by coagulopathy → in which case consider transjugular)

Treatment
- ICU care at liver transplant center to provide hemodynamic & ventilatory support, CVVH for ARF, D_{10} drip for hypoglycemia, etc.
- Cerebral edema: consider ICP monitoring (stage III/IV enceph); head of bed >30°, hyperventilation, mannitol, barbiturates, ? induction of hypothermia
- Coagulopathy: SC/IV vit K; FFP/plts/cryoprecipitate if active hemorrhage; ? rec. factor VIIa
- Infection: low threshold for abx (broad spectrum; IV vancomycin & 3rd-gen ceph.)
- Treatment of specific causes: N-acetylcysteine for acetaminophen, corticosteroids for autoimmune hepatitis, chelation therapy for Wilson's disease, IV acyclovir for HSV, gastric lavage and charcoal ± penicillin and silymarin for *Amanita phalloides*
- If unclear etiology: acetaminophen levels unreliable, esp in cases w/ unintentional OD (*Gastro* 2006;130:687); ∴ low threshold for NAC Rx (regardless of acetaminophen levels)
- Liver transplantation if poor prognosis (see below)
- Extracorporeal liver assist devices under evaluation as "bridge" to transplant

Prognosis
- Survival 10-50%
- Predictors of poor outcome (*Gastro* 1989;97:439)
  age <10 or >40 y; cause other than acetaminophen, HAV, or HBV
  grade III or IV encephalopathy (onset >7 d after onset of jaundice)
  PT >50, bilirubin >17.5
- Liver transplantation 1-y survival rate >60%

CIRRHOSIS

Definition
- Definition: **fibrosis and nodular regeneration** resulting from hepatocellular injury

Etiologies
- **Alcohol**
- **Viral hepatitis** (chronic HBV, HCV, HDV infection)
- **Autoimmune hepatitis** (female, ↑ IgG, ⊕ ANA, anti-smooth muscle Ab)
- **Metabolic diseases**: hemochromatosis, Wilson's disease, α_1-antitrypsin deficiency
- **Biliary tract diseases**: primary biliary cirrhosis, secondary biliary cirrhosis (calculus, neoplasm, stricture, biliary atresia), primary sclerosing cholangitis
- **Vascular diseases**: Budd-Chiari syndrome, R-sided CHF, constrictive pericarditis
- **Nonalcoholic fatty liver disease (NAFLD)**
- **Cryptogenic**: may reflect terminal progression of nonalcoholic fatty liver disease

Clinical manifestations
- Subclinical or may present as progressive liver dysfunction (jaundice, coagulopathy, encephalopathy) and/or portal hypertension (ascites, varices)

Physical exam
- Liver: enlarged, palpable, firm, nodular → shrunken and nodular
- Signs of liver failure: jaundice, spider angiomata, palmar erythema, Dupuytren's contractures, white nail lines (Muehrcke's lines) & proximal nail beds (Terry's nails), ↑ parotid & lacrimal glands, gynecomastia, testicular atrophy, asterixis, encephalopathy, fetor hepaticus, clubbing, hypertrophic osteoarthropathy
- Signs of portal hypertension: splenomegaly, ascites, dilated superficial abdominal veins (caput medusae), epigastric "Cruveilhier-Baumgarten" venous hum

Laboratory studies
- ↑ **bilirubin, ↑ PT, ↓ albumin**, ± ↑ aminotransferases and ↑ Aϕ (variable), ↓ Na
- Anemia (marrow suppression, hypersplenism, Fe and/or folate deficiencies), neutropenia (hypersplenism), thrombocytopenia (hypersplenism, ↓ Tpo production by liver)

Workup
- Abdominal U/S with Doppler: liver size, r/o HCC, ascites, assess patency of portal, splenic, and hepatic veins
- Hepatitis serologies (HBsAg, anti-HBs, anti-HCV), autoimmune hepatitis studies (IgG, ANA, anti-smooth muscle Ab), Fe and Cu studies, α_1-AT, anti-mitochondrial Ab, echocardiogram (if concerned about right-sided heart failure)
- ± Liver biopsy (percutaneous or transjugular)
- AFP to screen for hepatocellular carcinoma

Complications
- **Portal hypertension** = hepatic venous pressure gradient (HVPG) >5 mmHg
  ascites (60% w/in 10 y) ± spontaneous bacterial peritonitis (19%)
  gastroesophageal varices (if HVPG >12 mmHg) ± **UGIB**
    1° prevention UGIB (indicated if mod-large varices):
      nonselective β-blockers (titrate to 25% ↓ HR): ~50% ↓ bleeding (NEJM 1991;324:1532)
        optimal response defined as HVPG ↓ to <12 mmHg or ↓ ≥20% addition of nitrates may further ↓ bleeding (Lancet 1996;348:1677)
      βB no benefit for preventing development of varices (NEJM 2005;353:2254), but have been shown to ↓ progression from small → large varices (Gastro 2004;127:476)
      endoscopic band ligation: similar ↓ in bleeding and mortality as c/w with βB reserve for intolerance, ↓ response, or contraindications to βB (Hepatology 2001;33:802)
    2° prevention UGIB (indicated in all): β-blocker ± nitrates (goal 25% ↓ HR) (NEJM 2001;345:669), or band ligation, or combination; if rebleed → TIPS or transplant
- **Hepatic encephalopathy**: failure of liver to detoxify noxious agents (NH_3 and others) precipitated by excess dietary protein, constipation, GIB, medication noncompliance, infection, azotemia, hypokalemia, hepatic failure, HCC, portosystemic shunt, hypotension, alkalosis, dehydration, sedative/psychoactive meds
  clinical manifestations: subtle changes → asterixis & ΔMS → decerebrate posturing, coma
  treatment: identify/correct precipitants, restrict dietary protein acutely, but only modestly (60-80 g/d) long-term, lactulose (acidification of colon leading to NH_3 → NH_4^+; titrate to 2-4 stools per day); gut decontamination with rifaximin or neomycin (Δ gut flora → ↓ NH_3-producing organisms)

- **Hepatorenal syndrome:** progressive azotemia (Cr >1.5 mg/dl; note, often *overestimate* renal fxn in cirrhotics b/c ↓ muscle mass, ↑ Cr renal tubular secretion, and ↓ conversion of creatine → creatinine) and oliguria, U_{Na} <10 mEq/L, no response to volume challenge, exclusion of other causes of renal failure (drugs, ATN, obstruction) (*Lancet 2003;362:1819*)
  Type I: rapidly progressive, doubling of Cr to >2.5 in < 2 wks; usually occurs in Pts w/ severe liver failure, often following precipitating event (see below)
  Type II: more indolent course, median survival 6 mos; liver failure present, but less so than Type I; usually occurs in Pts w/ severe ascites w/ poor or no response to diuretics
  Precipitants: GIB, overdiuresis, infection, paracentesis, drugs (aminoglycosides, NSAIDs)
  Treatment: octreotide (200 mcg SC tid) + midodrine (12.5 mg PO tid) beneficial (*Hepatology 1999;29:1690*); albumin + vasoconstrictor (norepi, midodrine, terlipressin; *Hepatology 2002;36:374*)) and/or TIPS may be beneficial; definitive treatment → liver transplantation
- **Hepatopulmonary syndrome:** pulm gas exchange abnl (↑ A-a gradient ± hypoxia), evidence of intrapulmonary vascular shunting and absence of intrinsic cardiopulmonary disease
  may see platypnea-orthodeoxia, clubbing, cyanosis; CXR normal
  Diagnosis: contrast echocardiography (R → L shunt)
  Treatment: supportive ($O_2 \to P_aO_2$ >60 mmHg); liver transplant only definitive Rx
- **Portopulmonary hypertension:** ↑ PAP; unclear pathogenesis; poor prognosis
- **Liver failure:** precipitated by progressive hepatic damage or stressors (infxn, surgery)
- **Infections:** relative immunosuppression, thus susceptible to broad range of infxn
- **Hepatocellular carcinoma** (*Lancet 2003;362:1907*): consider if ↑ liver size, ↑ ascites, abdominal pain, ↑ encephalopathy, ↓ weight, ↑ AFP, or hepatic mass on U/S, CT, MRI

Prognosis
- Correlates with Child-Turcotte-Pugh class (A>B>C)

Modified Child-Turcotte-Pugh Classification			
	Points scored		
	1	**2**	**3**
Ascites	None	Easily controlled	Poorly controlled
Encephalopathy	None	Grade I or II	Grade III or IV
Bilirubin (mg/dl)	< 2	2-3	>3
Albumin (g/dl)	>3.5	2.8-3.5	<2.8
PT (sec > control)	< 4	4-6	>6
	Classification		
	A	**B**	**C**
Total points	5-6	7-9	10-15

(*Brit J Surg 1973;60:646*)

- **MELD** (Model for End-Stage Liver Disease): used to stratify Pts on liver transplant list; based on Cr, INR, & total bilirubin to predict 3-mo survival in Pts w/ variety of underlying forms of liver disease; to calculate: http://www.mayoclinic.org/gi-rst/mayomodel6.html hyponatremia worsens prognosis

Liver transplantation
- Evaluate ± list when Child class B and MELD ≥10
- Indications: recurrent or severe encephalopathy, refractory ascites, SBP, recurrent variceal bleeding, hepatorenal or hepatopulmonary syndrome, hepatocellular carcinoma (if no single lesion is >5 cm or ≤3 lesions with largest ≤3 cm), fulminant hepatic failure
- Contraindic.: advanced HIV, active substance abuse, sepsis, extrahepatic malignancy, severe comorbidity (cardiopulmonary in particular), persistent noncompliance
- Survival: 1-year survival up to 90%, 5-year survival up to 80%

OTHER ETIOLOGIES OF CIRRHOSIS

Hemochromatosis (*NEJM 2004;350:2383*)
- Definition: **iron overload** due to genetic disorder or ↑ ineffect. erythropoiesis (eg, thal.)
- Epidemiology (hereditary): 1 in 300; usually manifests in middle age and in men
- Manifestations of advanced disease: bronzing of the skin (melanin + iron, 90%), hypogonadism, diabetes mellitus (65%), arthritis (2nd & 3rd MCPs, 25-50%), CHF, infections (*Vibrio, Listeria, Yersinia*)
- Dx: ↑ iron saturation >45% (iron/TIBC × 100%; earliest sign, more Se & Sp than ferritin), ↑ ferritin (acute phase reactant, can be elevated in inflammatory conditions; can be normal in young Pts w/ hemochromatosis); "black liver" noted on MRI is suggestive

if ↑ iron saturation → ✓ *HFE* gene mutation (C282Y/C282Y or C282Y/H63D)
  liver biopsy if HFE mutation ⊕ and ferritin >1000 ng/ml, ↑ LFTs, or hepatomegaly to
    discern liver damage (can quantify using hepatic iron concentration)
• Treatment: phlebotomy (500 cc ≈ 1 unit) qwk until Fe sat <30% and ferritin <50, then as
  needed to keep in range; deferoxamine if cardiac involvement or unable to undergo
  phlebotomy; genetic counseling

Wilson's disease *(Lancet 2007;369:397)*
• Definition: autosomal recessive disorder (mutation in *ATP7B*) of **copper overload**
• Epidemiology: 1 in 40,000, usually manifests before age 30; almost always before 40
• Extrahepatic: neuro ψ disorders, Kayser-Fleischer rings, hemolytic anemia, renal dis.
• Dx: ↑ serum & 24-h urinary copper, ↓ serum ceruloplasmin, hepatic copper content
  >250 µg/g dry wt; Aφ often low in fulminant Wilson's disease (Aφ/bili <2 suggestive
  of Wilson's), AST/ALT >1 reflecting damage to hepatocellular mitochondria
• Treatment: chelation therapy with penicillamine + pyridoxine; alternative is trientine,
  which is ↓ toxic and prob. ~ effective; oral zinc if asymptomatic (must be given 4-5 h
  apart from chelators as they will neutralize each other and be rendered ineffective)

α₁-antitrypsin deficiency (α₁-AT)
• Abnormal α₁-AT → polymerization in liver (cirrhosis) & uninhibited protease activity in lung
  (emphysema)
• Additional clinical manifestations: emphysema, necrotizing panniculitis
• Dx: absence of α₁-AT globulin on SPEP, ⊕ PAS inclusion bodies on liver bx;
  gold standard = abnl protease inhibitor (Pi) phenotype (usually ZZ, null/null, or null/Z)
• Treatment: liver transplantation (for cirrhosis); α₁-AT replacement (for emphysema)

Primary biliary cirrhosis (PBC) *(NEJM 2005;353:1261; Lancet 2003;362:53)*
• Definition: autoimmune destruction of *intrahepatic* bile ducts
• Epidemiology: middle-aged *women*, concomitant autoimmune diseases
• Clinical manifestations: often asx; fatigue, pruritus, jaundice, fat malabsorption,
  xanthelasma, xanthoma
• Dx: ↑ Aφ, ↑ bilirubin, ⊕ anti-mitochondrial Ab (AMA) in 95%, ↑ cholesterol
• Treatment: ursodeoxycholic acid (13-15 mg/kg/d); fat-soluble vitamins; cholestyramine for
  pruritus; transplantation; colchicine ± methotrexate if incomplete response to UDCA

Primary sclerosing cholangitis (PSC) *(NEJM 1995;332:924)*
• Definition: idiopathic cholestasis with fibrosis, stricturing and dilatation of *intra- and
  extrahepatic* bile ducts
• Epidemiology: young *men* (age 20-50), associated with IBD in 70% of cases (UC >> CD)
• Clinical manifestations: fatigue, pruritus, jaundice, fevers, RUQ pain, cholangiocarcinoma
• Dx: ↑ bilirubin, ↑ Aφ, ⊕ p-ANCA in 70%, MRCP/ERCP → *multifocal beaded bile duct
  strictures*; "onion-skin" appearance of fibrosis around bile ducts on liver bx
• Treatment
  ? high dose ursodeoxycholic acid (20-30 mg/kg/d), ? cholestyramine, fat-soluble vit.
  endoscopic dilation and short-term stenting of dominant bile duct strictures
  liver transplantation (↑ risk of posttransplant duct strictures)

Budd-Chiari syndrome *(NEJM 2004;350:578)*
• Definition: occlusion of the hepatic veins or IVC → sinusoidal congestion and portal HTN
• Etiologies: hypercoagulable states (typically MPD, PNH, OCP, APLA, protein C/S def, JAK2
  mutation), tumor invasion (HCC, renal, adrenal), membranous webs, trauma, idiopathic
• Clinical manifestations: hepatomegaly, RUQ pain, ascites, dilated venous collaterals (if IVC)
• Dx: ± ↑ aminotransferases & Aφ; Doppler U/S of hepatic veins (85% Se & Sp); CT (I⁺)
  or MRI/MRA; "spider-web" pattern on hepatic venography; liver bx showing
  congestion (in Pt w/o evidence of right-sided CHF)
• Treatment: anticoagulation (heparin → warfarin), thrombolysis if acute thrombosis;
  TIPS (portocaval gradient <10) or surgical shunt (gradient >10); liver transplantation

Sinusoidal obstruction syndrome (SOS) *(Mayo 2003;78:589)*
• Previously known as **veno-occlusive disease (VOD)**
• Definition: occlusion of hepatic venules and sinusoids
• Etiology: stem cell transplant (SCT), chemotherapy, XRT, Jamaican bush tea
• Clinical manifestations: hepatomegaly, RUQ pain, ascites, weight gain, ↑ bilirubin
• Dx: U/S usually not helpful; dx made clinically or, if necessary, by liver bx
• Treatment: supportive; diuresis, analgesia, paracentesis for tense ascites;
  ursodeoxycholic acid prophylaxis in high risk SCT population

Etiologies	
Portal hypertension related **SAAG ≥1.1**	**Nonportal hypertension related** **SAAG <1.1**
Sinusoidal	**Peritonitis**: TB, ruptured viscus (↑ amy)
cirrhosis (81%), including SBP	**Peritoneal carcinomatosis**
acute hepatitis	Pancreatitis
extensive malignancy (HCC or mets)	Vasculitis
Postsinusoidal	Hypoalbuminemic states: nephrotic
right-sided CHF incl. constriction & TR	syndrome, protein-losing enteropathy
Budd-Chiari syndrome, SOS	Meigs' syndrome (ovarian tumor)
Presinusoidal	Bowel obstruction/infarction
portal or splenic vein thrombosis	Postoperative lymphatic leak
schistosomiasis	

Pathophysiology
- "Underfill" theory: portal hypertension → transudation of fluid into peritoneum → ↓ plasma volume → renal Na retention
- "Overflow" theory: hepatorenal reflex → Na retention
- Peripheral vasodilatation theory (favored): portal hypertension → systemic vasodilatation (? due to release of NO) → ↓ effective arterial volume → renal Na retention
- Hypoalbuminemia → ↓ serum oncotic pressure
- ↑ hepatic lymph production

Workup
- **Detection:** flank dullness (>1500 cc must be present), shifting dullness; **ultrasound** detects if >100 cc
- **Paracentesis** (*NEJM* 2006;355:e21): indicated in all Pts w/ new-onset ascites, as well as s/s of infxn (abd pain, fever, ΔMS, leukocytosis, acidosis); coagulopathy not a contraindic.
- **Serum-ascites albumin gradient (SAAG)** (*Annals* 1992;117:215): >95% accuracy ≥1.1 g/dl → portal hypertension related; <1.1 g/dl → nonportal hypertension related
- Ascites fluid total protein (AFTP): useful when SAAG ≥1.1 to distinguish cirrhosis (AFTP <2.5 g/dl) from cardiac ascites (AFTP >2.5 g/dl)
- If portal hypertensive etiology, consider standard cirrhosis w/u (see "Cirrhosis")
- Rule out infection: cell count with differential (infection if WBC >500/mm³ or PMN >250/mm³), culture → *bedside inoculation* of blood culture bottles (yield 90%) (*Gastro* 1988;95:1351), gram stain (less Se; most helpful w/ free perforation)
- Other tests as indicated: amylase (pancreatitis, gut perforation), triglycerides (chylous ascites), AFB/adenosine deaminase (TB), bilirubin (biliary/upper gut perforation), cytology (peritoneal carcinomatosis)

Treatment (portal hypertension related) (*NEJM* 2004;350:1646)
- ↓ **Na intake** (1-2 g/d); free H₂O restriction if hyponatremic
- **Diuretics** (effective in 80% of cases)
  spironolactone (start 100 mg PO qd) ± furosemide (start 40 mg PO qd); ↑ in proportion
  goals: diurese ~1L/d, steady wt loss (~0.5-1.0 kg/d), urinary Na/K ratio >1 (indicating effective blockade of endogenous aldosterone)
- Options for refractory ascites (ensure diet & medicine compliance)
  Large volume paracentesis: remove 4-6 L; ± albumin replacement (fewer asx chemical abnl; no Δ in mortality) (*Gastro* 1988;94:1493)
  TIPS: ↓↓ ascites in 75%, ↑ CrCl, ↑ transplantation-free survival (*NEJM* 2000;342:1701), but ↑ encephalopathy, 40% need TIPS revision, no Δ quality-of-life (*Gastro* 2003;124:634) consider if refractory ascites, Child's class A or B, minimal encephalopathy
  Liver transplantation if Pt is a candidate
- Treatment for nonportal HTN-related ascites depends on cause (TB, malignancy, etc)

Complications
- Spontaneous bacterial peritonitis (see below)
- Hepatorenal syndrome (see "Cirrhosis")
- Pleural effusions (usually unilateral and R >L; hepatic hydrothorax 2° diaphragmatic defect); chest tube contraindicated as → ↑ complications
- Other complications: cellulitis, tense ascites, abdominal wall hernias

Bacterial peritonitis
- Definitions and diagnosis

Type	Ascites cell count/mm³	Ascites culture
Sterile	<250 polys	⊖
Spontaneous bacterial peritonitis (SBP)	>250 polys	⊕ (one organism)
Culture-negative neutrocytic ascites (CNNA)	>250 polys	⊖
Nonneutrocytic bacterascites (NNBA)	<250 polys	⊕ (one organism)
Secondary	>250 polys	⊕ (polymicrobial)
Peritoneal dialysis-associated	>100 with poly predom.	⊕

- **SBP**
  epidemiology: occurs in 19% of cirrhotics; risk factors = AFTP < 1 g/dl, history of prior SBP, current GI hemorrhage
  clinical manifestations: fever, abdominal pain, rebound tenderness, Δ MS
    clinical signs may be unreliable; ∴ have a low threshold for diagnostic paracentesis
  pathogens: 70% GNR (*E. coli*, *Klebsiella*), 30% GPC (*S. pneumoniae*, other streptococci, *Enterococcus*)
  treatment: cefotaxime 2 gm IV q8h × 5 d; IV albumin 1.5 g/kg at time of diagnosis and 1 g/kg on day 3 results in survival benefit (*NEJM* 1999;341:403)
    repeat paracentesis after 48 h if w/o significant improvement
  prophylaxis (if h/o SBP, current GIB, or AFTP <1 g/dl)
    norfloxacin 400 mg PO qd or Bactrim DS qd
    however, selects for resistant gut flora, ∴ limit use of prophylactic abx as follows:
      inpatients w/ AFTP <1 g/dl, with discontinuation of abx at time of discharge
      acute variceal hemorrhage: norfloxacin 400 mg PO *bid*, Bactrim DS PO *bid*, or ceftriaxone 1g *IV* qd × 7 d
      h/o one or more episodes of SBP: indefinite treatment
- **CNNA**: variant of SBP w/ similar clinical course; Rx same as for SBP
- **NNBA**: often resolves w/o Rx; follow closely → Rx only if sx or persistently culture ⊕
- **Secondary** (intraabdominal abscess or perforated viscus)
  polymicrobial
  usually AFTP >1 g/dl, ascitic fluid glucose <50 mg/dl, or ascitic fluid LDH >225 U/L
  treatment: 3rd-gen. cephalosporin + metronidazole
    plains films (supine/upright), CT scan, and likely exploratory laparotomy for definitive diagnosis and treatment
- **Peritoneal dialysis-associated**
  clinical manifestations: cloudy abdominal fluid, abdominal pain, rebound, fever, nausea
  pathogens: 70% GPC, 30% GNR
  treatment: vancomycin + gentamicin (IV load then administer in PD)

Portal vein thrombosis (PVT)
- Thrombosis, constriction, or invasion of portal vein → portal HTN → splenomegaly and formation of portosystemic collaterals (esophageal, gastric, duodenal, jejunal varices)
- Etiologies: cirrhosis, neoplasm (pancreas, HCC), intra-abdominal inflammation/infection, hypercoagulable state (including MPS), surgery, trauma
- Clinical manifestations:
  acute PVT: can p/w pain, but usually clinically silent; dx as incidental finding on U/S or CT performed for other reasons
  chronic PVT: can present as incidental finding or as hematemesis 2° variceal bleeding; splenomegaly; occasionally ascites
- Diagnostic studies: LFTs usually normal; U/S with Doppler, MRA, CT (I⁺), angiography
- Treatment: as for portal hypertension; anticoagulation for acute portal vein thrombosis; consider surgical shunts or TIPS if refractory or recurrent bleeding

BILIACY TRACT DISEASE

CHOLELITHIASIS ("GALLSTONES")

Epidemiology
- >10% adults in the U.S. have gallstones
- Risk factors: women, Native Americans, ↑ age (usually >40 y), obesity, pregnancy, TPN, rapid weight loss, drugs (OCPs, estrogen, clofibrate, octreotide, ceftriaxone)

Pathogenesis
- Bile = bile salts, phospholipids, cholesterol; ↑ cholesterol saturation in bile + accelerated nucleation + gallbladder hypomotility → gallstones

Types of gallstones
- Mixed (80%): multiple stones, mostly cholesterol, may calcify (15-20%)
- Cholesterol (10%): usually single stone, large, uncalcified
- Pigment (10%)
  Black: unconjugated bilirubin (hence seen in chronic hemolysis) and calcium
  Brown: anaerobic infection of bile leading to ↑ unconjugated bilirubin and calcium

Clinical manifestations
- History: may be asymptomatic (symptoms develop in ~2%/y)
  biliary pain = episodic RUQ or epigastric abdominal pain that begins abruptly, is continuous, resolves slowly, and lasts for 30 min to 3 h associated **nausea**; may be precipitated by **fatty foods**
- Physical exam: afebrile, ± RUQ tenderness or epigastric pain

Diagnostic studies
- RUQ U/S: Se & Sp >90-95%, can show complications (cholecystitis); should be performed only after fasting ≥8 h to ensure distended, bile-filled gallbladder

Treatment
- Cholecystectomy (usually laparoscopic) if symptomatic
- Oral dissolution therapy with ursodeoxycholic acid (rare) for mild, uncomplicated biliary pain or Pts who are not surgical candidates

Complications
- Cholecystitis (30% of symptomatic biliary pain → cholecystitis within 2 y)
- Choledocholithiasis → cholangitis or gallstone pancreatitis
- Cholecystoenteric fistula (stone erodes through gallbladder into bowel), Mirizzi's syndrome (stone in cystic duct compresses common hepatic duct → jaundice, biliary obstruction)
- Gallbladder carcinoma (~1%)

CHOLECYSTITIS

Definition
- Inflammation of the gallbladder

Pathogenesis
- Stone impaction in the cystic duct causing obstruction
- Acalculous cholecystitis due to gallbladder stasis and ischemia → inflammatory response; occurs mainly in ill, hosp. Pts [TPN, sepsis, trauma, burns, opiates, immunosuppression, infxn (eg, CMV, Crypto, Campylobacter, typhoid fever)]

Clinical manifestations
- History: RUQ/epigastric pain ± radiation to R shoulder or back, nausea/vomiting, fever
- Physical examination: **RUQ tenderness, Murphy's sign =** ↑ RUQ pain and inspiratory arrest with deep breath during palpation of R subcostal region, ± palpable gallbladder
- Laboratory evaluation: ↑ WBC, ± mild ↑ bilirubin, Aφ, ALT/AST, and amylase; AST/ALT >500 U, bili >4 mg/dl, or amylase >1000 U/L → choledocholithiasis

Diagnostic studies (*JAMA* 2003;289:80)
- RUQ U/S: high Se and Sp for gallstones; specific signs of cholecystitis include pericholecystic fluid, gallbladder wall thickening, and a sonographic Murphy's sign
- Cholescintigraphy (**HIDA scan**): most sensitive test for acute cholecystitis. IV injection of radiolabeled HIDA is selectively secreted into biliary tree. In acute cholecystitis, HIDA enters CBD but not the gallbladder.

Treatment
- NPO, IV fluids, nasogastric tube if intractable vomiting, analgesia
- **Antibiotics** (*E. coli*, *Klebsiella*, enterococcus, and *Enterobacter* are usual pathogens)
  3rd-generation cephalosporin (or quinolone) + metronidazole; or piperacillin-tazobactam
- Semiurgent cholecystectomy (usually w/in 72 h)
- Cholecystostomy and percutaneous drainage if too sick for surgery
- Intra-operative cholangiogram or ERCP to r/o choledocholithiasis in Pts w/ jaundice, cholangitis, or stone in CBD on U/S

Complications
- Perforation
- Empyema
- Emphysematous gallbladder due to infection by gas-forming organisms
- Cholecystoenteric fistula (to duodenum, colon, or stomach): can see air in biliary tree
- Gallstone ileus: bowel obstruction (usually at terminal ileum) due to stone in intestine that passed through a fistula

---

CHOLEDOCHOLITHIASIS

Definition
- Gallstone lodged in the common bile duct (CBD)

Epidemiology
- Occurs in 15% of Pts with gallstones

Clinical manifestations
- Asymptomatic (50%)
- Biliary pain, RUQ/epigastric pain, jaundice, pruritis, nausea

Diagnostic studies
- Labs: ↑ bilirubin, A$_\phi$; transient spike in ALT or amylase suggests passage of stone
- RUQ U/S: CBD stones seen ~50% of cases; usually inferred from dilated CBD (>6 mm)
- ERCP preferred dx modality; cholangiogram (percutaneous, operative) when ERCP unavailable or unsuccessful; EUS/MRCP to exclude CBD stones when suspicion low

Treatment
- ERCP and papillotomy with stone extraction

Complications
- Cholangitis
- Pancreatitis
- Cholecystitis
- Stricture

CHOLANGITIS

Definition
- Common bile duct (CBD) obstruction → infection proximal to the obstruction

Etiologies
- CBD stone (~85%)
- Stricture
- Neoplasm (biliary or pancreatic)
- Infiltration with flukes (*Clonorchis sinensis*, *Opisthorchis viverrini*)

Clinical manifestations
- Charcot's triad: RUQ pain, jaundice, fever/chills; present in ~70% of Pts
- Reynold's pentad: Charcot's triad + shock and Δ MS; present in ~15% of Pts

Diagnostic studies
- Labs: ↑WBC, bilirubin, A$_\phi$, amylase; ⊕ blood cultures
- ERCP or percutaneous transhepatic cholangiogram (if ERCP unsuccessful)

Treatment
- **Antibiotics** (broad spectrum) to cover common bile pathogens (see above)
  ampicillin + gentamicin (or levofloxacin) ± MNZ (if severe); carbapenems; pip/tazo
- ~80% Pts respond to conservative mgmt and abx → biliary drainage on elective basis
- ~20% Pts require urgent **biliary decompression** via ERCP (papillotomy, stone extraction, and/or stent insertion), percutaneous transhepatic biliary drainage, or surgery

Definitions
- **Acidemia** → pH <7.36, **alkalemia** → pH >7.44
- **Acidosis** → process that increases [H^+]; **alkalosis** → process that decreases [H^+]
- Primary disorders: metabolic acidosis or alkalosis, respiratory acidosis or alkalosis
- Compensation

  respiratory: hyper- or hypoventilation alters P_aCO_2 to counteract 1° metabolic process
  renal: excretion/retention of H^+/HCO_3 by kidneys to counteract 1° respiratory process
  respiratory compensation occurs in min; renal compensation takes hrs to days
  compensation never fully corrects pH; if pH normal, consider mixed disorder

Workup
- Determine **primary disorder**: ✓ pH, P_aCO_2, HCO_3
- Determine if **degree of compensation** is appropriate

Primary Disorders				
Primary disorder	**Problem**	**pH**	**HCO₃**	**PₐCO₂**
Metabolic acidosis	gain of H^+ or loss of HCO_3	↓	⇓	↓
Metabolic alkalosis	gain of HCO_3 or loss of H^+	↑	⇑	↑
Respiratory acidosis	hypoventilation	↓	↑	⇑
Respiratory alkalosis	hyperventilation	↑	↓	⇓

Compensation for Acid/Base Disorders	
Primary disorder	**Expected compensation**
Metabolic acidosis	↓ $P_aCO_2 = 1.25 \times \Delta HCO_3$ (also, $PaCO_2$ = last two digits of pH)
Metabolic alkalosis	↑ $P_aCO_2 = 0.75 \times \Delta HCO_3$
Acute respiratory acidosis	↑ $HCO_3 = 0.1 \times \Delta P_aCO_2$ (also, ↓ pH = .008 × ΔP_aCO_2)
Chronic respiratory acidosis	↑ $HCO_3 = 0.4 \times \Delta P_aCO_2$ (also, ↓ pH = .003 × ΔP_aCO_2)
Acute respiratory alkalosis	↓ $HCO_3 = 0.2 \times \Delta P_aCO_2$ (also, ↑ pH = .008 × ΔP_aCO_2)
Chronic respiratory alkalosis	↓ $HCO_3 = 0.4 \times \Delta P_aCO_2$

Mixed disorders (more than one primary disorder at the same time)
- If compensation less or greater than predicted, may be 2 disorders:
  P_aCO_2 too low → concomitant 1° resp. alk.
  P_aCO_2 too high → concomitant 1° resp. acid.
  HCO_3 too low → concomitant 1° met. acid.
  HCO_3 too high → concomitant 1° met. alk.
- Normal pH *but* ...
  ↑ P_aCO_2 + ↑ HCO_3 → resp. acid. + met. alk.
  ↓ P_aCO_2 + ↓ HCO_3 → resp. alk. + met. acid.
  normal P_aCO_2 & HCO_3, *but* ↑ AG → AG met. acid. + met. alk.
  normal P_aCO_2, HCO_3, & AG → no disturbance *or* non-AG met. acid. + met. alk.
- *Cannot* have resp. acid. (hypoventilation) and resp. alk. (hyperventilation) simultaneously

Figure 4-1 Acid-Base nomogram

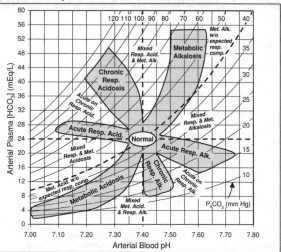

N.B., If ABG not available, can use VBG, but note that pH ~0.04 ↓, PaCO₂ ~8 mmHg ↑, and
HCO₃ ~2 mEq ↑. (Adapted from Brenner BM, ed. *Brenner & Rector's The Kidney*, 5th ed., 1996; Ferri F, ed.
Practical Guide to The Care of the Medical Patient, 5th ed., 2001)

Consequences of Severe Acid-Base Disturbances		
Organ System	Acidosis (pH <7.20)	Alkalosis (pH >7.60)
Cardiovascular	↓ contractility, arteriolar vasodilation ↓ MAP & CO; ↓ response to catecholamines ↑ risk of arrhythmias	Arteriolar vasoconstriction ↓ coronary blood flow ↑ risk of arrhythmias
Respiratory	Hyperventilation, ↓ resp muscle strength	Hypoventilation
Metabolic	↑ K	↓ K, ICa, Mg, PO₄
Neurologic	Δ MS	Δ MS, seizures

(*NEJM* 1998;338:26, 107)

METABOLIC ACIDOSIS

Initial workup
- ✓ **anion gap** (AG) = Na - (Cl + HCO₃) = unmeasured anions - unmeasured cations
  if ↑ glc, use measured *not* corrected Na
  expected AG is [albumin] × 2.5 (ie, 10 if albumin is 4 g/dl, 7.5 if albumin is 3 g/dl)
  ↑ AG → ↑ unmeasured anions such as organic acids, phosphates, sulfates
  ↓ AG → ↓ alb or ↑ unmeasured cations (Ca, Mg, K, Li, immunoglobulin)
- If ↑ AG, ✓ **delta-delta** (ΔΔ = ΔAG/ΔHCO₃) to assess if there is an additional metabolic
  acid-base disturbance; ΔAG = (calculated AG - expected AG), ΔHCO₃ = (24 - HCO₃)
  ΔΔ = 1-2 → pure AG metabolic acidosis
  ΔΔ < 1 → AG metabolic acidosis *and* simultaneous non-AG acidosis
  ΔΔ > 2 → AG metabolic acidosis *and* simultaneous metabolic alkalosis

Etiologies of AG Metabolic Acidosis	
Ketoacidosis	**Diabetes mellitus**, alcoholism, starvation
Lactic acidosis	**Type A**: impairment in tissue oxygenation, eg, **circulatory or respiratory failure, sepsis**, ischemic bowel, carbon monoxide **Type B**: no impairment in tissue oxygenation, eg, malignancy, alcoholism, meds (metformin, NRTIs, salicylates) **D-lactic acidosis**: short bowel syndrome → glc metab by colonic bacteria to D-lactate, which is absorbed; not detected by standard lactate assay
Renal failure	Accumulation of organic anions such as phosphates, sulfates, etc.
Ingestions	**Methanol**: manifestations include blurred vision **Ethylene glycol**: manifestations include ΔMS, cardiopulmonary failure, calcium oxalate crystals and renal failure **Paraldehyde** **Salicylates**: metabolic acidosis (from lactate, ketones) + respiratory alkalosis due to stimulation of CNS respiratory center **Acetaminophen**: glutathione depletion → accumulation of the endogenous organic acid 5-oxoproline in susceptible host

Workup for AG metabolic acidosis
- ✓ for **ketonuria** (dipstick acetoacetate) or plasma β-hydroxybutyrate (βOHB)
  nb, urine acetoacetate often not present in early ketoacidosis due to shunting to βOHB; ∴ acetoacetate may later turn ⊕, but does not signify worsening disease
- If ⊖ ketones, ✓ **renal function, lactate, toxin screen**, and **osmolal gap**
- **Osmolal gap** (OG) = measured osmoles - calculated osmoles
  calculated osmoles = $(2 \times Na) + (glucose/18) + (BUN/2.8) + (EtOH/4.6)$
  OG >10 → suggests ingestion (methanol, ethylene glycol)

Etiologies of Non-AG Metabolic Acidosis	
GI losses of HCO_3	Diarrhea, intestinal or pancreatic fistulas or drainage
RTAs	*See section on renal tubular acidoses below*
Early renal failure	Impaired generation of ammonia
Ingestions	Acetazolamide, sevelamer, cholestyramine, toluene
Dilutional	Due to rapid infusion of bicarbonate-free intravenous fluids
Post-hypocapnia	Respiratory alkalosis → renal wasting of HCO_3; rapid correction of resp. alk. → transient acidosis until HCO_3 regenerated
Ureteral diversion	Colonic Cl^-/HCO_3^- exchange, ammonium reabsorption

Workup for non-AG metabolic acidosis
- Evaluate history for causes (see above)
- ✓ **urine anion gap** (UAG) = $(U_{Na} + U_K) - U_{Cl}$
  UAG = unmeasured anions - unmeasured cations; as NH_4^+ is primary unmeasured cation, UAG is indirect assay for renal NH_4^+ excretion (NEJM 1988;318:594)
- ⊖ UAG → ↑ renal NH_4^+ excretion → appropriate renal response to acidemia
  GI causes, type II RTA, ingestions or dilutional
- ⊕ UAG → failure of kidneys to secrete NH_4^+
  type I or IV RTA, early renal failure; plasma K usually ↓ in type I and ↑ in type IV
- UAG interpretation assumes Pt not volume deplete and w/o AG met. acidosis → ⊕ UAG

Renal tubular acidoses (RTAs)
- **Type I (distal)**: defective distal H^+ secretion
  1°, autoimmune (Sjögren's, RA), nephrocalcinosis, meds (ampho, Li, ifosfamide), associated with ↑ K (sickle cell, obstruction, SLE, renal transplant)
- **Type II (proximal)**: ↓ proximal reabsorption of HCO_3
  1° (Fanconi's syndrome), paraprotein (multiple myeloma, amyloidosis), meds (acetazolamide, heavy metals, ifosfamide), renal transplant
- **Type IV (hypoaldo)**: ↑K → ↓ NH_3 synthesis/delivery → ↓ urine acid carrying capacity
  ↓ renin: diabetic nephropathy, NSAIDs, chronic interstitial nephritis, HIV
  normal renin, ↓ aldo synthesis: 1° adrenal disorders, ACEI, ARBs, heparin
  ↓ response to aldosterone
     meds: K-sparing diuretics, TMP-SMX, pentamidine, calcineurin inhibitors
     tubulointerstitial disease: sickle cell, SLE, amyloid, diabetes

Renal Tubular Acidosis						
Type	Location	Acidosis	UAG	U pH	FeHCO₃[†]	Serum K
I	Distal	severe	⊕	>5.3	<3%	↓[‡]
II	Proximal	moderate	±	<5.3*	>15%	↓
IV	Hypoaldo	mild	⊕	<5.3	<3%	↑

*urine pH will rise above 5.3 in the setting of HCO_3 load
[†]$FeHCO_3$ should be checked after an HCO_3 load
[‡]see above for causes of type I RTA associated with hyperkalemia

Figure 4-2 Approach to metabolic acidosis

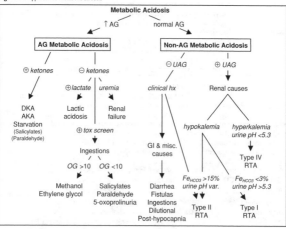

Treatment of severe metabolic acidoses (pH <7.2) (NEJM 1998;338:26)
- DKA: insulin, IVF; AKA: dextrose, IVF, replete K, Mg, PO_4 as needed
- Lactic acidosis: treat underlying condition, avoid vasoconstrictors
- Renal failure: hemodialysis
- Methanol & ethylene glycol: saline diuresis, thiamine, vit. B_6, fomepizole, hemodialysis
- Alkali therapy: $NaHCO_3$ (eg, 3 50-mmol amp in 1 L D_5W) to get serum HCO_3 >8 and pH >7.2 (estimate mmol of HCO_3 needed as $8-[HCO_3]_{serum} \times wt \times 0.5$) side effects: volume overload, hypernatremia, ↓ ICa, ↑ P_aCO_2 (and ∴ possibly intracellular acidosis), overshoot; no proven benefit in lactic acidosis (Annals 1990;112:492)

METABOLIC ALKALOSIS

Pathophysiology
- Saline-responsive etiologies require *initiating event* and *maintenance factors*, whereas saline-resistant etiologies develop from a variety of causes
- *Initiating event*
  loss of H^+ from GI tract or kidneys
  exogenous alkali
  contraction alkalosis: diuresis → excretion of HCO_3-poor fluid → extracellular fluid "contracts" around fixed amount of HCO_3 → ↑ HCO_3 concentration.
  posthypercapnia: respiratory acidosis → renal compensation with HCO_3 retention; rapid correction of respiratory disorder (eg, with intubation) → transient excess HCO_3
- *Maintenance factors*
  volume depletion → ↑ proximal reabsorption of $NaHCO_3$ and ↑ aldosterone (see next)
  hyperaldosteronism (either 1° or 2°) → distal Na reabsorption in exchange for K^+ and H^+ excretion (and consequent HCO_3 retention)
  hypokalemia → transcellular K^+/H^+ exchange; intracellular acidosis in renal proximal tubular cells promotes bicarbonate reabsorption and ammoniagenesis

Etiologies of Metabolic Alkalosis	
Saline-responsive	**GI loss of H⁺**: vomiting, NGT drainage, villous adenoma **Diuretic use** posthypercapnia

Saline-resistant	*Hypertensive* **(mineralocorticoid excess)**
	  1° hyperaldosteronism (eg, Conn's)
	  2° hyperaldosteronism (eg, renovascular dis. renin-secreting tumor)
	  non-aldo (eg, Cushing's, Liddle's, exogenous mineralocorticoids)
	Normotensive
	  severe hypokalemia
	  exogenous alkali load
	  Bartter's syndrome, Gitelman's syndrome

Workup

- Check **volume status** and U_{Cl}
   U_{Cl} <20 mEq/L → saline-responsive
   U_{Cl} >20 mEq/L → saline-resistant (unless currently receiving diuretics)
   (U_{Na} unreliable determinant of volume status as alkalemia → ↑HCO_3 excretion →
   ↑Na excretion; negatively charged HCO_3 "drags" Na^+ along)
   If U_{Cl} >20 and volume replete, ✓ **blood pressure**

Figure 4-3 Approach to metabolic alkalosis

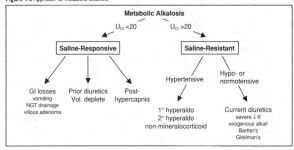

RESPIRATORY ACIDOSIS

Etiologies

- **CNS depression**: sedatives, CNS trauma, O_2 in chronic hypercapnia (↓ hypoxemic drive)
- **Neuromuscular disorders**: myasthenia gravis, Guillain-Barré, poliomyelitis, ALS, muscular dystrophy, severe hypophosphatemia
- **Upper airway abnormalities**: acute airway obstruction, laryngospasm, obstructive sleep apnea, esophageal intubation
- **Lower airway abnormalities**: asthma, COPD
- Lung parenchyma abnormalities (often cause hypoxia → ↑ RR → resp. alk., but eventual muscle fatigue → resp. acid.): pneumonia, pulmonary edema, restrictive lung disease
- Thoracic cage abnormalities: pneumothorax, flail chest, kyphoscoliosis

---

RESPIRATORY ALKALOSIS

Etiologies (*NEJM* 2002;347:43)

- **Hypoxia → hyperventilation**: pneumonia, pulm. edema, PE, restrictive lung disease
- **Primary hyperventilation**
   CNS disorders, pain, anxiety
   drugs: salicylates, progesterone, methylxanthines
   pregnancy
   sepsis
   hepatic failure

SODIUM AND WATER HOMEOSTASIS

OVERVIEW

General
- Disorders of serum sodium are generally due to Δs in *total body water*, not sodium
- Hyper - or hypoosmolality → rapid water shifts → Δs in brain cell volume → Δ MS, seizures

Key hormones
- **Antidiuretic hormone (ADH)**: primary hormone that regulates *sodium concentration*
  stimuli for secretion: hyperosmolality, $\downarrow\downarrow$ effective arterial volume (EAV)
  action: open water channels in collecting ducts → passive water reabsorption
  urine osmolality is an indirect functional assay of the ADH-renal axis
  U_{osm} range: 60 mOsm/L (no ADH) to 1200 mOsm/L (maximal ADH)
- **Aldosterone**: primary hormone that regulates *total body sodium* (and ∴ volume)
  stimuli for secretion: hypovolemia (via renin and angiotensin II), hyperkalemia
  action: isoosmotic reabsorption of sodium in exchange for potassium or H^+

HYPONATREMIA

Pathophysiology
- **Excess of water relative to sodium**; almost always due to ↑**ADH**
- ↑ ADH may be *appropriate* (eg, hypovolemia or hypervolemia with ↓ EAV)
- ↑ ADH may be *inappropriate* (SIADH)
- Rarely, ↓ ADH (appropriately suppressed), but kidneys unable to maintain nl [Na]$_{serum}$
  primary polydipsia: ingestion of massive quantities (usually >12 L/d) of free H_2O
  overwhelms diluting ability of kidney (normal solute load ~750 mOsm/d, min U_{osm}
  = 60 mOsm/L → excrete in ~12 L; if H_2O ingestion exceeds this, H_2O retention)
  "tea & toast" and "beer potomania": $\downarrow\downarrow$ daily solute load, ↑ free H_2O → insufficient
  solute to excrete H_2O intake (eg, if only 250 mOsm/d, minimum U_{osm} = 60
  mOsm/L → excrete in ~4 L; if H_2O ingestion exceeds this, H_2O retention)

Workup (NEJM 2000;342:1581)
- Measure **plasma osmolality**
  Hypotonic hyponatremia most common scenario; true excess of free H_2O relative to Na
  Hypertonic hyponatremia: excess of another effective osmole (eg, glc, mannitol) that
    draws H_2O intravascularly; each 100 mg/dl ↑ glc >100 mg/dl → ↓ [Na] by 2.4 mEq/L
  Isotonic hyponatremia: rare lab artifact from hyperlipidemia or hyperproteinemia
- For hypotonic hyponatremia, ✓ **volume status** (vital signs, orthostatics, JVP, skin
  turgor, mucous membranes, peripheral edema, BUN, Cr, uric acid)
- U_{osm} diagnostically useful in limited circumstances, because almost always >300
  exceptions: U_{osm} <100 in 1° polydipsia & ↓ solute intake
  moreover, U_{osm} >300 ≠ SIADH; must determine if ↑ADH appropriate or inappropriate
  however, U_{osm} important when deciding on *treatment* (see below)
- If euvolemic and ↑ U_{osm}, evaluate for glucocorticoid insufficiency and hypothyroidism

Figure 4-4 Approach to hyponatremia

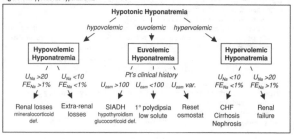

Hypovolemic hypotonic hyponatremia
- **Renal losses** (U_{Na} >20 mEq/L, FE_{Na} >1%): diuretics (espec. thiazides, as loop diuretics ↓ tonicity of medullary interstitium and impair urine concentrating ability), salt-wasting nephropathy, cerebral salt wasting, mineralocorticoid deficiency
- **Extrarenal losses** (U_{Na} <10 mEq/L, FE_{Na} <1%): GI losses (eg, diarrhea), third-spacing (eg, pancreatitis), inadequate intake, insensible losses

Euvolemic hypotonic hyponatremia
- **SIADH** (eu- or mild hypervolemia, inappropriately ↑ U_{osm}, **normal U_{Na}**, ↓ BUN & uric acid)
  pulmonary: pneumonia, asthma, COPD, SCLC, PTX, ⊕ pressure ventilation
  intracranial: trauma, stroke, hemorrhage, tumors, infxn, hydrocephalus
  drugs: antipsychotics, antidepressants, chemotherapy, vasopressin, dDAVP
  miscellaneous: pain, nausea, postoperative state
- **Endocrinopathies**: ↑ ADH activity seen in *glucocorticoid deficiency* (co-secretion of ADH & CRH) and *hypothyroidism* (↓ CO & ↓ GFR)
- **Psychogenic polydipsia** (U_{osm} <100, ↓ uric acid): usually requires intake >12 L/d
- **Low solute**: "tea & toast"; "beer potomania"
- Reset osmostat: chronic malnutrition (↓ intracellular osmoles) or pregnancy (hormonal effects) → ADH physiology reset to regulate a lower [Na]$_{serum}$

Hypervolemic hypotonic hyponatremia
- **CHF** (↓ CO → ↓ EAV; U_{Na} <10 mEq/L, FE_{Na} <1%)
- **Cirrhosis** (splanchnic arterial vasodilation and ascites → ↓ EAV; U_{Na} <10 mEq/L, FE_{Na} <1%)
- **Nephrotic syndrome** (hypoalbuminemia → edema → ↓ EAV; U_{Na} <10 mEq/L, FE_{Na} <1%)
- **Advanced renal failure** (U_{Na} >20 mEq/L)

Treatment
- **Goals of treatment**
  Asymptomatic hyponatremia: correct [Na]$_{serum}$ at rate of ≤0.5 mEq/L/h
  Symptomatic hyponatremia: *initial rapid correction of Na* (2 mEq/L/h for the first 2-3 h) until sx resolve
  Rate of ↑ Na *should not exceed 10-12 mEq/L/d* to avoid osmotic demyelination syndrome (spastic quadriplegia, dysarthria, dysphagia), espec if hypoNa chronic
- **Effect of IV fluids**

$$\text{initial } \Delta[\text{Na}]_{serum} \text{ per L infusate} = \frac{[\text{Na}]_{infusate} - [\text{Na}]_{serum}}{\text{TBW} + 1}$$

  TBW = 0.60 × IBW (× 0.85 if female and × 0.85 if elderly)

  eg, 1 L hypertonic saline (513 mEq Na) given to 70 kg (IBW) man
  w/ [Na] = 110 mEq/L will ↑ [Na]$_{serum}$ by 9.4 mEq
  however, above assumes entire infusate retained *without any output of Na or H_2O*
  if Pt is euvolemic, as in SIADH, then infused Na will be excreted
  eg, 1L NS (154 mEq of Na or 308 mOsm of solute in 1L H_2O) given to Pt with
  SIADH with U_{osm} = 616 → 308 mOsm solute excreted in 0.5 L H_2O →
  net gain 0.5 L H_2O → ↓ [Na]
  ∴ normal saline can *worsen* hyponatremia 2° SIADH if U_{osm} > infusate$_{osm}$
- **Hypovolemic hyponatremia**: volume repletion with **normal saline**
  once volume replete → stimulus for ADH removed → kidneys will excrete free H_2O → serum Na will correct rapidly
- **SIADH** (NEJM 2007;356:2064): free water restrict + treat underlying cause
  hypertonic saline (± loop diuretic) if sx or Na fails to ↑ w/ free H_2O restriction
  1 L hypertonic saline will raise [Na]$_{serum}$ by ~10 mEq (see above)
  ~50 ml/h will ↑ [Na] by ~0.5 mEq/L/h; 100-200 ml/h will ↑ [Na] by ~1-2 mEq/L/h
  formula only provides estimate; ∴ recheck serum Na frequently
  demeclocycline or Li: cause nephrogenic DI
  aquaresis with conivaptan (V1a and V2 vasopressin receptor antagonist)
- **Hypervolemic hyponatremia**
  free water restrict
  ↑ EAV (eg, vasodilators and loop diuretics to ↑ CO in CHF, colloid infusion in cirrhosis)
  ? aquaresis with tolvaptan (V2 vasopressin antagonist) (SALT-1 & SALT-2, *NEJM* 2006;355:2099)

HYPERNATREMIA

Pathophysiology (*NEJM* 2000;342:1493)
- Deficit of water relative to sodium
- Usually **loss of hypotonic fluid**; occasionally infusion of hypertonic fluid
- *And* **impaired access to free water** (eg, intubation, Δ MS): hypernatremia is powerful thirst stimulus, ∴ usually only develops in Pts w/o access to H_2O
- By definition, all Pts are hypertonic; can be either hypo-, eu-, or hypervolemic

Hypovolemic hypernatremia
- **Renal H_2O losses** (U_{osm} 300-600): loop diuretics, osmotic diuresis (glc, mannitol, urea)
- **Extrarenal H_2O losses** (U_{osm} >600): diarrhea, insensible loss (fever, exercise)

Euvolemic hypernatremia
- **Diabetes insipidus** (U_{osm} <300-600): ADH defic. (central) or resist. (nephrogenic)
  Central: congenital, trauma/surgery, tumors, or infiltrative disease of hypothalamus or posterior pituitary; also idiopathic, hypoxic encephalopathy, anorexia
  Nephrogenic (*Annals* 2006;144:186)
  congenital
  drugs: **Li**, amphotericin, demeclocycline, foscarnet, cidofovir
  metabolic: **hypercalcemia**, severe hypokalemia, protein malnutrition, congenital
  tubulointerstitial: **postobstruction**, **recovery phase of ATN**, PKD, sickle cell, Sjögren's, amyloid, pregnancy
  DI usually presents as *severe polyuria* and *mild hypernatremia*
- Seizures, exercise (U_{osm} >600): ↑ intracellular osmoles → H_2O shifts → transient ↑ $[Na]_{serum}$

Hypervolemic hypernatremia
- Hypertonic saline administration: eg, cardiac arrest resuscitation with $NaHCO_3$
- Mineralocorticoid excess: usually mild hypernatremia caused by ADH suppression

Workup
- ✓ **volume status** (vital signs, orthostatics, JVP, skin turgor, mucous membranes, peripheral edema, BUN, Cr)
- If hypovolemic, ✓ U_{osm} & U_{Na} to determine whether **renal** (U_{osm} 300-600; U_{Na} >20 mEq/L) or **extrarenal** (U_{osm} >600; U_{Na} <20 mEq/L) **free water loss**
- If euvolemic, ✓ U_{osm} to evaluate for complete (U_{osm} <300) or partial (U_{osm} 300-600) **DI** see "Polyuria" below for full details of DI workup

Figure 4-5 Approach to hypernatremia

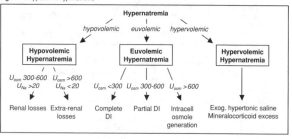

Treatment
- **Restore access to H_2O** or supply daily requirement of H_2O (≥ 1 L/d)
- **Hypovolemic hypernatremia:** replace volume and free H_2O deficits

$$\text{Free } H_2O \text{ deficit} = \frac{[Na]_{serum} - 140}{140} \times \text{TBW}$$

TBW $= 0.60 \times$ IBW ($\times 0.85$ if female and $\times 0.85$ if elderly)

for 70 kg (IBW) man, free H_2O deficit $\sim ([Na]_{serum} - 140)/3$

$$\Delta[Na]_{serum} \text{ per L infusate} = \frac{[Na]_{serum} - [Na]_{infusate}}{TBW + 1}$$

eg, 1 L D_5W given to 70 kg (IBW) man w/ [Na] = 160 mEq/L will ↓ [Na]$_{serum}$ by 3.7 mEq

rate of ↓ of Na *should not exceed* 0.5 mEq/L/h to avoid cerebral edema

in 70 kg (IBW) man, 125 ml/h of free H_2O will ↓ [Na] by ~0.5 mEq/L/h

can use $^1/_2$ NS (77 mEq) or $^1/_4$ NS (38 mEq) to simultaneously provide volume & free H_2O (which provide 500 ml or 750 ml of free H_2O per L, respectively)

can give free H_2O orally (via NGT/OGT) as well

formulas only provide estimates; ∴ recheck serum Na frequently

- **DI**

  central DI: desmopressin (dDAVP)

  nephrogenic DI: treat underlying cause if possible; Na restriction + thiazide (mild volume depletion → ↓ delivery of filtrate to dysfxnal diluting segment of kidney)

- **Hypervolemic hypernatremia:** D_5W + loop diuretic

POLYURIA

Definition and pathophysiology
- **Polyuria** defined as >3 L UOP per day
- Due to an *osmotic* or a *water diuresis*; almost always due to osmotic diuresis in inpatients

Workup
- Perform a timed urine collection (6 h sufficient) and measure U_{osm}
- 24-h osmole excretion rate = 24-h UOP (actual or estimate) $\times U_{osm}$
  - >1000 mOsm/d → osmotic diuresis
  - <800 mOsm/d → water diuresis

Osmotic diuresis
- Etiologies

  Glucose (uncontrolled diabetes mellitus)

  Mannitol

  Urea: recovering ARF, ↑ protein feeds, hypercatabolism (burns, steroids), GI bleed

  NaCl administration
- Treatment: address underlying cause, replace free-water deficit and ongoing losses

Water diuresis
- Etiologies: DI (Na$_{serum}$ >140) or 1° polydipsia (Na$_{serum}$ <140)

  see "Hypernatremia" above for list of causes of central and nephrogenic DI
- Workup of DI: U_{osm} <300 (complete) or 300-600 (partial)

  water deprivation test: deprive until P_{osm} >295 and U_{osm} <300, then administer vasopressin (5U SC) or dDAVP (10 μg intranasal):

  U_{osm} ↑ by >50% = central DI

  U_{osm} unchanged = nephrogenic DI
- Treatment of DI: see "Hypernatremia" above

POTASSIUM HOMEOSTASIS

Overview (*Lancet* 1998;352:135)

- Renal: potassium excretion regulated at **distal nephron** (collecting tubule)
  distal Na delivery & urine flow: Na absorption → lumen electronegative → K secretion
  aldosterone: increases Na absorption, K secretion
- Transcellular shifts: most common cause of acute change in serum potassium
  Acid-base disturbance: K^+/H^+ exchange across cell membranes
  Insulin → stimulates Na-K ATPase → hypokalemia
  Catecholamines → stimulate Na-K ATPase → hypokalemia; reversed by β-blockers
  Digoxin → blocks Na-K ATPase → hyperkalemia
  Massive necrosis (eg, tumor lysis, rhabdo, ischemic bowel) → release of intracellular K
  Hypo- or hyperkalemic periodic paralysis: rare disorders due to channel mutations

HYPOKALEMIA

Transcellular shifts

- Alkalemia, insulin, catecholamines, hypokalemic periodic paralysis (Ca channelopathy),
  acute ↑ in hematopoiesis (eg, megaloblastic anemia treated with B_{12}, AML crisis)

GI potassium losses (U_K <25 mEq/d or <15 mEq/L or TTKG <3)

- GI losses *plus* metabolic acidosis: diarrhea, laxative abuse, villous adenoma
- Vomiting & NGT drainage usually manifest as *renal losses* due to 2° hyperaldo & met. alk.

Renal potassium losses (U_K >30 mEq/d or >15 mEq/L or TTKG >7)

- Hypo- or normotensive
  acidosis: DKA, RTA (type IV RTA and some type I RTA cause hyperkalemia)
  alkalosis
    diuretics, vomiting/NGT drainage (via 2° hyperaldosteronism)
    Bartter's syndrome (loop of Henle dysfxn → furosemide-like effect; *NEJM* 1999;340:1177)
    Gitelman's syndrome (distal convoluted tubule dysfxn → thiazide-like effect)
  Mg depletion: mechanism unclear, variable acid-base
- Hypertensive: mineralocorticoid excess
  1° hyperaldosteronism (eg, Conn's syndrome)
  2° hyperaldosteronism (eg, renovascular disease, renin-secreting tumor)
  nonaldosterone mineralocorticoid (eg, Cushing's, Liddle's, exogenous mineralocort.)

Clinical manifestations

- Nausea, vomiting, weakness, muscle cramps
- ECG: U waves, ± ↑ QT interval, ventricular ectopy (PVCs, VT, VF)

Workup (*NEJM* 1998;339:451)

- Rule-out transcellular shifts
- ✓ 24-hr U_K and **transtubular potassium gradient** (TTKG) = $(U_K/P_K) / (U_{osm}/P_{osm})$
  U_K >30 mEq/d or >15 mEq/L or TTKG >7 → renal loss
  U_K <25 mEq/d or <15 mEq/L or TTKG <3 → extrarenal loss
- If renal losses, ✓ **BP** and **acid-base status**

Figure 4-6 Approach to hypokalemia

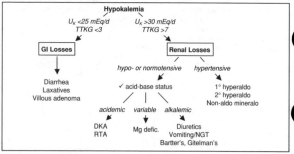

Treatment

- *If true potassium deficit:* potassium repletion ($\downarrow$ 1 mEq/L $\approx$ 200 mEq total body loss)
  KCl 40 mEq PO q4-6h if nonurgent, KCl 10 mEq/h IV if urgent, recheck K freq
- Beware of excessive potassium repletion if transcellular shift cause of hypokalemia
- Treat underlying cause (if hydration needed, avoid dextrose-containing solutions as
  dextrose $\rightarrow \uparrow$ insulin $\rightarrow$ intracellular potassium shifts)
- Replete Mg as necessary

HYPERKALEMIA

Transcellular shifts
- Acidosis, insulin defic. (DM), β-blockers, dig intox., massive cellular necrosis (tumor lysis, rhabdo, ischemic bowel), hyperkalemic periodic paralysis (Na channelopathy)

Decreased GFR
- Any cause of oligo- or anuric acute renal failure or any cause of end-stage renal disease

Normal GFR but with $\downarrow$ renal K excretion
- Normal aldosterone function (TTKG >7)
  $\downarrow$ EAV (K excretion limited by $\downarrow$ distal Na delivery & urine flow): CHF, cirrhosis
  excessive K intake: in conjunction with impairment in K excretion or transcellular shift
- **Hypoaldosteronism** (TTKG <7): same as etiologies of Type IV RTA
  $\downarrow$ renin: diabetic nephropathy, NSAIDs, chronic interstitial nephritis, HIV
  normal renin, $\downarrow$ aldo synthesis: 1° adrenal disorders, ACEI, ARBs, heparin
  $\downarrow$ response to aldosterone
    meds: K-sparing diuretics, TMP-SMX, pentamidine, calcineurin inhibitors
    tubulointerstitial disease: sickle cell, SLE, amyloid, diabetes

Clinical manifestations
- Weakness, nausea, paresthesias, palpitations
- ECG: peaked T waves, $\uparrow$ PR interval, $\uparrow$ QRS width, sine wave pattern, PEA

Workup
- Rule out pseudohyperkalemia (IVF with K, hemolysis during venipuncture, $\uparrow$ plt or WBC)
- Rule out transcellular shift
- **Assess GFR**
- If normal GFR, calculate **transtubular potassium gradient** (TTKG) = $(U_K/P_K)/(U_{osm}/P_{osm})$
    TTKG >7 $\rightarrow$ normal aldosterone function
    TTKG <7 $\rightarrow$ hypoaldosteronism

Treatment of Hyperkalemia			
Intervention	Dose	Onset	Comment
Calcium gluconate **Calcium chloride***	1-2 amps IV	few min	transient effect stabilizes cell membrane
Insulin	reg. insulin 10 U IV + 1-2 amps $D_{50}W$	15-30 min	transient effect drives K into cells
Bicarbonate	1-3 amps IV	15-30 min	transient effect drives K into cells in exchange for H
β2 agonists	albuterol 10-20 mg inh. or 0.5 mg IV	30-90 min	transient effect drives K into cells
Kayexalate†	30-90 g PO/PR	1-2 h	$\downarrow$ total body K exchanges Na for K in gut
Diuretics	furosemide $\geq$40 mg IV	30 min	$\downarrow$ total body K
Hemodialysis			$\downarrow$ total body K

*calcium chloride contains more calcium and is typically reserved for use in codes
†increased risk of intestinal necrosis with postoperative ileus

- *Rate of onset* important to note when establishing a treatment plan
- Calcium helps prevent cardiac complications; $\therefore$ should be initial Rx, esp. if ECG Δs
- Insulin, bicarbonate, and β2 agonists should follow to $\downarrow$ plasma K
- Treatments that eliminate total body K essential as other Rxs will wear off with time; kayexalate ± diuretics may be effective in many cases, but emergent hemodialysis should be considered in life-threatening situations

ACUTE RENAL FAILURE (ARF)

Definition (JAMA 2003;289:747; Lancet 2005;365:417)
- ARF: ↑ Cr ≥0.5 mg/dl or ↑ Cr ≥20% if baseline Cr >2.5 mg/dl in ≤2 wks
- Oliguria: UOP 100–400 ml/24 h; anuria: UOP <100 ml/24 h

Workup
- **History and physical:** recent procedures and medications, vital signs, volume status, signs and symptoms of obstruction, vascular disease or systemic disease
- **Urine evaluation:** output, urinalysis, sediment, electrolytes and osmolality
- **Fractional excretion of sodium (FE$_{Na}$)** = $(U_{Na}/P_{Na})/(U_{Cr}/P_{Cr})$
  <1% → prerenal, contrast, or glomerulonephritis; >2% → ATN
  In setting of diuretics, ✓ FE$_{UN}$ = $(U_{UN}/P_{UN})/(U_{Cr}/P_{Cr})$; <35% → prerenal
- Renal U/S: r/o obstruction & eval kidney size to estimate chronicity of renal failure
- Serologies (if indicated): see "Glomerular Disease"
- Renal biopsy: may be necessary if cause remains unclear

Etiologies and Diagnosis of Acute Renal Failure	
Etiologies	**U/A, Sediment, Indices**
Prerenal ↓ **Effective arterial volume** Hypovolemia Decreased cardiac contractility (eg, CHF) Systemic vasodilatation (eg, sepsis) **Renal vasoconstriction** NSAIDs, ACEI/ARB (↓ intraglomerular pressure), calcineurin inhibitors, hepatorenal, hypercalcemia **Large vessel:** RAS (bilateral + ACEI), thrombosis, embolism, dissection, vasculitis	Bland Transparent hyaline casts FE$_{Na}$ <1% BUN/Cr >20
Intrinsic **Acute tubular necrosis (ATN)** *Ischemia:* progression of prerenal disease *Toxins* Drugs: AG, amphotericin, cisplatin Pigments: myoglobin, hemoglobin Proteins: Ig light chains *Contrast-induced ARF (CIARF):* ↓ RBF + toxin	Pigmented granular "muddy brown" casts in ~75% (± in CIARF) ± RBCs & protein from tubular damage FE$_{Na}$ >2% (except pigment & CIARF)
Acute interstitial nephritis (AIN) *Allergic:* β-lactams, sulfa drugs, NSAIDs *Infection:* pyelonephritis *Infiltrative:* sarcoid, lymphoma, leukemia	WBCs, WBC casts, ± RBCs ⊕ eos in abx ⊕ lymphs in NSAIDs
Small vessel: cholesterol emboli, thrombotic microangiopathy (HUS/TTP, DIC, preeclampsia, malignant HTN, scleroderma renal crisis)	± RBCs ⊕ eos in cholesterol emboli
Glomerulonephritis (see "Glomerular Disease")	Dysmorphic RBCs & RBC casts
Postrenal **Bladder neck:** BPH, prostate cancer, neurogenic bladder, anticholinergic meds	Bland ± RBCs if nephrolithiasis
Ureteral: malig., LAN, retroperitoneal fibrosis, bilateral nephrolithiasis	
Tubular: precipitation of crystals	

Contrast-induced acute renal failure (CIARF)
- Risk factors: CKD, DM, CHF, age, hypotension, ↑ contrast volume (JACC 2004;44:1393)
- Clinical: Cr ↑ w/in 24 h, peaks in 3–5 d, resolves in 7–10 d
- Prevention (NEJM 2006;354:379; JAMA 2006;295:2765; Circ 2006;113:1799)
  N-acetylcysteine 600 mg PO bid on day prior to and day of contrast (Lancet 2003;362:598)
  Pre/post-hydration (NEJM 1994;331:1416) unless contraindication to IVF (eg, CHF)
  isotonic NaHCO$_3$: 3mL/kg/h × 1 h before, 1 mL/kg/h × 6 h after (JAMA 2004;291:2328)
  benefit additive to N-acetylcysteine (Circ 2007;115:1211)
  Hold ACEI/ARB, NSAIDs, diuretics
  Minimize contrast volume and consider isosmolar contrast (JACC 2006;48:692)
  ? Higher NAC dose (1200 mg IV) in acute MI undergoing PCI (NEJM 2006;354:2773)
  ? Hemofiltration (before & after if Cr >2.0 (NEJM 2003;349:1333)
- Gadolinium: can be cause of ARF in CKD (Neph Dial Trans 2006;21:697)
  prevention measures listed above for iodinated contrast are of no proven benefit

Treatment

- Treat underlying disorder (see relevant sections); consider steroids if AIN
- Avoid nephrotoxic insults; review dosing of renally cleared drugs
- Optimize hemodynamics (both MAP & CO)
- Watch for and correct volume overload, electrolyte ($\uparrow$ K, $\uparrow$ PO$_4$), & acid/base status
- If obstruction is diagnosed and relieved, watch for:
  Hypotonic diuresis (2° buildup of BUN, tubular damage); Rx with IVF (eg, $1/2$ NS)
  Hemorrhagic cystitis (rapid Δ in size of bladder vessels); avoid by decompressing slowly
- Indications for urgent dialysis (when condition refractory to conventional therapy)
  Acid-base disturbance: acidemia
  Electrolyte disorder: generally hyperkalemia; occasionally hypercalcemia; tumor lysis
  Intoxication: methanol, ethylene glycol, lithium, salicylates
  Overload of volume (CHF)
  Uremia: pericarditis, encephalopathy, bleeding
- No benefit to dopamine (Annals 2005;142:510), diuretics (JAMA 2002;288:2547), or mannitol

---

CHRONIC KIDNEY DISEASE (CKD)

Definition and Etiologies (Annals 2003;139:137)

- ≥ 3 months of **reduced GFR** (<60 ml/min/1.73 m^2) and/or **kidney damage** (abnormal pathology, blood/urine markers, or imaging)
- Prevalence 11% in U.S.; Cr poor estimate of GFR; $\therefore$ use prediction equation, eg, MDRD equation: www.kidney.org/professionals/KDOQI/gfr_calculator.cfm
  nb, equation may underestimate GFR in Pts w/ normal renal function
- Etiologies include diabetes HTN, PKD (Lancet 2007;369:1287), glomerulonephritis, congenital disease, drug-induced, myeloma, progression of ARF
- Rates of all-cause mortality and CV events increase with each stage of CKD, and are significantly higher than the rate of progression to kidney failure (NEJM 2004;351:1296)

Stages of CKD		
Stage	GFR	Goals
1 (nl or $\uparrow$ GFR)	>90	Dx/Rx of underlying condition & comorbidities, slow progression; cardiovascular risk reduction.
2 (mild)	60-89	Estimate progression
3 (moderate)	30-59	Evaluate and treat complications
4 (severe)	15-29	Prepare for renal replacement therapy (RRT)
5 (kidney failure)	<15 or dialysis	Dialysis if uremic

Signs and Symptoms of Uremia	
General	Nausea, anorexia, malaise, fetor uremicus, metallic taste, pruritis, uremic frost (white crystals in & on skin), susceptibility to drug O/D
Neurologic	Encephalopathy (Δ MS, $\downarrow$ memory & attention), seizures, neuropathy
Cardiovascular	Pericarditis, accelerated atherosclerosis, hypertension, hyperlipidemia, volume overload, CHF, cardiomyopathy
Hematologic	Anemia, bleeding (due to platelet dysfunction)
Metabolic	$\uparrow$ K, $\uparrow$ PO$_4$, acidosis, $\downarrow$ Ca, 2° hyperparathyroidism, osteodystrophy

Treatment (Lancet 2005;365:331)

- **General:** early nephrology referral and access planning (avoid subclavian lines; preserve an arm for access by avoiding blood draws, BP measurements, IVs)
- **Dietary restrictions:** Na (if hypertensive), K (if oliguric or hyperkalemic), ? moderate protein restriction, strict glucose control in diabetics
- **BP Control:** goal <130/80
  start with ACEI, effective in diabetic & non-diabetic CKD (NEJM 1993;329:1456 & 1996;334:939)
  ACEI + ARB may be superior to either alone (COOPERATE, Lancet 2003;361:117)
  ACEI may be effective and safe in nondiabetic CKD (Cr 3–5, NEJM 2006;354:131)
- **Metabolic acidosis:** sodium bicarbonate or sodium citrate if HCO$_3$ <22
- **Anemia:** goal Hgb 11–12 mg/dl ($\uparrow$ death, HTN, and thrombosis w/ higher levels; NEJM 2006;355:2071 & 2085; Lancet 2007;369:381)
  epoetin (start 80–120 U/kg SC, divided 3x/wk) or darbepoetin (0.45 mcg/kg q wk)
  iron supplementation when indicated (often given IV in HD Pts)
  uremic bleeding: desmopressin (dDAVP) 0.3 μg/kg IV or 3 μg/kg intranasally

- **2° Hyperparathyroidism:** ↑ PO_4, ↓ Ca, ↓ calcitriol all stimulate PTH release

CKD Stage	3	4	5
Target PTH (pg/ml)	35–70	70–110	150–300

phosphorus binders
  if ↑ PO_4 and ↓ Ca → calcium acetate (PhosLo) or calcium carbonate
  if refractory ↑ PO_4 or in setting of ↑ Ca → sevelamer (Renagel), lanthanum (Fosrenol)
  if severe ↑ PO_4 → aluminum hydroxide (Amphojel), *short-term use only*
calcitriol or paricalcitol if Ca-PO_4 product <55 (? ↑ survival in HD Pts, *NEJM* 2003;349:446)
cinacalcet (parathyroid calcium sensing receptor agonist) if PTH remains elevated despite
  phosphorus binders ± vit D analogue (*NEJM* 2004;350:1516)
parathyroidectomy
- **Consider transplant evaluation**

DIALYSIS

Hemodialysis (HD) (*NEJM* 1998;338:1428 & 339:1054)
- Physiology: blood flows along one side of *semipermeable* membrane, dialysate along other.
  Fluid removal (ie, Na + H_2O) via transmembrane pressure (TMP) gradient.
  Solute removal via transmembrane concentration gradient and inversely proportional
  to size (∴ effective removal of K, urea, and Cr, but not PO_4).
- Typical orders: duration, volume removal goals, K and Ca in dialysate bath, anticoagulation
- Complications: hypotension, arrhythmia, access complications, disequilibrium syndrome

	Vascular Access	
	Advantages	**Disadvantages**
AV Fistula	Highest patency Lowest risk of bacteremia	Long maturation time (2-6 mo) Primary nonfunction (20%)
AV Graft	Easier to create than AVF Maturation time (2-3 wks)	Poor 1° patency, often requiring thrombectomy or angioplasty
Catheter	Immediate use Use as bridge to AVF/AVG	Highest risk of bacteremia ↓ blood flow → ↓ HD efficiency

Continuous Veno-Venous Hemofiltration (CVVH) (*NEJM* 1997;336:1303)
- Physiology: based on *ultrafiltration* rather than dialysis. Blood under pressure passes down
  one side of a *highly permeable* membrane allowing water and solutes to pass across the
  membrane via TMP gradient. Filtrate is discarded. Replacement fluid is infused (solute
  concentrations similar to plasma, except no K, urea, Cr, PO_4). Fluid balance precisely
  controlled by adjusting amounts of filtrate and replacement fluid.
- Access: double-lumen central venous catheter
- Typical orders: volume removal goals, replacement fluid buffer: **HCO_3** (requires heparin to
  prevent machine from clotting) **vs.** citrate (hepatically metabolized to HCO_3; provides
  anticoagulation w/ in machine via Ca chelation; ∴ need Ca infusion to maintain serum Ca)
- Complications: hypotension, ↓ PO_4, access complications; ↓ ICa (citrate toxicity in Pts with
  hepatic dysfunction → look for ↓ ICa but normal/↑ serum Ca and AG metabolic acidosis)
- Potential advantages over HD: less hypotension, better volume control, removal of
  inflammatory mediators; however, no survival advantage (*Lancet* 2006;368:379)

Peritoneal Dialysis (PD) (*Perit Dial Int* 2001;21:25)
- Physiology: peritoneum acts as membrane. Fluid balance controlled by choosing dialysate
  glucose concentration (higher concentrations pull more fluid into peritoneum); longer
  dwell times pull less fluid as glucose equilibrates across peritoneum
- Access: temporary catheter inserted midline, permanent catheter inserted in OR
- Typical orders for CAPD (continuous ambulatory peritoneal dialysis):
  PD fluid = 1.5%, 2.5%, or 4.25% dextrose
  buffer (lactate), Na^+, K^+, Ca^{2+}, Mg^{2+}
  infuse 10 min, dwell 30 min-5.5 h, drain 20 min
- Can use overnight cycler device that infuses & drains more rapidly, with shorter dwells,
  while Pt sleeps. Called automated or continuous cycling peritoneal dialysis (APD, CCPD).
- Complications
  Peritonitis (abdominal pain, tenderness, cloudy drainage)
    diagnosis: WBC >100 and >50% PMNs
    spectrum: 60-70% GPC, 15-20% GNR, remainder no bacteria or fungal
    Rx: abx IV or in PD, catheter removal for certain pathogens (eg, yeast, pseudomonas)
  Hyperglycemia: exacerbated by inflammation, long dwell times, and higher [glc]

GLOMERULAR DISEASE

OVERVIEW

Definitions
- **Glomerulonephritis** (GN) (NEJM 1998;339:888; Lancet 2005;365:1797)
  pathologically: intraglomerular inflammation (ranging from focal proliferative to diffuse proliferative to crescentic)
  clinically: hematuria w/ dysmorphic RBCs or RBC casts, ± subnephrotic proteinuria often w/ renal failure, HTN, edema; spectrum of progression tempo:
    acute GN = over days; rapidly progressive GN (RPGN) = wks; chronic GN = mos but can have asymptomatic glomerular hematuria
- **Nephrotic syndrome:** noninflammatory injury to glomerular filtration barrier proteinuria >3.5 g/d, alb <3.5 mg/dl, edema, ↑ cholesterol, lipiduria, hypercoag.

GLOMERULONEPHRITIS

ANCA ⊕ Vasculitis (pauci-immune or minimal staining)						
Disease	Gran	Renal	Pulm	Asthma	ANCA Type*	ANCA ⊕
Wegener's granulomatosis	⊕	80%	90%	–	c-ANCA (anti-PR3)	90%
Microscopic polyangiitis	–	90%	50%	–	p-ANCA (anti-MPO)	70%
Churg-Strauss syndrome	⊕	45%	70%	⊕	p-ANCA (anti-MPO)	50%

*Predominant ANCA type; either p- or c-ANCA can be seen in all three diseases. (NEJM 1997;337:1512)

Anti-GBM Disease (linear staining)			
Disease	Glomerulonephritis	Pulm hemorrhage	Anti-GBM
Goodpasture's	⊕	⊕	⊕
Anti-GBM disease	⊕	–	⊕

Immune Complex (IC) Disease (granular staining)	
Renal-limited diseases	**Systemic diseases**
Poststreptococcal GN (PSGN, ⊕ ASLO, ↓ C3)	SLE (⊕ ANA, anti-dsDNA, ↓ C3)
Membranoproliferative GN (MPGN, ↓ C3)	Endocarditis (fever, ⊕ BCx, valvular disease, ↓ C3)
Fibrillary glomerulonephritis (normal C3)	Cryoglobulinemia (⊕ cryocrit, ↓ C3, ↓ C4, HCV Ab)
IgA nephropathy (normal C3)	Henoch-Schönlein purpura (IgA nephropathy + systemic vasculitis, normal C3)

Workup (Archives 2001;161:25)
- AGN/RPGN ± lung hemorrhage is an emergency → requires early Dx and Rx
- ANCA (Lancet 2006;368:404), anti-GBM, complement levels (C3, C4)
- Depending on clinical hx: ANA, ASLO, blood cultures, cryocrit, hepatitis serologies
- Renal biopsy with immunofluorescence (IF) ± electron microscopy (EM)
- Consider GN mimics: thrombotic microangiopathy, cholesterol emboli, AIN, myeloma

Figure 4-7 Approach to glomerulonephritis

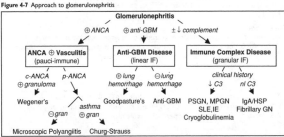

NEPHRITIC 4-15

Treatment

- ANCA ⊕, anti-GBM: immediate steroids + cyclophosphamide; ± plasmapheresis
- SLE nephritis: IV cyclophosphamide + steroids → azathioprine or MMF (JAMA 2005;293:3053); induction with MMF (no cyclophosphamide) may be as effective (NEJM 2005;353:2219)
- Other IC disease: ? steroids ± alkylating agents; treat underlying systemic disease

---

ASYMPTOMATIC GLOMERULAR HEMATURIA

Definition and Etiologies

- Hematuria ± proteinuria of glomerular origin w/o renal insufficiency or systemic disease (nonglomerular hematuria more common; see "Hematuria")
- Ddx: any cause of GN, especially IgA; also consider Alport's (X-linked, deafness, renal failure) and thin basement membrane nephropathy (autosomal dominant, benign course)

IgA Nephropathy (NEJM 2000;347:738; JASN 2005;16:2088)

- Most common cause of GN; male predominance w/ peak incidence 20-30s
- Wide range of clinical presentations: asx hematuria (30-40%), gross hematuria after URI (30-40%), chronic GN (10%), nephrotic syndrome (5%), RPGN (<5%)
- Though clinical presentation can be highly suggestive, definitive dx only with biopsy
- Prognosis: 25-30% will reach ESRD within 20-25 y of presentation
- Treatment: ACEI/ARB, ± fish oils (NEJM 1994;331:1194); steroids ± cytotoxic therapy for crescentic GN and nephrotic syndrome, consider for progressive chronic GN

NEPHROTIC SYNDROME

Primary glomerular diseases (grouped by pathology)

- **Focal segmental glomerulosclerosis (40%)**
  idiopathic, HIV (collapsing variant), pamidronate, heroin (acute nephrotic syndrome) sustained hyperfiltration due to prior nephron loss, obesity, vesiculoureteral reflux
- **Membranous nephropathy (30%)**
  idiopathic, infection (especially HBV, also HCV, syphilis), autoimmune (especially SLE) carcinomas, drugs (gold, penicillamine, NSAIDs)
- **Minimal change disease (20%, more common in children)**
  idiopathic, NSAIDs, Hodgkin's disease & other lymphoproliferative disorders
- **Membranoproliferative GN (5%, mixed nephrotic/nephritic features)**
  Type I: infection (especially HCV ± cryos; IE, HBV, other chronic infxns), immune complex disease (SLE, cryos, Sjögren's), lymphoproliferative disorders, idiopathic
  Type II: very rare; autoAb blocks inactivation of C3 convertase = C3 nephritic factor
- **Fibrillary-immunotactoid glomerulopathy (1%)**
- **Mesangial proliferative GN (likely atypical forms of MCD or FSGS, 5%)**

Systemic diseases

- **Diabetes mellitus:** nodular glomerulosclerosis (Kimmelstiel-Wilson lesion); large kidneys hyperfiltration → microalbuminuria → dipstick ⊕ → nephrotic range (10-15 y) concomitant proliferative retinopathy seen in 90% of type 1 and 60% of type 2
- **Amyloidosis:** primary (Ig light chain) or secondary (serum amyloid)
- **SLE:** typically with membranous nephropathy (WHO class V)
- **Cryoglobulinemia:** typically with membranoproliferative GN

Workup (Archives 2001;161:25)

- Urine sediment: usually benign w/o concurrent nephritis; ± oval fat bodies
- r/o secondary causes
  ↑ Hb$_{A1C}$ + retinopathy → presumpt. dx of diabetic nephropathy unless another suggested
  ANA, anti-dsDNA, C3, C4, SPEP/UPEP, fat pad bx, cryocrit, HBV, HCV, HIV, RPR
- Renal biopsy

Treatment

- General: protein supplementation; diuretics for edema; treat hyperlipidemia
- **ACEI/ARB:** decrease proteinuria → slow nonimmunologic progression of renal disease
- Primary glomerular disease: steroids ± cytotoxic therapy
- Secondary causes: treat underlying disease

Complications

- Malnutrition (protein loss)
- Thrombosis (especially renal vein, because loss of ATIII & other endogenous anticoags)
- Infection (especially encapsulated organisms, because loss of immunoglobulin)
- Accelerated atherosclerosis (hypercholesterolemia)

Urine Dipstick

Measurement	Significance and uses
Specific gravity	estimate U_{osm}; each 0.001 above 1 ≈30 osm (SG 1.010 → U_{osm} ≈300) S.G. and U_{osm} useful in evaluating ARF, dysnatremias, polyuria heavy substances (glucose, contrast) increase SG more than U_{osm}
pH	range: 4.5-8.5; useful in evaluation of stones and RTAs
Protein	detects albumin (marker for glomerular dysfxn); see "Proteinuria"
RBC	see "Hematuria"; also ⊕ with myoglobinuria (rhabdomyolysis)
WBC	suggests inflammation (UTI, interstitial nephritis, GN)
Ketones	detects acetoacetate (ie, ketoacidosis), but not β-hydroxybutyrate
Nitrite	suggests presence of Enterobacteriaceae
Bilirubin	↑ in biliary or hepatic disease
Glucose	⊕ in hyperglycemia, pregnancy, Fanconi's syndrome

Urine Sediment (microscopic examination)

Method: centrifuge test tube × 3-5 min at 1500-3000 RPM; pour off supernatant in one motion; resuspend pellet by agitating base of tube; pour suspension onto slide, place coverslip; view under "high - dry" power; phase contrast for RBC morphology.

Cells	RBCs: assess amount & morphology (many dysmorphic → glomerular) WBCs: PMNs (UTI) vs. eosinophils (AIN; may require special stain) Epithelial cells: tubular (ATN), transitional (bladder or ureters), squamous
Casts	Proteins molded in lumen of renal tubule ± entrapped cellular elements RBC → GN WBC → AIN, pyelonephritis, GN Granular ("muddy brown"): degenerating cellular casts → ATN Tubular cell → ATN Hyaline: Tamm-Horsfall protein (nonspecific) Waxy and broad → advanced renal failure
Crystals	Calcium oxalate monohydrate: spindle, oval, or dumbbell shaped Calcium oxalate dihydrate: envelope shaped or octahedral Uric acid: variable shape; polychromatic under polarized light Cystine: hexagon shaped Struvite: coffin-lid shaped; seen in chronic UTI with urea-splitting organisms

PROTEINURIA

Etiologies of Proteinuria

Category	Description	Etiologies
Glomerular (can be >3 g/d)	Disruption of filtration barrier → lose albumin	Glomerulonephritis Nephrotic syndrome
Tubulointerstitial (usually <1–2 g/d)	↓ reabsorption of freely filtered proteins → lose globulins	ATN AIN Fanconi's syndrome
Overflow	↑ production of freely filtered proteins	Multiple myeloma Myoglobinuria
Isolated	By def'n: asx, normal renal fxn, sed, & imaging, no h/o renal disease	Functional (fever, exercise, CHF) Orthostatic (only when upright) Idiopathic (transient or persistent)

- **Urine dipstick**
  1+ ≈30 mg/dl, 2+ ≈100 mg/dl, 3+ ≈300 mg/dl, 4+ >2 g/dl → interpretation depends on SG; eg, 3+ in very concentrated urine might not indicate heavy proteinuria
  Insensitive for microalbuminuria and myeloma light chains; false ⊕ with contrast
- **Spot urine:** protein (mg/dl)/creatinine (mg/dl) ≈ g/d of proteinuria (NEJM 1983;309:1543). Unlike urine dipstick, will detect myeloma light chains.

Etiologies of Hematuria	
Extrarenal (far more common)	**Intrarenal**
Nephrolithiasis	Nephrolithiasis or crystalluria
Neoplasm: transitional cell, prostate	Neoplasm
Infection: cystitis, urethritis, prostatitis	Trauma
Foley trauma	Vascular: renal infarcts, renal vein thrombosis
	Glomerulonephritis

Workup (NEJM 2003;348:2330)
- **Urine dipstick:** ⊕ if >3 RBCs; ⊕ dipstick and ⊖ sediment → myo- or hemoglobinuria
- **Urine sediment:** dysmorphic RBCs or RBC casts → GN → consider renal bx
- If no evidence of glomerulonephritis:
  r/o UTI
  Urine cytology
  Renal imaging: helical CT (r/o nephrolithiasis and neoplasia of upper tract), cystoscopy
  (r/o bladder neoplasia), ? U/S (r/o obstruction or parenchymal disease)

NEPHROLITHIASIS

Types of stones and risk factors (JAMA 2005;293:1107; Lancet 2006;367:333)
- **Calcium** (Ca oxalate > Ca phosphate): **70–90% of kidney stones**
  Urine characteristics: ↑ Ca, ↑ oxalate, ↑ urate, ↑ pH, ↓ citrate, ↓ volume
  2° hypercalciuria: 1° hyperparathyroidism, type 1 RTA, sarcoid
  2° hyperoxaluria: Crohn's or other ileal disease with intact colon
  Diet: ↑ animal protein, ↑ sucrose, ↓ K, ↓ fluid, ↓ fruits/vegetables
- **Uric acid:** 5–10% of kidney stones, radiolucent on plain film
  Urine characteristics: ↑ uric acid (eg, gout), ↓ pH (eg, from chronic diarrhea)
- **Magnesium ammonium phosphate** ("struvite" or "triple phosphate")
  Chronic UTI with urea-splitting organisms (eg, Proteus) → ↑ urine NH_3 and pH
- **Cystine:** inherited defects of tubular amino acid reabsorption

Clinical manifestations
- Hematuria (absence does not exclude diagnosis), flank pain, N/V, dysuria, frequency
- Ureteral obstruction (stones >5mm unlikely to pass spont.) → ARF if solitary kidney
- UTI: ↑ risk of infection proximal to stone; urinalysis of distal urine may be normal

Workup
- **Noncontrast helical CT scan**
- Strain urine for stone to analyze; U/A & UCx, electrolytes, BUN/Cr, Ca, PO_4, PTH, uric acid
- 24-h urine (>6 wks after acute setting) for Ca, PO_4, uric acid, oxalate, citrate, Na, Cr

Acute treatment (NEJM 2004;350:684)
- Analgesia (narcotics or NSAIDs), aggressive PO/IV hydration, antibiotics if UTI
- Consider CCB or alpha blocker to promote ureteral relaxation (Lancet 2006;368:1171)
- Indications for **immediate urologic evaluation and/or hospitalization:** obstruction
  (especially solitary or transplant kidney), urosepsis, intractable pain or vomiting, ARF
- Urologic Rx: lithotripsy, cystoscopic stent, percutaneous nephrostomy, stone removal

Chronic treatment
- Increase fluid intake (>2 L/d)
- Calcium stones: 24-h urine identifies **specific urinary risk factors to treat**
  ↓ Na and meat intake (NEJM 2002;346:77), thiazides: decrease urine Ca
  Depending on 24-h urine: K-citrate, dietary oxalate restriction, allopurinol
  High dietary Ca is likely beneficial, unclear role of Ca supplements
- Uric acid: urine alkalinization (K-citrate), allopurinol
- Magnesium ammonium phosphate: antibiotics to treat UTI, urologic intervention
- Cystine: urine alkalinization (K-citrate), D-penicillamine, tiopronin

↓ in RBC mass: Hct <41% or Hb < 13.5 g/dl (men); Hct <36% or Hb < 12 g/dl (women)

Clinical manifestations
- Symptoms: ↓ O_2 delivery → fatigue, exertional dyspnea, angina (if CAD)
- Signs: pallor (mucous membranes, palmar creases), tachycardia, orthostatic hypotension
- Other findings: **jaundice** (hemolysis), **splenomegaly** (thalassemia, neoplasm, chronic hemolysis), **petechiae/purpura** (bleeding disorder), **glossitis** (iron, folate, vitamin B_{12} defic.), **koilonychia** (iron defic.), **neurologic abnormalities** (B_{12} defic.)

Diagnostic evaluation
- History: bleeding, systemic illness, drugs, exposures, alcohol, diet (including **pica**), FHx
- CBC w/ differential; RBC parameters incl. reticulocyte count, MCV, RDW
- **Reticulocyte index** (RI) = [reticulocyte count × (Pt's Hct/nl Hct)]/maturation factor
  maturation factors for a given Hct: 45% = 1, 35% = 1.5, 25% = 2, 20% = 2.5
  RI >2% → adequate marrow response; RI <2% → hypoproliferation
- **Peripheral smear**: select area where RBCs evenly spaced and very few touch each other

	Peripheral Smear Findings
Feature	**Abnormalities and diagnoses**
Size	normocytic vs. microcytic vs. macrocytic → see below
Shape	**anisocytosis** → unequal RBC size; **poikilocytosis** → irregular RBC shape **spherocytes** → HS, AIHA; **sickle** cells → sickle cell anemia **stomatocyte** → central pallor appears as curved slit → liver disease, EtOH **tear drop** cells = dacryocytes → myelofibrosis, myelophthisic anemia, megaloblastic anemia, thalassemia **schistocytes**, helmet cells → MAHA (eg, DIC, TTP/HUS), mechanical valve echinocytes = **burr** cells (even, regular projections) → uremia, artifact acanthocytes = **spur** cells (irregular projections) → liver disease **target** cells → liver disease, hemoglobinopathies, splenectomy **bite** cells (removal of Heinz bodies by phagocytes) → G6PD deficiency **rouleaux** → hyperglobulinemia (eg, multiple myeloma)
Intra-RBC findings	**basophilic stippling** (ribosomes) → abnl Hb, sideroblastic, megaloblastic **Heinz bodies** (denatured Hb) → G6PD deficiency, thalassemia **Howell-Jolly bodies** (nuclear fragments) → splenectomy, sickle cell **nucleated** RBCs → hemolysis, extramedullary hematopoiesis
WBC findings	**hypersegmented** (>5 lobes) PMNs: megaloblastic anemia (B_{12}/folate def.) **toxic granules** (coarse, dark blue) and **Döhle bodies** (blue patches of dilated endoplasmic reticulum) → sepsis, severe inflammation **pseudo-Pelger-Huët anomaly** (bilobed nucleus, "pince-nez") → MDS **blasts** → leukemia, lymphoma; **Auer rods** → acute myelogenous leukemia

(NEJM 2005;353:498)

- Additional laboratory evaluations as indicated: hemolysis labs (if RI >2%), iron, folate, B_{12}, LFTs, BUN and Cr, TFTs, Hb electrophoresis, enzyme analyses, gene mutation screens
- **Bone marrow (BM) aspirate and biopsy (bx)** with cytogenetics as indicated

Figure 5-1 Approach to anemia

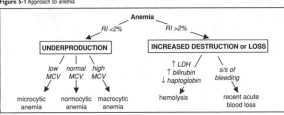

Iron deficiency *(NEJM 1999;341:1986)*
- ↓ marrow iron → ↓ heme synthesis → microcytosis → anemia
- Special clinical manifestations: angular cheilosis, atrophic glossitis, pica (consumption of nonnutritive substances such as ice, clay), koilonychia (nail spooning) Plummer-Vinson syndrome (iron deficiency anemia, esophageal web & atrophic glossitis)
- Etiologies: **chronic bleeding** (GI, menstrual, etc.), ↓ **supply** (malnutrition; ↓ absorp. due to celiac sprue, Crohn's, ↑ gastric pH, subtotal gastrectomy), ↑ **demand** (preg., epo)
- Diagnosis: ↓ Fe, ↑ TIBC, ↓ ferritin (espec. <15), ↓ Fe/TIBC (espec. <15%), ↑ soluble transferrin receptor; ↑ plt; unless history c/w a different source, *initiate workup for GIB*
- Treatment: Fe supplementation (~6 wks to correct anemia; ~6 mos to replete Fe stores)

Thalassemias *(NEJM 2005;353:1135)*
- ↓ synthesis of α- or β-globin chains of Hb → ≠ subunits → destruction of RBCs and erythroid precursors; ∴ anemia from hemolysis *and* ineffective erythropoiesis
- **α-thalassemia**: deletions in α-globin gene complex on chr. 16 (nl 4 α genes)
  - 3 α → α-thal-2 trait = silent carrier; 2 α → α-thal-1 trait or α-thal minor = mild anemia
  - 1 α → HbH (β_4) disease = severe anemia, hemolysis and splenomegaly
  - 0 α genes → Hb Barts (γ_4) = intrauterine hypoxia and hydrops fetalis
- **β-thalassemia**: mutations in β-globin gene on chr. 11 → absent or ↓ gene product
  - 1 mutated β gene → thal minor = mild anemia (no transfusions)
  - 2 mutated β genes → thal intermedia (occasional transfusions) or thal major (= Cooley's anemia; transfusion-dependent) depending on severity of mutations
- Special clinical manifestations (in severe cases): chipmunk facies, pathologic fractures, hepatosplenomegaly, high-output CHF, bilirubin gallstones, iron overload syndromes (from chronic transfusions)
- Diagnosis: MCV <70, **normal Fe, MCV/RBC count <13**, ± ↑ retics, basophilic stippling; **Hb electrophoresis**: ↑ HbA₂ ($\alpha_2\delta_2$) in β-thal; *normal pattern in α-thal trait*
- Treatment: folate; transfusions + deferoxamine, deferasirox (oral iron chelator); splenectomy if ≥50% ↑ in transfusions; consider allogeneic HSCT in children w/ severe β-thal major

Anemia of chronic inflammation (ACI; *NEJM 2005;352:1011*)
- Impaired iron utilization & ↓ epo-responsiveness due to ↑ hepcidin & cytokines in setting of autoimmune disorders, chronic infection, inflammation, HIV, malignancy
- Dx: ↓ Fe, ↓ TIBC, ± ↑ ferritin; usually normocytic but can be microcytic if prolonged
- ACI w/Fe-deficiency anemia: soluble transferrin receptor (sTFR) ↑ in Fe deficiency sTFR/log Ferritin: >2 → ACI w/ Fe deficiency; <1 → ACI alone (*Blood 1997;89:1052*)
- Treatment: treat underlying disease ± erythropoietin; for cancer- or chemo-related use epo for goal Hb 10-12 (11-12 if sx) g/dl. Iron if ferritin <100 or Fe/TIBC <20%.

Sideroblastic anemia
- Defective heme biosynthesis within RBC precursors
- Etiologies: **hereditary, idiopathic (MDS), reversible** (alcohol, lead, isoniazid, chloramphenicol, copper deficiency, hypothermia)
- Special clinical manifestations: hepatosplenomegaly, iron overload syndromes
- Diagnosis: can be micro-, normo-, or macrocytic; variable population of hypochromic RBCs; ↑ Fe, normal TIBC, ↑ ferritin, basophilic stippling, RBC **Pappenheimer bodies** (iron-containing inclusions), **ringed sideroblasts** (with iron-laden mitochondria) in BM
- Treatment: treat reversible causes; supportive transfusions for severe anemia; high-dose pyridoxine for some hereditary cases

Figure 5-2 Approach to microcytic anemias

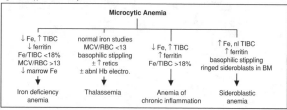

NORMOCYTIC ANEMIAS

Pancytopenia (see below)

Anemias of chronic disorders
- Anemia of chronic inflammation (see above)
- Renal failure: ↓ epo; may see burr cells; treat w/epo (see "Chronic Kidney Disease")
- Endocrine deficiencies: hypometabolism and ↓ O_2 demand with thyroid, pituitary, adrenal, or parathyroid disease → ↓ epo; can be normocytic or macrocytic

Sideroblastic anemia (see above)

Pure red cell aplasia
- Destructive antibodies or lymphocytes → ineffective erythropoiesis
- Associated with thymoma, CLL, and parvovirus infection
- Diagnostic studies: **lack of erythroid precursors on BM bx**, other lines normal
- Treatment: thymectomy if thymus enlarged; IVIg if parvovirus infection; immunosuppression if CLL or idiopathic; supportive care with PRBC transfusions

MACROCYTIC ANEMIAS

includes megaloblastic and nonmegaloblastic causes

Megaloblastic anemia
- **Impaired DNA synthesis** → cytoplasm matures faster than nucleus → ineffective erythropoiesis and macrocytosis; due to **folate** or **B_{12} deficiency**
- ✓ **folate** and **vitamin B_{12}**,↑ LDH & indirect bilirubin (due to ineffective erythropoiesis)
- Smear: **neutrophil hypersegmentation**, **macro-ovalocytes**, anisocytosis, poikilocytosis

Folate deficiency
- Folate present in leafy green vegetables and fruit; total body stores sufficient for **2-3 mos**
- Etiologies: **malnutrition** (alcoholics, anorectics, elderly), ↓ absorption (sprue), impaired metabolism (methotrexate, pyrimethamine, trimethoprim), ↑ requirement (chronic hemolytic anemia, pregnancy, malignancy, dialysis)
- Diagnosis: ↓ folate;↓ RBC folate, ↑ homocysteine but nl methylmalonic acid (unlike B_{12} defic.)
- Treatment: folate 1-5 mg PO qd; *important to r/o B_{12} deficiency*

Vitamin B_{12} deficiency
- B_{12} present only in foods of animal origin; total body stores sufficient for **2-3 y**
- Binds to **intrinsic factor** (IF) secreted by gastric parietal cells; absorbed in terminal ileum
- Etiologies: malnutrition (alcoholics, vegans), **pernicious anemia** (autoimmune disease against gastric parietal cells, associated with polyglandular endocrine insufficiency and ↑ risk of gastric carcinoma), other causes of ↓ absorption (gastrectomy, sprue, Crohn's disease), ↑ competition (intestinal bacterial overgrowth, fish tapeworm)
- Clinical manifestations: **neurologic** changes (**subacute combined degeneration**) affecting peripheral nerves, posterior and lateral columns of the spinal cord, and cortex → numbness, paresthesias, ↓ vibratory and positional sense, ataxia, dementia
- Diagnosis: ↓ B_{12}; ↑ homocysteine and methylmalonic acid; anti-IF Ab; Schilling test
- Treatment: 1 mg B_{12} IM qd × 7 d → q wk × 4-8 wks → q month for life
  neurologic abnormalities are reversible if treated w/ in 6 mos
  folate can reverse *hematologic* abnormalities of B_{12} deficiency but not *neurologic* changes
  oral supplementation (2 mg qd) appears feasible as well (*Blood* 1998;92:1191)

Nonmegaloblastic macrocytic anemias
- **Liver disease**: often macrocytic, may see target cells
- **Alcoholism**: BM suppression & macrocytosis independent of folate/B_{12} defic. or cirrhosis
- **Reticulocytosis**
- Hypothyroidism
- MDS
- Medications that impair DNA synthesis: zidovudine, 5-FU, hydroxyurea, Ara-C
- Metabolic disorders: hereditary orotic aciduria, Lesch-Nyhan syndrome

PANCYTOPENIA

Etiologies
- Hypocellular bone marrow: **aplastic anemia**, hypoplastic MDS
- Cellular bone marrow: **MDS**, aleukemic leukemia, PNH, severe megaloblastic anemia
- Marrow replacement (myelophthisis): **myelofibrosis**, metastatic solid tumors, granulomas
- Systemic diseases: hypersplenism, sepsis, alcohol

Clinical manifestations
- Anemia → fatigue
- Neutropenia → recurrent infections
- Thrombocytopenia → mucosal bleeding & easy bruisability

Aplastic anemia = stem cell failure (Lancet 2005;365:1647)
- Epidemiology: 2-5 cases/10^6/y; biphasic (major peak in adolescents, 2nd peak in elderly)
- Etiologies
  idiopathic ($^1/_2$-$^2/_3$ of cases)
  stem cell destruction: radiation, chemotherapy, chemicals (eg, benzene)
  idiosyncratic reaction to **medications** (eg, chloramphenicol, NSAIDs, sulfa drugs, gold, antiepileptics, antithyroid)
  viruses (HHV-6, HIV, EBV, parvovirus B19); also **post-hepatitis** (non A, B, or C)
  immune disorders (SLE, GVHD post HSCT, thymoma)
  PNH (see below); Fanconi's anemia (congenital disorder w/ pancytopenia, macrocytic anemia, ↑ risk of MDS, AML, & SCC of head & neck, and multiple physical anomalies)
  telomerase (hTERT) mutation (NEJM 2005;352:1413)
- Treatment and prognosis
  allogeneic HSCT: for *young* Pts → ~80% long-term survival and significantly ↓ risk of malignant evolution, but has risk of transplant-related morbidity & mortality; if possible avoid transfusions (and alloimmunization) pre-transplant
  immunosuppression (CsA, ATG): 70-80% respond, with 80-90% 5-y survival in responders; 15-20% 10-y incidence of clonal disorders (mostly MDS, AML, PNH)
  supportive care: transfusions, antibiotics, possible utility of G-CSF and epo

Myelodysplastic syndromes (MDS)
- Acquired clonal stem cell disorder → ineffective hematopoiesis → **cytopenias, dysmorphic blood cells and precursors**, variable risk of **leukemic transformation**
- Epidemiology: <100 cases/10^6/y; median age ~65 y
- Mechanisms/etiologies: **idiopathic** or 2° to chemotherapy with **alkylating agents, topoisomerase II inhibitors**; ↑ risk with radiation, benzene
- Clinical manifestations: **anemia** (85%), neutropenia (50%), thrombocytopenia (25%)
- Diagnosis: dysplasia (usually multilineage) in peripheral smear (ovalomacrocytes, **pseudo-Pelger-Huët anomaly**, Auer rods) and bone marrow (blasts ± RS)

Comparison of FAB and WHO Classification Systems for MDS		
FAB Classification	**Marrow**	**WHO Classification**
Refractory anemia (RA)	<5% blasts <15% RS	RA: isolated erythroid dysplasia RA with 5q-syndrome: isolated del(5q)
		Refractory cytopenias with multilineage dysplasia (RCMD): dysplasia in ≥2 lines
Refractory anemia with ringed sideroblasts (RARS)	<5% blasts ≥15% RS	RARS: RA with ≥15% RS RCMD with RS: RCMD with ≥15% RS
Refractory anemia with excess of blasts (RAEB)	5-20% blasts	RAEB-1: 5-9% blasts in BM RAEB-2: 10-19% blasts in BM
RAEB in transform. (RAEB-T)	21-30% blasts	Reclassified: AML w/ multilineage dyspl.
Chronic myelomonocytic leukemia (CMML)	>1000/μl periph. monos	MDS/MPD: new category for CMML Includes atypical CML and juvenile CMML
t(15;17), t(8;21), inv16, t(16;16) or MLL rearrang.		Should be classified as AML regardless of bone marrow blast count

- Treatment: intensity based on risk category (see below), age, performance status (PS)
  Poor PS, any risk → supportive care = transfusions, G-CSF, epo, abx if needed
  Low/intermediate risk → lenalidomide (esp for 5q- syndrome; NEJM 2005;352:549); DNA demethylating agents (azacitidine or decitabine; Cancer 2000;15:1794 & JCO 2002;20:2429)
  Intermediate/high risk → DNA demethylating agents, combination **chemotherapy** (akin to AML therapy) or **allogeneic HSCT** if age <60
  Hypoplastic MDS → **immunosuppressive regimen** (CsA, ATG, prednisone)

- Prognosis: IPSS correlates with **survival** and **progression to AML**

International Prognostic Scoring System (IPSS) Score						Risk group	Total score	Median survival
	0	0.5	1	1.5	2	Low	0	5.7 y
Blasts (%)	<5	5-10	–	11-20	21-30	Int-1	0.5-1	3.5 y
Karyotype	Good	Int.	Poor	–	–	Int-2	1.5-2	1.2 y
Cytopenias	0 or 1	2 or 3	–	–	–	High	≥2.5	0.4 y

(Blood 1997;89:2079)

Paroxysmal nocturnal hemoglobinuria (PNH)
- Acquired clonal stem cell disorder = inactivating somatic mutation of *PIG-A* gene → inability to form GPI-anchor for CD55 & CD59 (inhib of complement) → complement-mediated RBC lysis, plt aggreg. & hypercoagulability
- Clinical manifestations: intravascular **hemolytic anemia**, **venous thrombosis** (esp. intraabdominal, cerebral); **deficient hematopoiesis** (cytopenias); associated with aplastic anemia, MDS and evolution into AML
- Diagnosis: peripheral blood **flow cytometry** (↓ CD55 & CD59)
- Treatment: supportive care (iron, folate, transfusions)
    allogeneic HSCT for hypoplasia or severe thrombosis
    eculizumab (Ab inactivates terminal complement C5): ↓ hemolysis (NEJM 2004;350:552)

Myelophthisic anemia (see "Agnogenic Myeloid Metaplasia with Myelofibrosis")
- Infiltration of bone marrow
- Etiologies: agnogenic myeloid metaplasia with myelofibrosis, tumors, granulomas

HEMOLYTIC ANEMIAS

Causes of Hemolytic Anemia by Mechanism			
Location	Mechanism	Examples	Mode
Intrinsic	Enzyme deficiency	G6PD deficiency	**Hereditary**
	Hemoglobinopathies	Sickle cell anemia, thalassemia	
	Membrane abnormalities	Hereditary spherocytosis	
		PNH	
Extrinsic	Immune-mediated	Autoimmune; drug-induced, tx rxn	**Acquired**
	Traumatic	MAHA; prostheses	
	Direct infections, toxins	Malaria, babesiosis; snake & spider venoms; Wilson's; hypotonic infusions	
	Entrapment	Hypersplenism	

(Lancet 2000;355:1169 & 1260)

Diagnostic evaluation
- ↑ reticulocyte count (RI >2%), ↑ LDH, ↓ haptoglobin (83% Se, 96% Sp), ↑ indirect bili
- Autoimmune hemolysis: Coombs' test = direct antiglobulin test (DAT) → ⊕ if agglutination occurs when antisera against Ig or C3 are applied to patient RBCs
- Intravascular: ↑↑ LDH, ↓↓ haptoglobin; hemoglobinemia, hemoglobinuria, hemosiderinuria
- Extravascular: splenomegaly
- Family h/o anemia; personal or family h/o cholelithiasis

Glucose-6-phosphate dehydrogenase (G6PD) deficiency (NEJM 1991;324:169)
- X-linked defect of metabolism causing ↑ susceptibility to oxidative damage
- Most common in males of African or Mediterranean descent
- Hemolysis precipitated by **drugs** (dapsone, primaquine, sulfamethoxazole, doxorubicin, methylene blue), **infection**, **DKA**, or **foods** (fava beans in children)
- Diagnosis: smear may show RBC **Heinz bodies** (oxidized Hb) that result in **bite cells** once removed by spleen; ↓ G6PD levels (may be normal after acute hemolysis as older RBCs have already lysed and young RBCs may still have near normal levels)

Sickle cell anemia (NEJM 1999;340:1021)
- Recessive β-globin mutation → structurally abnl hemoglobin (HbS)
    ~8% of African-Americans are heterozygotes and ~1 in 400 are homozygotes
- Deoxygenated HbS polymerizes → RBC sickles and ↓ RBC deformability → **hemolysis** and **microvascular occlusion**
- **Anemia**: chronic hemolysis ± acute aplastic (parvo. B19) or splenic sequestration crises
- **Vaso-occlusion and infarction**: painful crises, acute chest syndrome, CVA, splenic sequestration, hand-foot syndrome, renal papillary necrosis, aseptic necrosis, priapism
- **Infection**: splenic infarction → overwhelming infection by **encapsulated organisms**; infarcted bone → **osteomyelitis** (Salmonella, Staph. aureus)

- Diagnosis: sickle-shaped RBCs and Howell-Jolly bodies on smear; Hb electrophoresis
- Treatment: **hydroxyurea** causes ↑ HbF → ↓ painful crises, acute chest episodes (*NEJM* 1995;332:1317) and may ↓ mortality (*JAMA* 2003;289:1645); allogeneic HSCT may have a role in young Pts with severe disease (*Blood* 2000;95:1918)
- Supportive care: folic acid qd; pneumococcal, meningococcal, *H. flu* & HBV vaccination; pain crises treated with **hydration**, **oxygen**, and **analgesia**; simple or exchange transfusion for CVA, severe acute chest syndrome, and preop (goal Hb 10 g/dl)

Hereditary spherocytosis (HS) (*Br J Hematology* 2004;126:455)
- Defect in a cytoskeletal protein of RBC membrane → membrane loss mutations in ankyrin, α- and β- spectrin, band 3, and pallidin have been identified
- Most common in N. European populations (1 in 5000 births); ⊕ FHx (75% of Pts)
- Anemia, jaundice, splenomegaly, pigmented gallstones
- Diagnosis: spherocytes on smear, ⊕ osmotic fragility test (~80% Se), ↓ eosin-5-maleimide (EMA) binding (92% Se; 99% Sp)
- Treatment: folate, splenectomy for moderate and severe HS

Paroxysmal nocturnal hemoglobinuria (see above)

Autoimmune hemolytic anemia (AIHA)
- Acquired, antibody-mediated RBC destruction
- **Warm AIHA: IgG** Abs opsonize RBCs *at body temp* → removal by spleen
  Etiologies: idiopathic, lymphoproliferative disorders (CLL), autoimmune diseases (SLE), drugs (see below)
- **Cold AIHA: IgM** Ab bind to RBCs *at temp <37°C* → **complement fixation** → intravascular hemolysis and acrocyanosis upon exposure to cold
  Etiologies: idiopathic, lymphoproliferative disorders (monoclonal), *Mycoplasma pneumoniae* infection and infectious mononucleosis (polyclonal)
- Diagnosis: spherocytes on smear, ⊕ **Coombs**; ✓ cold agglutinin titer
- Treatment: treat underlying disease; **warm AIHA**: corticosteroids ± splenectomy, IVIg, cytotoxic agents, rituximab; **cold AIHA**: cold avoidance, steroids often ineffective, rituximab (*Blood* 2004;103:2925)

Drug-induced hemolytic anemia
- Acquired, antibody-mediated, RBC destruction precipitated by a medication:
  abx: cephalosporins, sulfa drugs, rifampin
  CV: methyldopa, procainamide, quinidine, thiazides
  other: TCAs, phenothiazines, NSAIDs, sulfonylureas, MTX, 5-FU
- Diagnosis: Coombs' usually negative

Microangiopathic hemolytic anemia (MAHA)
- Intra-arteriolar fibrin which damages RBCs → acquired intravascular hemolysis
- Etiologies: **hemolytic-uremic syndrome** (HUS), **thrombotic thrombocytopenic purpura** (TTP), **disseminated intravascular coagulation** (DIC), malignancy, malignant HTN, eclampsia/HELLP, mech. cardiac valves, infected vascular prostheses
- Diagnosis: **schistocytes** ± thrombocytopenia ± abnormalities associated with specific disorders, eg, ↑ PT in DIC, ↑ Cr in HUS, ↑ LFTs in HELLP
- Treatment: treat underlying abnormality, consider plasma exchange for TTP

Hypersplenism
- Splenomegaly → stasis and trapping in the spleen → macrophagic attack and remodeling of RBC surface → spherocytosis → hemolysis

Causes of Splenomegaly	
Etiology	**Comments**
Reticuloendothelial system hyperplasia	Hemolytic anemia, sickle cell disease, **thalassemia major**
Immune hyperplasia	Infection (HIV, EBV, CMV, TB, **malaria**, **kala-azar**, *Mycobacterium avium* complex), autoimmune disorders (SLE, RA with Felty's syndrome), sarcoidosis, serum sickness
Congestion	Cirrhosis, CHF, portal/splenic vein thrombosis, **schistosomiasis**
Infiltration (nonmalignant)	Lysosomal storage disorders (**Gaucher's**, Niemann-Pick), glycogen storage diseases, histiocytosis X
Neoplasm	MPD (**CML, AMM/MF, PV, ET**), CMML, leukemia/lymphoma (**NHL, HL, hairy cell leukemia, CLL**), multiple myeloma, amyloid

(**boldface** = causes of massive splenomegaly)

Clinical Characteristics of Bleeding Disorders		
Feature	Platelet/Vascular Defect	Coagulation Defect
Site	Skin, mucous membranes	Deep in soft tissues (muscles, joints)
Lesions	Petechiae, ecchymoses	Hemarthroses, hematomas
Bleeding	After minor cuts: yes	After minor cuts: unusual
	After surgery: immediate, mild	After surgery: delayed, severe

Purpura
- **Nonblanching** purple/red lesions due to extravasation of RBCs into dermis
- **Nonpalpable** (macular; ≤3 mm in diameter = petechiae; >3 mm = ecchymoses)
  platelet disorder: thrombocytopenia, defect in platelet function
  thromboemboli: DIC, TTP, cholesterol or fat emboli
  vascular fragility: amyloidosis, Ehlers-Danlos, scurvy
  trauma
- **Palpable** (papular)
  vasculitis: leukocytoclastic, HSP, PAN, RMSF
  infectious emboli: meningococcemia, bacterial endocarditis

Figure 5-3 Approach to abnormal hemostasis

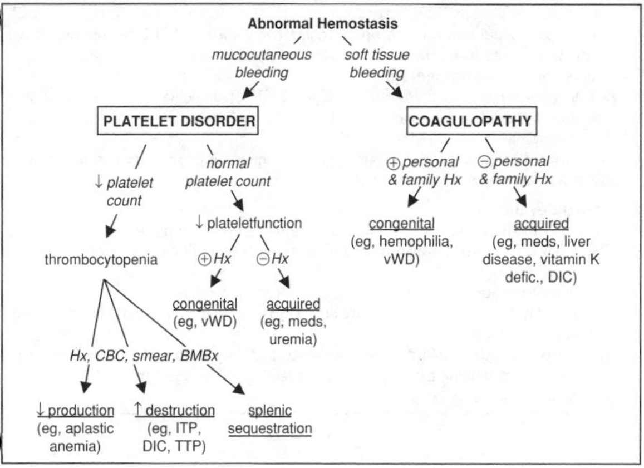

THROMBOCYTOPENIA (Plt count <150,000/μl)

Thrombocytopenia and Risk of Bleeding	
Platelet count (cells/μl)	**Risk**
>100,000	No ↑ risk
50,000-100,000	Risk with major trauma; can proceed with general surgery
20,000-50,000	Risk with minor trauma or surgery
<20,000	Risk of *spontaneous* bleeding (less so with ITP)
<10,000	Risk of severe, life-threatening bleeding

Etiologies
- ↓ production
  hypocellular bone marrow: aplastic anemia (see "Aplastic anemia"), drugs (eg, thiazides, antibiotics), and alcohol
  cellular bone marrow: MDS, leukemia, severe megaloblastic anemia
  marrow replacement: myelofibrosis, hematologic and solid malignancies, granulomas
- ↑ **destruction**
  immune-mediated
  Primary (idiopathic): immune thrombocytopenic purpura (**ITP**, see below)
  Secondary: infections (HIV, herpes viruses, HCV), collagen vascular diseases (**SLE**),
  antiphospholipid syndrome, lymphoproliferative disorders (**CLL**, lymphoma), drugs
  (*many*, including **heparin**, abciximab, quinidine, sulfonamides, vancomycin),
  alloimmune (posttransfusion)
  non-immune-mediated: MAHA (DIC, HUS,TTP), ticlopidine/clopidogrel, vasculitis,
  preeclampsia/HELLP syndrome, cardiopulmonary bypass, CVVH, IABP, cavernous
  hemangioma
- **Abnormal distribution or pooling**: splenic sequestration, dilutional, hypothermia
- **Unknown**: Ehrlichiosis, Babesiosis, RMSF

Diagnostic evaluation
- H&P: meds, infxns, underlying conditions, splenomegaly, lymph nodes, bleeding
- **CBC with differential**: isolated thrombocytopenia vs. multilineage involvement
- **Peripheral smear**
  ↑ destruction → look for large platelets, **schistocytes**
  ↓ production → rarely limited to platelets → look for **blasts**, hypersegmented PMNs,
  leukoerythroblastic Δs
  rule out **pseudothrombocytopenia** due to platelet clumping (✓ platelet count in
  non-EDTA-containing tube, eg citrate-containing yellow top tube)

Figure 5-4 Approach to thrombocytopenia

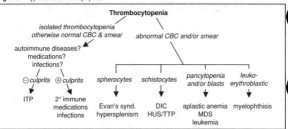

- Additional laboratory evaluations as indicated
  if anemia: ✓ reticulocyte count, LDH, haptoglobin, bilirubin to detect hemolysis
  if hemolytic anemia: ✓ PT, PTT, fibrinogen, D-dimer, Coombs, ANA
  BM bx for unexplained thrombocytopenia, esp. if associated with splenomegaly

Immune thrombocytopenic purpura (ITP)
- ITP refers to *primary* immune platelet destruction; *a diagnosis of exclusion*
- Clinical manifestations: insidious onset of mucocutaneous bleeding; female:male = 3:1
- Diagnosis of exclusion: *rule out other etiologies*
  CBC: isolated ↓ platelets; 10% have ITP + AIHA = Evans syndrome
  peripheral smear: large platelets
  BM bx: ↑ megakaryocytes; perform in adults >60 y to r/o myelodysplasia
  consider ANA, viral serologies (eg HIV, EBV, hepatitis), *H. pylori* Ab
  antiplatelet antibody tests are not useful
- Treatment: 50-75% respond to steroids, but <20% have sustained remission after taper
  ~65% have long-term remission with splenectomy
  plts for bleeding or ? if plt <20,000/μl; limited benefit w/o concurrent IVIg or anti-Rh(D)

Treatment of ITP in Adults		
Approach	Treatment	Notes
Initial	**Steroids** (prednisone 1-1.5 mg/kg/d PO tapered over wks vs. dexamethasone 40 mg PO × 4 d)	Useful acutely, but long-term s/e ↓ Fc receptor on Mφ ↓ anti-plt Ab production
	Anti-Rh(D) Ig 75 μg/kg/d IV	For Rh(D) ⊕ Pts Ab-coated RBCs overwhelm Mφ Fc receptors
	IVIg (1 g/kg/d IV × 2-3 d)	If plts <5000 despite steroids Blocks Fc receptors on Mφ ↓ anti-plt Ab production
Refractory	**Splenectomy**	↓ plt clearance
	Rituximab (anti-CD20)	↓ plt clearance, Ab against B-cell
	Danazol, vincristine	↓ plt clearance
	Azathioprine, cyclophosphamide	Immunosuppressants ↓ anti-plt Ab production
	AMG531, AKR-501, eltrombopag	Thrombopoiesis stim. proteins
Bleeding	Aminocaproic acid	Inhibits plasmin activation
	Methylprednisolone 1 g/d IV × 3 d	See above
	IVIg	See above
Chronic Refractory	Autologous HSCT	Investigational

(NEJM 2002;346:995 & 2003;349:831 & 2006;355:1672)

Overview of Heparin-Induced Thrombocytopenias		
Feature	Type I	Type II
Mechanism	Direct effect of heparin	Immune (Ab)-mediated IgG vs. platelet factor 4 – heparin complex
Incidence	20%	1-3%
Onset	After 1-4 d of heparin therapy	After 4-10 d; but can occur early (<24 h) with h/o prior exposure w/in last 100 d (felt to be secondary to persistent Ab). Can occur after heparin d/c.
Platelet nadir	>100,000/μl	30-70,000/μl, ↓ >50%
Sequelae	None	Thrombotic events (HITT) in 30-50% Rare hemorrhagic complications
Management	Can continue heparin and observe	**Discontinue heparin** Alternative anticoagulation

(JACC 1998;31:1449; NEJM 2001;344:1286)

- Pathophysiology (type II): Ab binds heparin-PF4 → immune complex binds to platelets
  → **platelet activation**, further PF4 release → platelet aggregates removed from
  circulation → **thrombocytopenia**; procoagulants released by platelets and tissue factor
  released by endothelial cells damaged by HIT Abs → **prothrombotic state**
- Diagnosis: need to meet clinical *and* pathologic criteria
  Clinical: plt <100,000 or ↓ 50% from baseline; or **venous** (DVT, PE) or **arterial** (limb
  ischemia, CVA, MI) thrombosis (4:1 ratio); or heparin-induced skin lesions
  (may also manifest ↑ heparin resistance)
  Pathologic: ⊕ HIT Ab using PF4-heparin ELISA (~90% Se, rev if high suspicion), may
  be confirmed by a functional platelet aggregation (serotonin-release) assay (>90% Sp)

- Treatment of type II (NEJM 2006;355:809)
  discontinue heparin (including flushes, LMWH prophylaxis, heparin-impregnated lines)
  avoid plt transfusions
  ⊕ thrombosis: alternative anticoag. (lepirudin or argatroban), overlap w/ warfarin
  (✓ chromogenic Xa to titrate), treat for ≥3 mos
  ⊖ thrombosis: consider screening for DVT; nonheparin anticoag. at least until plt count
  nl; no consensus on duration of subsequent anticoag. (likely ~1 mo if no clot)
- Use of heparin if h/o HIT: if disappearance of PF4 Ab (usually >100 d after dx), risk of HIT
  recurrence low (NEJM 2001;344:1286)

Hemolytic-uremic syndrome (HUS) & thrombotic thrombocytopenic purpura (TTP)
- Definition: vascular occlusive disorders w/ systemic (TTP) or intrarenal (HUS) plt aggreg.
  → thrombocytopenia & mechanical injury to RBCs (MAHA) (NEJM 2002;347:589)
  HUS triad = thrombocytopenia + MAHA + renal failure
  TTP pentad = thrombocytopenia + MAHA ± Δ MS ± renal failure ± fever
- Pathophysiology: mechanism in most HUS cases is distinct from TTP (NEJM 1998;339:1578)
  HUS: Shiga toxin binds & activates renal endothelial cells & plts → intrarenal thrombi
  TTP: ↓ ADAMTS13 protease activity → persistence of large vWF multimers on endothelial
  surface → adhesion and aggregation of passing platelets → thrombosis
- Clinical manifestations and associations
  HUS: usually in children; prodrome of bloody diarrhea due to enterohemorrhagic E. coli
  TTP: usually in adults; **idiopathic**, **drugs** (CsA, gemcitabine, mitomycin C, ticlopidine,
  clopidogrel, quinine), HIV, pregnancy, HSCT, autoimmune disease, familial
- Diagnosis: unexplained thrombocytopenia (typically <20k) + MAHA → *sufficient for dx*
  ⊕ **schistocytes**, ⊖ Coombs, normal PT/PTT & fibrinogen
  ↑↑ LDH (tissue ischemia + hemolysis), ↑ indirect bili., ↓↓ haptoglobin, ↑ Cr (esp. in HUS)
  Biopsy: arterioles filled with platelet hyaline thrombi
  Ddx: DIC, vasculitis, malignant hypertension, preeclampsia/HELLP syndrome
- Treatment: **plasma exchange** ± glucocorticoids in all adults w/suspected TTP-HUS;
  FFP if delay to plasma exchange;
  platelet transfusions contraindicated → ↑ microvascular thrombosis (NEJM 2006;354:1927)

Disseminated intravascular coagulation (DIC): see "Disorders of Coagulation"

DISORDERS OF PLATELET FUNCTION

Mechanisms and Etiologies of Platelet Function Abnormalities		
Function	**Inherited**	**Acquired**
Adhesion	Bernard-Soulier; vWD	Uremia; acquired vWD
Aggregation	Afibrinogenemia Glanzmann's thrombasthenia	Ticlopidine, clopidogrel, GP IIb/IIIa Dysproteinemias (myeloma)
Granule release	Chediak-Higashi syndrome Hermansky-Pudlak syndrome	Drugs (ASA, NSAIDs); liver disease; MPD; cardiopulmonary bypass

Tests of platelet function
- Bleeding time: global screen of platelet function; *not reliable and rarely used*
- Platelet aggregation tests: measure aggregation in response to agonists (eg, ADP)

von Willebrand's disease (vWD)
- Most common inherited bleeding disorder
- von Willebrand's factor (vWF) function = platelet glue & plasma carrier of factor VIII
- Classification of inherited vWD
  Type 1 (autosomal dominant; 85% of cases): partial quantitative deficiency in vWF
  Type 2 (autosomal dominant; 15% of cases): qualitative deficiency of vWF (4 types:
  A = defective multimers, B = excessive GPIbIX binding, M = defective GPIbIX binding,
  N = defective factor VIII binding)
  Type 3 (autosomal recessive; rare): near complete deficiency of vWF
- Acquired vWD: associated with many disorders (malignancy, autoimmune, hypothyroidism,
  drugs) and caused by different mechanisms (anti-vWF Abs, ↑ clearance, ↓ synthesis)
- Diagnosis: ↓ **vWF:Ag**, ↓ **vWF activity** (measured by ristocetin cofactor assay), ↓ **factor
  VIII**, ± ↑ PTT, ± ↓ platelets; confirm with **vWF multimer analysis**
- Treatment: **desmopressin** (IV/IN) → ↑ endothelial cell release of vWF; variable efficacy
  depending on type, ∴ ✓ response before use w/ subseq. bleeding or procedures;
  vWF replacement: cryoprecipitate, factor VIII concentrates rich in vWF, recomb. vWF
  (NEJM 2004;351:683)

COAGULOPATHIES

Screening Test Abnormalities in Inherited and Acquired Coagulopathies

PT	PTT	Inherited	Acquired
↑	↔	FVII defic.	Vit. K defic.; liver disease; FVII inhib.
↔	↑	Hemophilias, vWD	Factor inhibs.; antiphospholipid Ab
↑	↑	Fbgn, FII, or FV defic.	DIC; liver disease; fgbn, FII, FIV, or FX inhib.

Further coagulation tests
- Mixing study: useful if ↑ PT or PTT; mix Pt's plasma 1:1 w/ normal plasma and retest
  PT/PTT normalizes → factor **deficiency**; PT/PTT remains elevated → factor **inhibitor**
- Coagulation factor levels: useful if mixing study suggests factor deficiency
  DIC → all factors consumed; ∴ ↓ factor V and VIII
  liver disease → ↓ all factors except VIII; ∴ ↓ factor V, normal factor VIII
  vitamin K deficiency → ↓ factors II, VII, IX, X (and protein C, S); ∴ normal V and VIII
- **DIC screen**: fibrinogen (consumed), fibrin degradation products (FDPs), ⊕ due to intense
  fibrinolysis), D-dimer (more specific FDP test that detects degradation of X-linked fibrin)

Hemophilias (NEJM 2001;344:1773)
- X-linked **factor VIII** (hemophilia A) or **factor IX** (hemophilia B) **deficiency**
- Classification: mild (5-25% normal factor activity), moderate (1-5%), or severe (<1%)
- Clinical manifestations: hematomas, hemarthroses, bruising, bleeding (mucosal, GI, GU)
- Diagnosis: ↑ PTT (normalizes w/mixing study), normal PT & vWF, ↓ factor VIII or IX
- Treatment: purified/recomb. factor VIII or IX concentrate, desmopressin (mild disease),
  aminocaproic acid; recomb. factor VIIa if factor inhib., cryo (only has factor VIII)

Coagulation factor inhibitors
- Etiologies: hemophilia (treated with factor replacement); postpartum; lymphoproliferative
  disorders and other malignancies; autoimmune diseases; most commonly anti-factor VIII
- Diagnosis: ↑ PTT (does *not* normalize w/mixing study); Bethesda assay quantitates titer
- Treatment: high titer → **recomb. factor VIIa**, porcine factor concentrates, activated
  prothrombin complex; others → high-purity human factor, plasmapheresis, immune tol.

Disseminated intravascular coagulation (DIC) (NEJM 1999;341:586)
- Etiologies: trauma, shock, infection, malignancy, obstetrical complications
- Pathogenesis: *massive* activation of coagulation that overwhelms control mechanisms
  thrombosis in microvasculature → ischemia + microangiopathic hemolytic anemia
  acute consumption of coagulation factors and platelets → **bleeding**
  chronic DIC → able to replete factors and platelets → **thrombosis**
- Diagnosis: ↑ PT, ↑ PTT, ↓ **fibrinogen** (may be *nl* b/c acute phase), ⊕ **FDP/D-dimer**, ↓
  plts, ⊕ schisto, ↑ LDH, ↓ hapto; *chronic DIC*: ⊕ FDP/D-dimer, variable plts, other labs nl
- Treatment: treat underlying process; support with **FFP**, **cryoprecipitate** (goal fibrinogen
  >100 mg/dl), and **platelets**; consider activated protein C in severe sepsis

Vitamin K deficiency
- Etiologies: malnutrition, ↓ absorption (**antibiotic** suppression of vitamin K-producing
  intestinal flora or malabsorption), liver disease (↓ stores), **warfarin**

Properties and Antidotes for Anticoagulants & Fibrinolytics

Anticoag.	t_{1/2}	Labs	Rx for O/D w/ serious bleeding*
UFH	60-90′ RES	↑ PTT	**Protamine** IV 1 mg/100 U UFH (max 50 mg). For infusions, dose to reverse 2 × UFH given per h.
Bivalirudin	25′, K	↑ PTT	Dialysis
Lepirudin	80′, K	↑ PTT	Dialysis
Argatroban	45′, L	↑ PTT	? Dialysis
Enoxaparin	8°, K	(anti-Xa)	? Protamine (reversal incomplete)
Fondaparinux	24°, K	(anti-Xa)	? Dialysis
Warfarin	36°, L	↑ PT	*No bleeding*: INR >5: **vit. K** 1-5 mg PO (superior to SC, ≈IV at 24°); 2.5 mg for INR 6-10; 5 mg for INR>10 (Archives 2003;163:2469) *Bleeding*: **vit. K** 10 mg IV + **FFP** 2-4 units IV q 6-8°
Fibrinolytic	20-90′ LK	↓ fbgn ↑ FDP	**Cryoprecipitate**, **FFP**, ± aminocaproic acid

*Initial step should be immediate d/c of anticoag. Decision to dialyse should take into account time for anticoag. to
be metabolized (noting any renal or liver insufficiency) w/o dialysis vs. potential sequelae of bleeding while waiting.
Rx for warfarin O/D w/o bleeding is also given. K = kidney, L = liver, RES = reticuloendothelial system.

HYPERCOAGULABLE STATES

Suspect in Pts with venous or arterial thrombosis at young age or unusual locations, recurrent thromboses or pregnancy loss, ⊕ FHx

Inherited Hypercoagulable States			
Risk factor	**Prevalence** (Caucasians)	**VTE risk**	**Comments**
Factor V Leiden	4%	7×	Activated protein C (APC) resist.
Prothrombin mutation	2%	2.8×	G20210A → ↑ prothrombin level
Hyperhomocysteinemia	5-10%	2.5×	Inherited or acquired
Protein C or S deficiency	0.3%	10×	Warfarin-induced skin necrosis risk
Antithrombin III deficiency	0.04%	25×	May be relatively heparin-resistant

(NEJM 2001;344:1222)

	Vascular Beds Affected by Inherited and Acquired Hypercoagulable States	
	Venous	**Venous and arterial**
Inher.	Factor V Leiden Prothrombin mutation ↓ protein C, S, or AT III	? factor V Leiden + smoking Hyperhomocysteinemia (inherited or acquired) Dysfibrinogenemia
Acquired	Stasis: immobilization, surgery, CHF Malignancy Hormonal: OCPs, HRT, tamoxifen, pregnancy Nephrotic syndrome	Platelet defects: myeloproliferative disorders, HIT, PNH Hyperviscosity: polycythemia vera, Waldenström's macroglobulinemia, sickle cell, acute leukemia Vessel wall defects: vasculitis, trauma, foreign bodies Others: antiphospholipid syndrome, IBD

Diagnostic evaluation
- APC resistance screen; prothrombin PCR test; functional assays for protein C and S, ATIII; homocysteine level; anticardiolipin and lupus anticoagulant antibody assays
- Proteins C & S and ATIII levels are affected by acute thrombosis and anticoagulation; ∴ levels best assessed ≥2 weeks after completing anticoagulation course
- Age-appropriate malignancy screening (⊕ in 12% with "idiopathic" DVT; Annals 1996;125:785)

Treatment
- Asx w/inherited risk factor: consider prophylactic anticoag. if develops acquired risk factor
- Thrombosis w/ inherited risk factor: see "Venous Thromboembolism"

Antiphospholipid syndrome (APS) (NEJM 2002;346:752)
- Definition: ≥1 clinical & ≥1 laboratory criteria
  - Clinical: thrombosis (any) or complication of pregnancy (≥3 spont. abortions before 10 wks or ≥1 fetal loss after 10 wks or premature birth before 34 wks)
  - Laboratory: ⊕ moderate-high titer anticardiolipin (ACL) or lupus anticoagulant (LA) antibodies on ≥2 occasions at least 6 wks apart
- Clinical manifestations: **DVT/PE/CVA**, recurrent fetal loss, **thrombocytopenia**, hemolytic anemia, livedo reticularis; "**catastrophic APS**" = widespread acute thrombotic microangiopathy with multiorgan visceral damage → high mortality
- Etiologies: primary (idiopathic) or secondary due to **autoimmune syndromes** (eg, SLE), **malignancy**, **infections**, drug reactions
- Diagnosis: **antiphospholipid antibodies** are classified by method of detection
  - ACL: Ab against cardiolipin, a mitochondrial phospholipid; IgG more specific than IgM
  - LA: Ab that prolongs phospholipid-dependent coagulation reactions; ∴ ↑PTT that does *not* correct with mixing study but does correct with excess phospholipids or platelets; standard PT is not affected because the reaction contains much more phospholipid
  - false ⊕VDRL: nontreponemal test for syphilis in which cardiolipin is part of Ag complex
- Treatment: lifelong warfarin after a thrombotic event; goal INR ≥3 (NEJM 1995;332:993) or 2-3 (NEJM 2003;349:1133); consider ASA prophylaxis for high-risk asx Pt (eg, SLE)

Neutrophilia (>7500-10,000/μl)	
Infection	Usually bacterial; ± toxic granulations, Döhle bodies
Inflammation	Burn, tissue necrosis, MI, PE, collagen vascular disease
Drugs and toxins	Corticosteroids, β-agonists, lithium, G-CSF; cigarette smoking
Stress	Release of endogenous glucocorticoids and catecholamines
Marrow stimulation	Hemolytic anemia, immune thrombocytopenia
Asplenia	Surgical, acquired (sickle cell), congenital (dextrocardia)
Neoplasm	Can be 1° (MPD) or paraneoplastic (eg, carcinomas of lung, GI)
Leukemoid reaction	>50,000/μl + left shift, not due to leukemia; unlike CML, ↑ LAP

Lymphocytosis (>4000-5000/μl)	
Infection	Usually viral; "atypical lymphocytes" with mononucleosis syndromes Other: pertussis, toxoplasmosis
Hypersensitivity	Drug-induced, serum sickness
Stress	Cardiac emergencies, trauma, status epilepticus, postsplenectomy
Autoimmune	Rheumatoid arthritis (large granular lymphocytes), malignant thymoma
Neoplasm	Leukemia (ALL, CLL, others), lymphoma

Monocytosis (>500/μl)	
Infection	Usually TB, SBE, Listeria, Brucella, rickettsiae, fungi, parasites
Inflammation	IBD, sarcoidosis, collagen vascular diseases
Neoplasm	Hodgkin's disease, leukemias, MPD, carcinomas

Eosinophilia (>500/μl)	
Infection	Usually parasitic (helminths)
Allergic	Drugs; asthma, hay fever, eczema; ABPA
Collagen vascular disease	RA, Churg-Strauss syndrome, eosinophilic fasciitis, PAN
Endocrine	Adrenal insufficiency
Neoplasm	Hodgkin's lymphoma, CML, mycosis fungoides, carcinomas, mastocytosis
Atheroembolic disease	Cholesterol emboli syndrome
Hypereosinophilic syndrome	Multiorgan system involvement including heart and CNS, associated with FIP1L1-PDGFRA fusion (NEJM 2003;348:1201)

Basophilia (>150/μl)	
Neoplasm	MPD, Hodgkin's disease
Alteration in BM or reticuloendothelial compartment	Hemolytic anemia, splenectomy
Inflammation or allergy	IBD, chronic airway inflammation

Lymphadenopathy	
Viral	HIV, EBV, CMV, HSV, VZV, hepatitis, measles, rubella
Bacterial	Generalized (brucellosis, leptospirosis, TB, atypical mycobacteria, syphilis) Localized (streptococci, staphylococci, cat-scratch disease, tularemia)
Fungal and parasitic	Histoplasmosis, coccidioidomycosis, paracoccidioidomycosis Toxoplasmosis
Immunologic	Collagen vascular disease, drug hypersensitivity (eg, phenytoin), serum sickness, histiocytosis X, Castleman's and Kawaski disease
Neoplasm	Lymphoma, leukemia, amyloidosis, metastatic carcinoma
Other	Sarcoidosis; lipid storage diseases
Factors that favor biopsy	Age (>40), size (>2 cm), location (supraclavicular is always abnormal), duration (>1 m). Consistency (hard vs. rubbery vs. soft) & tenderness are not reliable.

TRANSFUSION THERAPY

Blood Products and Indications	
Packed red blood cells (PRBCs)	For acute blood loss or to ↑ O_2-carrying capacity if end-organ ischemia. In critical illness, Hb goal 7-9 g/dl adequate; consider 10-12 g/dl if coronary ischemia (*NEJM* 1999;340:409 & 2001;345:1230). 1 U PRBC → ↑ Hb by ~1 g/dl. Tx large # PRBCs can → ↓ Ca & ↑ K.
Platelets (plts)	Plts <10,000/μl or <20,000/μl with infection or ↑ bleeding risk *or* <50,000/μl with active bleeding or preprocedure. *Contraindicated in* TTP/HUS, HELLP, HIT. 6U → ↑ plt count by ~30-60,000/μl. Refractory = ↑ <5000/μl 30-60 min posttransfusion. Suggests *alloimmunization* → trial ABO matched plts. If still refractory ✓ panel reactive Abs (PRA) to determine utility of HLA-matched plts.
Fresh frozen plasma (FFP)	Contains all coagulation factors. For bleeding due to deficiency of multiple coagulation factors (e.g. DIC, TTP/HUS, liver disease, warfarin excess, dilution) or PT >17 sec preprocedure.
Cryoprecipitate	Enriched for fibrinogen, vWF, VIII, and XIII. For bleeding in vWD, factor XIII deficiency or fibrinogen <100 mg/dl.
Irradiated	Prevents donor T-cell proliferation in recipient. For Pts with risk of transfusion associated GVHD (HSCT, hematologic malignancies, congenital immunodeficiency).
CMV-negative	From CMV-negative donors. For CMV-seronegative pregnant women, transplant candidates/recipients, SCID, AIDS Pts.
Leukoreduced	WBCs cause HLA alloimmunization and fever (cytokine release) and carry CMV. For chronically transfused Pts, potential transplant recipients, h/o febrile nonhemolytic transfusion reaction, cases in which CMV-negative products are desired but unavailable.
Intravenous immune globulin (IVIg)	Polyvalent IgG from >1000 donors. For postexposure prophylaxis (e.g. HAV), certain autoimmune disorders (eg, ITP, Guillain-Barré, ? CIDP), congenital or acquired hypogammaglobulinemia (CVID, CLL).
Plasmapheresis and cytapheresis	Removes Ig molec wt subst. (eg, cryoglobulinemia, Goodpasture's, Guillain-Barré, hyperviscosity syndrome, TTP) or cells (eg, leukemia w/ hyperleukocytosis, sx thrombocytosis, sickle cell) from plasma.

Transfusion Complications			
Noninfectious	Risk (per unit)	Infectious	Risk (per unit)
Febrile	1:100	CMV	common
Allergic	1:100	Hepatitis B	1:220,000
Delayed hemolytic	1:1000	Hepatitis C	1:1,600,000
Acute hemolytic	<1:250,000	HIV	1:1,800,000
Fatal hemolytic	<1:100,000	Bacteria (PRBCs)	1:500,000
TRALI	1:5000	Bacteria (platelets)	1:12,000

(*NEJM* 1999;340:438; *JAMA* 2003;289:959)

Transfusion reactions

- For all reactions (except minor allergic): **stop transfusion**; send remaining blood product and fresh blood sample to blood bank
- **Acute hemolytic**: fever, hypotension, flank pain, renal failure <24 h after transfusion
  Due to ABO incompatibility → preformed Abs against donor RBCs
  Treatment: vigorous IVF, maintain UOP with diuretics, mannitol, or dopamine
- **Delayed hemolytic**: generally less severe than acute hemolytic; 5-7 d after transfusion
  Due to undetected allo-Abs against minor antigens → anamnestic response
  Treatment: usually no specific therapy required; dx is important for future transfusion
- **Febrile nonhemolytic**: fever and rigors 0-6 h after transfusion
  Due to Abs against donor WBCs and cytokines released from cells in blood product
  Treatment: acetaminophen ± meperidine; rule out infection and hemolysis
- **Allergic**: urticaria; rarely, **anaphylaxis**: bronchospasm, laryngeal edema, hypotension
  Reaction to plasma proteins in blood product; anaphylaxis is usually seen in IgA-deficient Pts who have preformed anti-IgA Abs
  Treatment: urticaria → diphenhydramine; anaphylaxis → epinephrine ± glucocorticoids
- **Transfusion-related acute lung injury** (TRALI): noncardiogenic pulmonary edema
  Due to donor Abs that bind recipient WBCs, which then aggregate in pulmonary vasculature and release mediators causing ↑ capillary permeability
  Treatment: see "ARDS"

MYELOPROLIFERATIVE DISORDERS (MPD)

General (NEJM 2006;355:2452)
- Results from clonal expansion of multipotent hematopoietic stem cell
- Different from MDS in that the cells are not dysplastic (ie, normally developed)
- Gain of fxn mutations in **JAK2** (Janus kinase) present in most cases of MPD (PV ~95%, ET 23-57%, AMM 43-57%, NEJM 2005;352:1779) and **Bcr-Abl fusion** in **all** cases of CML; useful diagnostic tool

POLYCYTHEMIA VERA (PV)

Definition
- ↑ in RBC mass ± ↑ granulocytes and platelets in the absence of physiologic stimulus

Etiologies of erythrocytosis
- Relative ↑ RBC (↓ plasma): dehydration; "stress" erythrocytosis (Gaisböck's syndrome)
- Absolute ↑ RBC: 1° (PV, other MPD) or 2° due to **hypoxia; carboxyhemoglobinemia; inappropriate erythropoietin** (renal, hepatic, cerebellar tumors); Cushing's syndrome

Clinical manifestations (common between PV and ET)
- Symptoms → often termed "vasomotor symptoms"
  hyperviscosity (erythrocytosis): headache, dizziness, tinnitus, blurred vision
  thrombosis (hyperviscosity, thrombocytosis): transient visual disturbances (amaurosis, ocular migraine); Budd-Chiari syndrome; erythromelalgia = intense burning, pain, and erythema of extremities due to microvascular thrombi
  bleeding (abnormal platelet function): easy bruising, epistaxis, GI bleeding
  ↑ histamine from basophils → **pruritus**, peptic ulcers; ↑ uric acid (cell turnover) → gout
- Signs: **plethora, splenomegaly**, hypertension, engorged retinal veins

Diagnostic evaluation
- ✓ Epo to rule out secondary causes of erythrocytosis; If epo ↓, PV likely
  If epo ↑, then ✓ SaO_2 or PaO_2, carboxyhemoglobin
- Red cell mass is diagnostic "gold standard" test but not commonly done
- ± ↑ WBC, platelets, basophils; ↑ uric acid, leukocyte alkaline phosphatase, vitamin B_{12}
- Peripheral smear → no morphologic abnormalities
- BM bx → hypercellular, megakaryocytic hyperplasia, ↓ iron, absence of Ph chromosome

Treatment
- **Phlebotomy** to moderate degree of Fe deficiency → Hct <45% (men) or <42% (women)
- **Low-dose ASA** in all Pts (NEJM 2004;350:114)
- **Hydroxyurea** if high risk of thrombosis (age ≥60, prior thrombosis) or symptomatic thrombocytosis (plt >1.5 × 10⁶/μl)
- Supportive: allopurinol (gout), H_2-blockers/antihistamines (pruritus)

Prognosis
- Median survival 9-12 y with transformation into acute leukemia in 2% of cases
- Post-PV myeloid metaplasia (spent phase) occurs in 15% of cases, usually after 10 y

ESSENTIAL THROMBOCYTOSIS (ET)

Definition
- ↑ in platelets (>600,000/μl) ± ↑ RBC and granulocytes

Etiologies of thrombocytosis
- 1° = ET or other MPD; myelodysplastic syndromes (5q-syndrome)
- 2° = **reactive thrombocytosis**: inflammation (RA, IBD, vasculitis), infection, acute bleeding, iron deficiency, postsplenectomy, neoplasms (particularly Hodgkin's disease)
- Of Pts w/ plt >10⁶/μl, <1 in 6 will have ET

Clinical manifestations (see "Polycythemia Vera")
- Thrombosis with erythromelalgia (risk of thrombosis highest in Pts with WBC >8700), bleeding, pruritus; mild splenomegaly

Diagnostic evaluation
- Peripheral smear: large hypogranular platelets
- BM bx: megakaryocytic hyperplasia; absence of Philadelphia chromosome and lack of collagen fibrosis; normal iron stores

Treatment of ET			
Risk	Features	ASA 81 mg qd	Cytoreduction
Low	Age <60 and no h/o thrombosis and plt <1.5 x 10^6/µl and no CV risk factors	Consider for vasomotor symptoms	No
Int.	Neither low nor high risk	±	Consider if plt >1.5 x 10^6/µl
High	Age ≥60 or h/o thrombosis or plt >1.5 x 10^6/µl	⊕	**Hydroxyurea** superior to **anagrelide** (NEJM 2005;353:33) Goal plt <400,000/µl

Prognosis
- Overall survival similar to control population with low rate of transformation into PV, AMM/MF or acute leukemia; ∴ low-risk Pts (see below) do not need treatment

AGNOGENIC MYELOID METAPLASIA WITH MYELOFIBROSIS (AMM/MF)

Definition
- Clonal myeloproliferation with reactive marrow fibrosis & extramedullary hematopoiesis

Etiologies of myelophthisis (marrow replacement)
- 1° = agnogenic myeloid metaplasia with myelofibrosis; post-PV/ET myeloid metaplasia
- 2° = hematologic (eg, leukemia, MDS) or metastatic malignancies (eg, breast, prostate)
  collagen vascular disorders (eg, SLE)
  toxins (eg, benzene, radiation)
  granulomas from infection (eg, TB, fungal) or sarcoid
  deposition diseases (eg, Gaucher's disease)

Clinical manifestations (NEJM 2000;342:1255)
- Ineffective erythropoiesis → anemia; extramedullary hematopoiesis → **massive splenomegaly** (abdominal pain, early satiety) ± hepatomegaly
- Tumor bulk and ↑ cell turnover → fatigue, weight loss, fever, sweats

Diagnostic evaluation
- Anemia with variable WBC and platelet counts
- Peripheral smear → **"leukoerythroblastic"** (**teardrop cells**, nucleated RBCs, immature WBCs); large abnormal platelets
- BM aspirate → **"dry" tap**; BM bx → **severe fibrosis**, replacement by reticulin & collagen
- Need to r/o CML (absence of Ph chromosome, BCR-ABL translocation)

Treatment
- Allogeneic HSCT only potential cure → consider in young Pts with poor prognosis
- Supportive care: **transfusions**; inconsistent benefit from androgens or epo; splenectomy for blood counts refractory to transfusion or painful splenomegaly
- Hydroxyurea for significant leukocytosis or thrombocytosis

Complications and prognosis
- Median survival ~5 y; transformation into AML occurs at a rate of ~8%/y
- Worse prognosis with Hb <10 g/dl or with either WBC >30,000/µL or WBC <4,000/µL

CHRONIC MYELOGENOUS LEUKEMIA

(SEE "LEUKEMIA")

LEUKEMIA

ACUTE LEUKEMIA

Definition
- Clonal proliferation of hematopoietic precursor with ↓ ability to differentiate into mature elements → ↑ blasts in bone marrow and periphery → ↓ RBCs, platelets, and neutrophils

Epidemiology and risk factors
- Acute myelogenous leukemia (AML): ~12,000 cases/y; median age 65 y; >80% of adult acute leukemia cases
- Acute lymphocytic leukemia (ALL): ~4000 cases/y; median age 10 y; bimodal with 2nd peak in elderly
- Risk factors: **radiation**, **chemotherapy** (alkylating agents and topoisomerase II inhibitors), benzene, smoking
- Acquired hematopoietic diseases: MDS, MPD (especially CML), aplastic anemia, PNH
- Inherited: Down's & Klinefelter's, Fanconi's anemia, Bloom syndrome, ataxia telangiectasia

Clinical manifestations
- Cytopenias → **fatigue** (anemia), **infection** (neutropenia), **bleeding** (thrombocytopenia)
- More common in **AML**:
  leukostasis (when blast count >50,000/μl): occluded microcirculation → local hypoxemia and hemorrhage → headache, blurred vision, TIA/CVA, dyspnea, hypoxia; look for *hyperviscosity retinopathy* (vascular engorgement, exudates, hemorrhage)
  DIC (especially with APML)
  leukemic infiltration of skin, gingiva (especially with monocytic subtypes M4 and M5)
  chloroma: extramedullary tumor of leukemic cells, virtually any location
- More common in **ALL**:
  bone pain, lymphadenopathy, hepatosplenomegaly (also seen in monocytic AML)
  CNS involvement (~15%): cranial neuropathies, nausea and vomiting, headache
  anterior mediastinal mass (especially in T-cell ALL)
  tumor lysis syndrome (see "Oncologic Emergencies")

Diagnostic evaluation
- **Peripheral smear**: anemia, thrombocytopenia, variable WBC (50% p/w ↑ WBC, 50% p/w normal or ↓ WBC) + circulating **blasts** (seen in >95%)
- **Bone marrow**: hypercellular w/ >20% blasts; cytogenetics, flow cytometry
- Tumor lysis syndrome (rapid cell turnover): ↑ UA, ↑ LDH, ↑ K, ↑ PO₄, ↓ Ca
- Coagulation studies to r/o DIC: PT, PTT, fibrinogen, D-dimer
- LP (w/ co-admin of **intrathecal chemotherapy** to avoid seeding CSF w/ circulating blasts) for *all* Pts (CNS is sanctuary site) and for AML w/ CNS sx
- **TTE** if prior cardiac history or before use of anthracyclines
- **HLA typing** of Pt, siblings, and parents for potential allogeneic HSCT candidates

ACUTE MYELOGENOUS LEUKEMIA (AML)

Classification (NEJM 1999;341:1051)
- Features used to confirm myeloid lineage and subclassify AML to guide treatment:
  morphology: ⊕ **granules**, ± **Auer rods** (eosinophilic needle-like inclusions)
  cytochemistry: ⊕ **myeloperoxidase** and/or **nonspecific esterase**
  FAB class. based on morphology & cytochem., but falling out of favor (except for M3)
  immunophenotype: CD13 & CD33 are myeloid antigens; ⊕ CD41 associated with M7
  cytogenetics: important for prognosis, eg, t(15;17) associated with M3 subtype. Other favorable cytogenetics include t(8;21) associated with M2, and inv16 with M4Eo.

FAB Classification of AML					
Type	Freq	Description	Type	Freq	Description
M0	<5%	No differentiation (maturation)	M4 M4Eo	20%	Myelomonocytic Eo = eosinophilic var.
M1	20%	Myeloblastic w/ min. diff.	M5	20%	Monoblastic
M2	25%	Myeloblastic w/ diff.	M6	5%	Erythroleukemia
M3	10%	Promyelocytic (APML)	M7	<5%	Megakaryoblastic

WHO Classification of AML	
Subtype	Examples
With recurrent genetic abnormalities	t(8;21); inv(16); t(15;17); 11q23 anomalies
With multilineage dysplasia	With or without antecedent MDS or MPD
Therapy-related	Alkylating agents or topoisomerase inhibitors
Not otherwise categorized	Other entities as defined in FAB system

Treatment
- **Induction chemo** (non-M3): "3 + 7" = ida/daunorubicin × 3 d + cytarabine × 7 d
- ✓ for complete remission (CR) = normal peripheral counts, <5% BM blasts
  CR ≠ cure ∴ must always f/u induction with **consolidation Rx**
- If ⊕ CR: consolidation Rx based on risk stratification: chemotherapy or allogeneic or autologous HSCT *(NEJM 1995;332:217; Lancet 1998;351:700; NEJM 1998;339:1649)*
- If ⊖ CR: reinduction with similar chemotherapy
- If relapse after CR: salvage chemotherapy followed by allogeneic or autologous HSCT
- **M3 subtype = APML**: defined by t(15;17) translocation (>95% of cases), biologically distinct; responds to **all-trans-retinoic acid (ATRA)**, which induces differentiation; induction chemotherapy is anthracycline + ATRA ± cytarabine; both untreated and refractory M3 AML also respond to arsenic trioxide; consolidation Rx is followed by prolonged maintenance Rx
- **Supportive care**: hydration + allopurinol or raspuricase for tumor lysis prophylaxis; transfusions ± erythropoietin and G-CSF; antibiotics for fever and neutropenia; hydroxyurea ± leukophoresis for leukostasis

Prognosis
- CR achieved in 70-80% of Pts <60 y and in 40-50% for Pts >60 y
- Overall survival depends on prognostic factors: ranges from ~50% for Pts <60 y w/o poor prognostic factors to <10% for Pts >60 y w/ poor prognostic factors
- Poor prognostic factors: **age >60**, unfavorable cytogenetics (eg, monosomy or del. of chr. 5 or 7, complex karyotype), poor performance score, antecedent MDS/MPD
- Gene expression profiling may be useful *(NEJM 2004;330:1605, 1617; Blood 2007;109:431)*
- APML is the most favorable subtype b/c of response to ATRA (70-80% cure rate)

ACUTE LYMPHOCYTIC LEUKEMIA (ALL)

Classification
- Morphology: **no granules** (granules seen in myeloid lineage)
- Cytochemistry: ⊕ terminal deoxynucleotidyl transferase (TdT) in 95% of ALL
- Cytogenetics: t(9;22) = Philadelphia chromosome (Ph) in ~25% of adults w/ ALL
- Immunohistochemistry distinguishes 3 major phenotypes (Burkitt's usually treated differently)

WHO Immunophenotype Classification of ALL			
WHO Type	FAB	Adult Freq	Immunohistochemistry
Precursor B-cell	L1, L2	75%	⊕ TdT, ⊕ CD19; variable CD10, CD20
Precursor T-cell	L1, L2	20%	⊕ TdT, ⊕ T-cell Ag (CD2, 3, 5, 7) ⊖ CD10, ⊖ mature T-cell Ag (CD4, 8)
B-cell	L3	5%	⊖ TdT, ⊕ surface Ig

Treatment *(NEJM 2006;354:166)*
- **Induction chemo**: combination of cyclophosphamide, doxorubicin, vincristine, methotrexate, steroids, ± asparaginase
- **CNS prophylaxis**: intrathecal MTX/cytarabine ± either cranial irradiation or systemic MTX
- **Postremission therapy** options:
  consolidation/intensification chemo followed by maintenance chemo
  high-dose chemo w/ allo or auto HSCT; survival benefit in high-risk pts w/ allo HSCT
- If relapse → allogeneic HSCT if able
- Ph + t(9;22) → add imatinib & consider for allogeneic HSCT
- MLL-AF4 t(4;11) → consider for allogeneic HSCT

Prognosis
- CR achieved in >90% of children, 80% of adults
- Cure achieved in 50-70% if good prog. factors vs. in 10-30% w/ poor prog. factors
- Good prognostic factors: younger age, WBC <30,000/μl, T-cell immunophenotype, absence of Ph chromosome or t(4;11), early attainment of CR
- Gene expression patterns may be useful in predicting chemo resistance *(NEJM 2004;351:533)*

CHRONIC MYELOGENOUS LEUKEMIA (CML)

Definition (Mayo Clin Proc 2006;81:973)
- **Myeloproliferative disorder** with overproduction of myeloid cells that can differentiate
- **Philadelphia chromosome** (Ph) = t(9;22) → **Bcr-Abl** fusion → ↑ Abl kinase activity
  2-5% of Pts have a cryptic Ph chr., but are *BCR-ABL* PCR ⊕ and respond to imatinib
  5% of Pts are Ph chr. & *BCR-ABL* ⊖; likely distinct disease & does not respond to imatinib

Epidemiology and risk factors
- ~4300 new cases/y in U.S.; median age ~50 at presentation; 15% of adult leukemias
- ↑ risk with irradiation; no clear relation to cytotoxic drugs

Clinical manifestations
- Triphasic clinical course; 85% present in the chronic phase
- **Chronic phase**: often asymptomatic but common features are fatigue, malaise, weight loss, night sweats, abdominal fullness (**splenomegaly** 50%)
- **Accelerated phase**: refractory leukocytosis and worsening symptoms → fever, weight loss, progressive splenomegaly, bone pain, bleeding, infections, pruritus (basophilia)
- **Blastic phase** ≈ acute leukemia → severe constitutional symptoms, infection, bleeding, and possible **leukostasis** (see "Acute Leukemia")

Diagnostic evaluation
- **Peripheral smear**: **leukocytosis** (often >100,000/μl), left-shifted with *all stages of myeloid maturation*; anemia, thrombocytosis, basophilia
- **Bone marrow**: hypercellular, ↑ myeloid to erythroid ratio, ↓ leuk alkaline phosphatase
- **Chronic**: <10% blasts (peripheral or BM)
- **Accelerated**: 10-20% blasts, >20% basos, plts <100k, ↑ spleen size, karyotypic prog.
- **Blastic**: >20% blasts (2/3 myeloid, 1/3 lymphoid), may see extramedullary leukemia

Treatment (NEJM 2003;349:1451 & 2006;355:2408)
- **Imatinib**, a selective inhibitor of the Bcr-Abl tyrosine kinase
  active in chronic, accelerated, and blastic phases (but less as disease advances)
  higher response rates than prior standard of IFN + ara-C (NEJM 2003;348:994, 1423)
  consider for all Pts in chronic phase
- Imatinib resistance associated with *BCR-ABL* mutation or amplification
  newer tyrosine kinase inhibitors such as dasatinib and nilotinib inhibit most imatinib resistance mutations in Bcr-Abl except for T315I (NEJM 2006;354:2531, 2542)
- **Allogeneic HSCT**: consider for Pts w/ available donor who present in accelerated or blastic phase; reasonable option for Pts with relapsed/refractory disease to imatinib

Goals of Imatinib Therapy		
Response	**Definition**	**Goal time**
Hematologic	WBC <10K, Plt <450, <5% myelocytes & metamyelocytes, <20% basos, no immature cells in blood, no extramedullary involvement	3 mo
Cytogenetic	Absence of the Ph chromosome in metaphase cells	12 mo
Molecular	3-log reduction by quantitative PCR	12-18 mo

Prognosis
- Chronic phase CML Rx'd w/ imatinib: 89% overall survival, 7% progression to blast phase at 5 y (NEJM 2006;355:2408)
- Accelerated phase CML Rx'd w/ imatinib: ~50% overall survival at 4 y (Cancer 2005;103:2099)
- Poor prognostic factors: ↑ age, ↑ platelet count, ↑ spleen size, ↑ percentage of blasts

CHRONIC LYMPHOCYTIC LEUKEMIA (CLL)

Definition *(NEJM 2005;352:804)*
- Monoclonal accumulation of immunologically incompetent mature B-lymphocytes
- CLL & small lymphocytic lymphoma (SLL) now classified as same disease (WHO)

Epidemiology and risk factors
- ~10,000 new cases/y; median age at dx is 65 y; most common adult leukemia
- ↑ incidence in 1st-degree relatives; no known association with radiation, chemicals, drugs

Clinical manifestations
- Symptoms: **often asx** & identified when CBC reveals lymphocytosis; 10-20% p/w fatigue, malaise, night sweats, weight loss (ie, lymphoma "B" sx)
- Signs: **lymphadenopathy** (80%) and **hepatosplenomegaly** (50%)
- **Autoimmune hemolytic anemia** (AIHA) or **thrombocytopenia** (ITP)
- Hypogammaglobulinemia ± neutropenia → ↑ susceptibility to **infections**
- Bone marrow failure
- Monoclonal gammopathy in ~5%
- Aggressive transformation: ~5% develop **Richter's syndrome** = transformation into high-grade lymphoma (usually DLBCL) and sudden clinical deterioration

Diagnostic evaluation (see "Lymphoma" for general approach)
- **Peripheral smear**: **lymphocytosis** (>5000/μl, mature-appearing small cells) "smudge" cells from damage to abnl lymphs from shear stress of making blood smear
- **Bone marrow**: normo- or hypercellular; infiltrated w/ small B-cell lymph (≥30%)
- **Lymph nodes**: infiltrated w/ small lymphocytic or diffuse small cleaved cells = SLL
- **Flow cytometry**: dim surface Ig (sIg); CD5+, CD19+, CD20+, CD23+. CD38+ or ZAP70+ a/w unmutated Ig variable heavy chain region & worse prognosis
- **Cytogenetics**: 11q22-23 & 17p13 are unfavorable, trisomy 12 is neutral, while 13q14 is favorable *(NEJM 2000;343:1910)*

	CLL Staging			
Rai System		**Median survival**	**Binet System**	
Stage	**Description**		**Description**	**Stage**
0	Lymphocytosis *only*	>10 y	<3 node areas	A
I	⊕ lymphadenopathy	7 y	>3 node areas	B
II	⊕ hepatosplenomegaly			
III	⊕ anemia (not AIHA)	1-2 y	Anemia or thrombocytopenia	C
IV	⊕ thrombocytopenia (not ITP)			

Treatment
- Treatment is *palliative* → early stage disease can be followed w/o Rx
- Indications for treatment: Rai stages III/IV, Binet stage C, disease-related sx, progressive disease, AIHA or ITP refractory to steroids, recurrent infections
- Options for treatment
  purine analogs: fludarabine ("F"), pentostatin ("P")
  alkylating agents: cyclophosphamide ("C"), CVP, CHOP; chlorambucil for elderly
  monoclonal Ab against CD20 (rituximab, "R") or CD52 (alemtuzumab)
  ≈ survival w/ single agents, although higher response rate w/ F *(NEJM 2000;343:1750)*
  combination regimens most popular (ie, FR, FC, FCR, PCR)
- Role of autologous and allogeneic HSCT being studied
- Supportive care: PCP, HZV, VZV prophylaxis; CMV monitoring for Pts receiving CD52; AIHA/ITP → steroids; recurrent infections → IVIg; bulky disease with compressive symptoms → XRT; splenomegaly with refractory cytopenias → splenectomy

Prognostic Factors & Median Survival in CLL			
Factor	**Years**	**Factor**	**Years**
Cytogenetics		*CD38 expression*	
17p-	2.5	Low (<20-30%)	8
11q-	6.6	High (>20-30%)	Unclear
Trisomy 12 or Normal	9	*Zap-70 expression*	
13q-	11	Low (<20-30%)	24.3
IgVH gene status		High (>20-30%)	9.3
Mutated (>2%)*	>24	*% difference c/w germline	
Unmutated (<2%)*	<8		

(NEJM 2004;351:893 & 2005;353:1793)

LYMPHOMA

Definition
- Malignant disorder of lymphoid cells that reside predominantly in lymphoid tissues
- **Hodgkin's lymphoma** (HL) is distinguished from **non-Hodgkin's lymphoma** (NHL) by the presence of **Reed-Sternberg** (RS) **cells**

Clinical manifestations
- Lymphadenopathy (nontender)

    HL: superficial (usually **cervical/supraclavicular**) ± mediastinal lymphadenopathy; **nodal** disease with **orderly, anatomic spread** to adjacent nodes

    NHL: diffuse; **nodal and extranodal** disease with **noncontiguous spread**; symptoms reflect involved sites (abdominal fullness, bone pain)
- Constitutional ("B") symptoms: **fever** (>38°), **sweats**, **weight loss** (>10% over 6 mos)

    HL: periodic, recurrent "Pel-Ebstein" fever; 10-15% have pruritus

    NHL: "B" symptoms less common than in HL

Diagnostic and staging evaluation
- History: "B" symptoms
- Physical exam: lymph nodes, liver/spleen size, Waldeyer's ring, testes (1% of NHL), skin
- Pathology: **excisional lymph node bx** (not FNA, need surrounding architecture) with immunophenotyping and cytogenetics; **BM bx** (except in HL clinical stage IA/IIA with favorable features); LP if CNS involvement is clinically suspected
- Laboratory tests: CBC, BUN/Cr, LFTs, ESR, LDH, uric acid, Ca, albumin

    Consider HIV, HBV, HCV, HTLV, & EBV serologies and connective tissue diseases autoAbs
- Imaging: **chest/abd/pelvic CT** (but don't reliably detect spleen/liver involvement) ∴ need 2nd modality: **gallium or PET scans**

    head CT/MRI if neurological symptoms; bone scan if bony pain or if Aϕ elevated

Ann Arbor Staging System with Cotswolds Modifications	
Stage	**Features**
I	Single lymph node (LN) region
II	≥2 LN regions on the same side of the diaphragm
III	LN regions on both sides of the diaphragm
IV	Disseminated involvement of one or more extralymphatic organs
Modifiers: A = no symptoms; B = fever, night sweats or weight loss; X = bulky disease = greatest transverse diam. of mediastinal mass / max diam. of chest wall >1/3 on CXR or >10 cm if in abd; E = involves single contiguous extranodal site; H = hepatic; S = splenic	

HODGKIN'S LYMPHOMA (HL)

Epidemiology and risk factors
- ~7,500 cases/y; bimodal distribution (15-35 & >50 y); ↑ male; ? role for EBV

Pathology
- Affected nodes show RS cells (<1%) in background of non-neoplastic inflammatory cells
- Classic RS cells: bilobed nucleus & prominent nucleoli with surrounding clear space ("owl's eyes"). RS cells are **clonal B-cells**: CD15+, CD30+, CD20- by flow cytometry.

Rye Histologic Classification of Classical HL		
Lymphocyte predominance	5%	Abundant normal-appearing lymphocytes; mediastinal LAN uncommon; male predominance; good prognosis
Nodular sclerosis	60-80%	Collagen bands; frequent mediastinal LAN; young adults; female predominance; usually stage I/II at dx
Mixed cellularity	15-30%	Pleomorphic; older age; male predominance; ≥50% stage III/VI at presentation; intermediate prognosis
Lymphocyte depletion	<1%	Diffuse fibrosis and large numbers of RS cells; older, male patients; disseminated at dx; seen in HIV; worst prognosis

- **Nonclassical** (5%): nodular lymphocyte predominant (NLP); involves peripheral LN 80% present in stage I-II and Rx can be RT alone or ABVD + RT w/ 80% 10-y progression-free survival, 93% overall survival (JCO 1997;15;3060)

    Consider rituximab as most NLP RS cells are CD20 +

    Stage III-IV treated as classical HL (see below)

Classical HL Stage I-II Disease Treatment	
Modalities	**Description**
Combined Modality Therapy (CMT)	Usually ABVD × 4-6 cycles ± involved field radiotherapy (IFRT)
	Stanford V + IFRT is an option as well
	XRT should be strongly considered for all bulky sites
Chemo Alone	Emerging modality given long-term toxicities of XRT
	2 cycles past best response (usually ABVD × 6)
	Slightly worse disease-free survival vs. CMT, but overall survival same
Radiation Alone	Historically came first; now rarely used given long-term toxicities
	Consider only for isolated stage IA disease

(JCO 2005;23:6400)

HL Stage III-IV International Prognostic Score (IPS) and Treatment			
Prognosis		**Chemotherapy regimens**	**Radiotherapy**
IPS	**5-y PFS**		
0	84%		Consider to initial bulky sites or if PET ⊕ after chemotherapy
1	77%	ABVD (preferred 1st line) (NEJM 1992;327:1478)	
2	67%	? Stanford V (JCO 2002;20:630)	
3	60%	Consider BEACOPP if IPS ≥4 (Blood 2004:104:91a)	
4	51%		
≥5	42%		

IPS (negative prognostic indicators): Alb <4 g/dl; Hb <10.5 g/dl; male; age ≥45 y; Stage IV; WBC ≥15k/μl; Lymph <600/μl or <8% of differential (NEJM 1998;339:1506)

- ABVD (doxorubicin, bleomycin, vinblastine, dacarbazine): usually 6-8 cycles
- Stanford V (doxorubicin, bleomycin, vinblastine, vincristine, mechlorethamine, etoposide, prednisone): usually 3 cycles
- BEACOPP (bleomycin, etoposide, doxorubicin, cyclophosphamide, vincristine, procarbazine, and prednisone) in regular and escalated doses
- Relapsed disease: salvage chemo, high-dose chemo + auto HSCT, allo HSCT
- Pts at risk for **second malignancies**: acute leukemia/MDS, NHL, lung cancer (related to both radiation and chemotherapy), breast cancer (radiation)

Non-Hodgkin's Lymphoma (NHL)

Epidemiology and risk factors
- ~53,000 new cases/y; median age at diagnosis ~65 y; male predominance
- Associated conditions: immunodeficiency (eg, HIV, posttransplant); autoimmune disorders (eg, Sjögren's, RA, SLE); infection (eg, EBV, HTLV-I, *H. pylori*)
- Burkitt's lymphoma: (1) endemic or African (jaw mass, 80-90% EBV-related); (2) sporadic or American (20% EBV-related); (3) HIV-related

WHO/REAL Classification System of NHL	
Aggressiveness	**Lymphomas** (90% B cell, 10% T cell or NK cell)
Indolent (35-40%)	**follicular lymphoma**
	small lymphocytic lymphoma (SLL) / CLL
	plasma cell myeloma, marginal zone lymphoma (includes MALT), mantle cell lymphoma, lymphoplasmacytic lymphoma (~ Waldenström's), hairy cell leukemia, T-cell/NK cell tumors (mycosis fungoides, T-cell large granular lymphocyte leukemia, T-cell prolymphocytic leukemia, NK cell large granular lymphocyte leukemia)
Aggressive (~50%)	**diffuse large B-cell lymphoma** (DLBCL)
	follicular lymphoma (grade III)
	peripheral T-cell lymphoma, anaplastic large cell lymphoma
Highly aggressive (~5%)	**Burkitt's lymphoma**
	precursor B lymphoblastic leukemia (= pre B-ALL) / **lymphoma**
	precursor T lymphoblastic leukemia (= T-ALL) / **lymphoma**
	adult T-cell lymphoma/leukemia

Treatment
- Treatment and prognosis determined by histopathologic classification rather than stage
- **Indolent**: goal is symptom management (bulky disease, cytopenias, "B" sx)
  Options include radiation for localized disease, single-agent chemotherapy (chlorambucil, cyclophosphamide, fludarabine), combination chemotherapy, and rituximab. Newer rituximab radioimmunotherapy (RIT) conjugates include I[131] tositumomab and Y[90] ibritumomab tiuxetan.

- **Aggressive** (DLBCL): goal is cure (JCO 2005;23:6387)
  - **CHOP-R** (cyclophosphamide, doxorubicin = hydroxydaunorubicin, vincristine = Oncovorin, prednisone, rituximab) (NEJM 2002;346:235); CHOP alone if CD20 negative
    5-y progression-free survival = 54%; overall survival = 58% (JCO 2005;23:4117)
    + **Radiation** for localized or bulky disease
  - **CNS prophylaxis** w/ intrathecal or systemic high-dose methotrexate if paranasal sinus, testicular, breast, periorbital, paravertebral, or bone marrow involved; ≥2 extranodal site + ↑ LDH may also warrant
  - Relapse: salvage chemo; high-dose chemo + auto-HSCT (NEJM 1995;333:1540); allo-HSCT if beyond 2nd relapse
- **Highly Aggressive**
  - Burkitt's: treat with short bursts of intensive chemotherapy (Blood 2004;104:3009)
  - Low risk defined as nl LDH & single focus of disease <10 cm; all others high risk
  - Low risk Rx = CODOX-M (cyclophosphamide, vincristine, doxorubicin, high-dose methotrexate ± rituximab) (Leuk Lymph 2004;45:761)
  - High risk Rx = CODOX-M/IVAC (above w/ ifosfamide, etoposide, high-dose cytarabine)
  - All Pts receive CNS prophylaxis and tumor lysis syndrome prophylaxis
  - Lymphoblastic lymphoma (B- or T-cell): treated like ALL (see "Acute Leukemia")

Prognosis
- Indolent: ↓ response to chemotherapy, but long median survival

Follicular Lymphoma International Prognostic Index (FLIPI)		
Factors: age >60, stage III/IV, Hb <12 g/dl, >4 nodal areas, LDH >nl		
# Factors	5-y Overall Survival	10-y Overall Survival
0-1	90%	71%
2	78%	51%
≥3	52%	35%

(Blood 2004;104:1258)

- Aggressive: ↑ chance of cure, but overall worse prognosis

International Prognostic Index (IPI) for Aggressive NHL		
Factors: age >60, stage III/IV, ≥2 extranodal sites, performance status ≥2, LDH >nl		
# Factors	Complete Response	5-y Overall Survival
0-1	87%	73%
2	67%	51%
3	55%	43%
4-5	44%	26%
Revised IPI Prognosis in Patients Rx'd with CHOP-R		
# Factors	% at dx	4-y Overall Survival
0	10%	94%
1-2	45%	79%
3-5	45%	55%

(NEJM 1993;329:987; Blood 2007;109:1857)

HIV-associated NHL (Blood 2006;107:13)
- HIV ⊕ imparts 60-100× relative risk
- NHL is an AIDS-defining malignancy along with Kaposi's, cervical CA, anal CA
- Concurrent HAART & chemotherapy likely provides survival benefit
- DLBCL & immunoblastic lymphoma (67%): CD4 <100, EBV associated
  Treat as non-HIV (CHOP-R), but avoid rituximab if CD4 <100
- Burkitt's and Burkitt's-like (20%): can occur with CD4 >200
  Treat as non-HIV disease, though prognosis is significantly worse
- Primary CNS lymphoma (16%): CD4 <50, EBV associated
  Treat with high-dose methotrexate + steroids ± RT
- Primary effusion lymphoma (<5%): HHV8 driven
  Treat with standard CHOP, but poor prognosis

PLASMA CELL DYSCRASIAS

MULTIPLE MYELOMA (MM)

Definition and epidemiology
- Malignant proliferation of **plasma cells** producing a monoclonal Ig = "**M component**"
- ~14,600 new cases and ~10,900 deaths/y in U.S.; median age at diagnosis 66 y
- African-American:Caucasian ratio ≈ 2:1

Clinical manifestations
- **Anemia** (normocytic) due to myelophthisis, ↓ bone marrow production, autoimmune Ab
- **Bone pain** and **hypercalcemia** due to ↑ osteoclast activity → lytic lesions, pathologic fx
- **Recurrent infections** due to hypogammaglobulinemia (excluding M component)
  pneumonia and pyelonephritis are the most common infections
- **Renal disease**: multiple mechanisms
  toxic effect of filtered light chains → **renal failure** (cast nephropathy) or **type II RTA**
  amyloidosis or light chain deposition disease → **nephrotic syndrome**
  hypercalcemia, urate nephropathy, type I cryoglobulinemia
- Neurologic: cord compression; POEMS (polyneuropathy, organomegaly,
  endocrinopathy, M protein, skin changes) syndrome
- Hyperviscosity: usually when IgM >4 g/dl, IgG >5 g/dl, or IgA >7 g/dl
- Coagulopathy: inhibition of or Ab against clotting factor; Ab-coated platelets
- Amyloidosis (see "Amyloidosis")

Diagnostic and staging evaluation
- **Criteria** = marrow plasmacytosis >10% (or presence of a plasmacytoma) and one of
  following: lytic bone lesions or M component in either serum (usually >3 g/dl) or urine
- **Variants:**
  smoldering MM (asx w/ M >3 g/dl and/or plasmacytosis >10%)
  solitary bone plasmacytoma (single lytic lesion w/o marrow plasmacytosis)
  extramedullary plasmacytoma (usually upper respiratory tract)
  plasma cell leukemia (plasma cell count >2,000/μl)
  nonsecretory MM (marrow plasmacytosis & lytic lesions, but no M component)
- Ddx of M component: MM, MGUS (see below), CLL, lymphoma, cirrhosis, sarcoidosis, RA
- Peripheral smear → rouleaux; ✓ Ca, alb, Cr; ↓ anion gap, ↑ globulin, ↑ ESR
- **Protein electrophoresis and immunofixation**
  serum protein electrophoresis (SPEP): quantitates M component; ⊕ in ~80% of Pts
  urine protein electrophoresis (UPEP): detects the ~20% of Pts who secrete only light
  chains (= Bence Jones proteins), which are filtered rapidly from the blood
  immunofixation: shows component is monoclonal and identifies Ig type → IgG (50%),
  IgA (20%), IgD (2%), IgM (0.5%), light chain only (20%), nonsecretors (<5%)
  serum-free light chain assay: important test for dx and to follow treatment response
- **Bone marrow biopsy**
- **Skeletal survey** (plain radiographs) to identify lytic bone lesions and areas at risk for
  pathologic fracture; bone scan is not useful for detecting lytic lesions
- **Staging**: International (JCO 2005;23:3412) vs. Durie-Salmon System (Cancer 1975;36:842)

ISS (↑ β2m most powerful independent poor prognostic factor)		
Stage	β2-microglobulin	Albumin
I	<3.5 mg/l *and*	>3.5 g/dl
II	3.6-5.4 mg/l *or*	<3.5 g/dl
III	>5.5 mg/l	Any

Durie-Salmon Staging System		
Stage	Criteria	Median survival
I	*all of the following:* Hb >10 g/dl; Ca ≤12 mg/dl; 0-1 lytic bone lesions IgG <5 g/dl or IgA <3 g/dl or urine light chain <4 g/24 h	61 mo
II	fulfilling criteria for neither I nor III	55 mo
III	*any of the following:* Hb <8.5 g/dl; Ca >12 mg/dl; >5 lytic bone lesions IgG >7 g/dl or IgA >5 g/dl or urine light chain >12 g/24 h	30 mo for IIIA 15 mo for IIIB
Subclassification by serum Cr: A <2 mg/dl; B ≥2 mg/dl		

Treatment (NEJM 2004;351:1860)
- Treatment not indicated for smoldering MM or asymptomatic stage I disease
- **Systemic chemotherapy**: ↑ median survival, but not curative
  regimens include melphalan, prednisone or dexamethasone, thalidomide or
  lenalidomide (NEJM 1999;341:1565), bortezomib (proteasome inhibitor; NEJM
  2003;348:2609; 2005;352:2487), or combinations
  melphalan + prednisone + thalidomide if auto-HSCT not an option (Lancet 2006;367:825)
- High-dose chemo + **auto-HSCT**: not curative, but ↑ survival c/w conventional chemo
  (NEJM 1996;335:91 & 2003;348:1875); ∴ offer to good candidates <70 y;
  + thalidomide → ↑ response rate but no Δ in overall survival (NEJM 2006;354:1021)
  double auto-HSCT ↑ survival, espec. if poor response to 1st auto (NEJM 2003;349:2495)
- Local radiation for solitary or extramedullary plasmacytoma
- Adjunctive treatment
  bone: **bisphosphonates** (NEJM 1996;334:488), XRT for sx bony lesions
  renal: *avoid NSAIDs & IV contrast*; consider plasmapheresis for acute renal failure
  hyperviscosity syndrome: plasmapheresis
  infections: consider IVIg for recurrent infections

MONOCLONAL GAMMOPATHY OF UNCERTAIN SIGNIFICANCE (MGUS)

Definition and epidemiology (NEJM 2006;355:2765)
- M component <3 g/dl, no urinary Bence Jones proteins, marrow plasmacytosis <10%,
  and no lytic bone lesions, anemia, hypercalcemia, or renal insufficiency
- Prevalence ~3% in population >50 y of age, ~5% in population >70 y of age, and
  7.5% in population >85 y of age (NEJM 2006;354:1362)

Management
- ✓ CBC, Ca, Cr, SPEP and UPEP with immunofixation to exclude MM
- Close observation: repeat SPEP in 6 mos and then yearly thereafter if stable

Prognosis (NEJM 2002;346:564)
- ~1%/y or ~25% lifetime risk → MM, WM, amyloidosis, or malign. lymphoproliferative dis.
- Abnormal serum-free light chain ratio associated w/ ↑ risk of progression to MM (Blood
  2005;105:812)

WALDENSTRÖM'S MACROGLOBULINEMIA (WM)

Definition (JCO 2005;23:1564)
- Low-grade NHL (lymphoplasmacytic lymphoma) that secretes IgM
- *No evidence of bone lesions* (IgM M component + lytic bone lesions = "IgM myeloma")

Clinical manifestations
- **Tumor infiltration**: BM (cytopenias), hepatomegaly, splenomegaly, lymphadenopathy
- **Circulating IgM**
  hyperviscosity syndrome (~15%)
  neurologic: blurred vision ("sausage" retinal veins on funduscopy), HA, dizziness, Δ MS
  cardiac: congestive heart failure
  pulmonary: pulmonary infiltrates
  type I **cryoglobulinemia** → **Raynaud's phenomenon**
  anemia (prominent **rouleaux**; 10% Coombs' ⊕ = AIHA)
  mucosal bleeding due to abnormalities in platelet fxn
- **IgM deposition**
  peripheral neuropathy: may be due to IgM against myelin-associated glycoprotein
  amyloidosis
  glomerulopathy

Diagnostic evaluation
- SPEP + immunofixation with IgM >3 g/dl; only 20% have ⊕ UPEP
- Bone marrow biopsy: ↑ plasmacytoid lymphocytes
- **Relative serum viscosity**: defined as ratio of viscosity of serum to H_2O (normal
  ratio 1.8) hyperviscosity syndrome when relative serum viscosity >5-6

Treatment
- Hyperviscosity: **plasmapheresis**
- Symptoms: systemic chemotherapy with chlorambucil, fludarabine, cladribine, rituximab,
  or combination therapy
- Thalidomide and HSCT are investigational modalities

Transplantation of donor pluripotent cells that can reconstitute all recipient blood lineages

Categories of Stem Cell Transplantation		
Feature	Allogeneic (Allo)	Autologous (Auto)
Donor-recipient relationship	Immunologically distinct	Donor is also recipient
Graft-versus-host disease	Yes	No
Graft-versus-tumor effect	Yes	No
Risk of graft contam. w/ tumor	No	Yes
Relapse risk (leukemia)	Lower	Higher
Transplant-related mortality	Higher	Lower

- **Graft-versus-host disease (GVHD)**: *undesirable* side effect of allo HSCT
  allogeneic T cells view host cells as foreign; ↑ incid. w/ mismatch or unrelated donors
  ∴ need post-transplant immunosuppression
- **Graft-versus-tumor (GVT)** effect: *desirable* consequence of allo HSCT;
  allogeneic T cells attack host tumor cells

Indications *(NEJM 2006;354:1813)*
- **Malignant disease**:
  Auto HSCT allows **higher doses of chemo** by rescuing hematopoietic system
    (used for lymphoma, multiple myeloma, testicular cancer)
  Allo HSCT produces **graft-versus-tumor** (GVT) effect, in addition to
    hematopoietic rescue (used for AML, ALL, CML, CLL, MDS, lymphoma)
- **Nonmalignant disease**: allo HSCT replaces abnormal lymphohematopoietic
  system with one from normal donor (eg, immunodeficiencies, aplastic anemia,
  hemoglobinopathies, possibly autoimmune disorders)

Transplantation procedure
- **Preparative regimen**: *eradication of disease* for which transplant is being performed and
  immunosuppression to prevent rejection of transplanted graft (allo only)
  myeloablative (traditional): chemotherapy and/or total body irradiation
  nonmyeloablative: low-intensity conditioning regimen → ↓ toxicity to allow Pts w/
    comorbidities or older Pts to tolerate HSCT. Allows mixed chimeric state in an
    attempt to temper GVHD while harnessing GVT effect.
- **Sources of stem cells**:
  bone marrow: original source, most experience
  peripheral blood stem cells (PBSC): faster engraftment, easier collection
  umbilical cord blood: less stringent HLA-matching requirements, though fewer
    available cells from donor (multiple donors can be combined), slower engraftment
- **Absolute neutrophil count (ANC)** recovers to 500/μl w/in ~3 wks w/ BM and
  ~2 wks w/ PBSC. G-CSF accelerates recovery by 3-5 d in both scenarios.

Complications
- Either **direct chemoradiotoxicites** associated with preparative regimen or consequences
  of **interaction between donor and recipient immune systems**

Timing and Mechanism of Noninfectious Complications of HSCT			
Timing	<30 d	30-90 d	>90 d
Regimen-related	Pancytopenia		Growth failure
	Mucositis, rash, alopecia		Hypogonadism/infertility
	Nausea, vomiting, diarrhea		Hypothyroidism
	Peripheral neuropathies		Cataracts
	Hemorrhagic cystitis		Avascular necrosis of bone
	Veno-occlusive disease		Second malignancy
	Interstitial pneumonitis		
Immune-mediated	Acute GVHD		Chronic GVHD
	Primary graft failure	Secondary graft failure	

- **Sinusoidal obstruction syndrome** (**SOS**; incidence ~10%, mortality ~30%)
  Previously known as **veno-occlusive disease** (**VOD**)
  Mech: direct cytotoxic injury to hepatic venules → *in situ* thrombosis
  Symptoms: tender hepatomegaly, ascites, jaundice, fluid retention
    with severe disease → liver failure, encephalopathy, hepatorenal syndrome
  Diagnosis: ↑ALT/AST, ↑ bilirubin; ↑ PT with severe disease; Doppler U/S *may* show
    reversal of portal vein flow; ↑ hepatic wedge pressure; abnl liver bx
  Treatment: supportive; prophylaxis with **ursodiol** or low-dose heparin; defibrotide
- **Idiopathic interstitial pneumonitis** (**IIP**, up to 70% mortality)
  Mech: alveolar injury due to direct toxicity → fever, hypoxia, diffuse pulmonary infiltrates
  Diffuse alveolar hemorrhage (**DAH**): subset of IIP
  Diagnosis: bronchoscopy to exclude infection; ↑ bloody lavage fluid seen with DAH
  Treatment: high-dose corticosteroids (limited data)
- **Acute GVHD** (within 3 mos of transplant)
  Clinical grade I-IV based on scores for **skin** (severity of maculopapular rash), **liver**
    (bilirubin level), and **GI** (volume of diarrhea); bx supports diagnosis
  Prevention: **immunosuppression** (MTX + CsA or tacrolimus) ± T-cell depletion of graft
  Treatment: grade I → none; grade II-IV-associated with ↓ survival and ∴ treated with
    immunosuppressants (corticosteroids, CsA, tacrolimus, rapamycin, rituximab)
- **Chronic GVHD** (developing or persisting beyond 3 mos posttransplant)
  Clinical: malar rash, sicca syndrome, arthritis, obliterative bronchiolitis, bile duct
    degeneration and cholestasis
  Treatment: immunosuppression as above; photopheresis
- **Graft failure**
  Primary = persistent neutropenia without evidence of engraftment
  Secondary = delayed pancytopenia after initial engraftment; either immune mediated due
    to attack by immunocompetent host cells in the allogeneic setting (termed **graft
    rejection**) or non-immune mediated (eg, CMV infection)
- **Infectious complications**
  due to regimen-induced pancytopenia and immunosuppression
  auto HSCT recipients do not require immunosuppression and ∴ remain at ↑ risk only
    during the pre-engraftment and immediate postengraftment phases
  both primary infections and reactivation events occur (eg, CMV, HSV, VZV)

Infectious Complications Following Allogeneic HSCT			
	Time after transplant and associated risk factors		
Class of pathogen and associated prophylaxis	**Days 0-30** Mucositis Organ dysfunction Neutropenia	**Days 30-90** Acute GVHD ↓ cellular immunity	**>90 days** Chronic GVHD ↓ cellular & humoral immunity
Viral acyclovir to d 365 (HSV/VZV); valganciclovir or ganciclovir if CMV ⊕ (monitor until d 100 or until no longer immunesupp.)	Respiratory and enteral viruses		
	HSV*	CMV*, HHV 6 & 7	
		EBV-related lymphoma	
			VZV*, BK/JC
Bacterial antibiotics (eg, fluoroquinolone) while neutropenic	Gram ⊕ cocci (coagulase-negative staph., S. aureus, S. viridans) GNRs (Enterobacteriaceae, Pseudomonas, Legionella, S. maltophilia)		Encapsulated bacteria
Fungal fluconazole to d 75 for Candida	Candida spp.		
	Aspergillus spp.		
Parasitic TMP-SMX to d 180 (or off immunosuppression) for PCP		T. gondii P. carinii S. stercoralis	T. gondii P. carinii

*Primarily among persons who are seropositive before transplant

LUNG CANCER

Epidemiology and risk factors
- Most common cause of cancer-related death for both men and women in U.S.
- **Cigarette smoking**: 85% of all lung cancers occur in smokers
  risk proportional to total pack-years; ↓ risk after quitting or reducing, but not to baseline (*JAMA* 2005;294:1505)
  squamous & small cell almost exclusively in smokers
  adenocarcinoma most common type in nonsmokers
  bronchioalveolar carcinoma associated with females, nonsmokers, EGFR mutations
- Asbestos: when combined with smoking, synergistic ↑ in risk of lung cancer
- Radon: risk to general population unclear

Pathology
- **Non-small cell lung cancer (NSCLC)**: ~85% of lung cancers in U.S.
  Peripheral: adenocarcinoma, large cell carcinoma
  Central: squamous cell carcinoma
  Bronchioalveolar carcinoma: track along airways, can be multifocal
- **Small cell lung cancer (SCLC)**: ~15% of lung cancers in U.S.; typically central

Clinical manifestations
- ~10% are asymptomatic at presentation and are detected incidentally by imaging
- **Endobronchial growth** of 1° tumor: cough, hemoptysis, dyspnea, wheezing, post-obstructive pneumonia; more common with squamous or small cell (central location)
- **Regional spread**
  pleural effusion, pericardial effusion, hoarseness (recurrent laryngeal nerve palsy), dysphagia (esophageal compression), stridor (tracheal obstruction)
  Pancoast's syndrome: apical tumor → brachial plexus involvement (C8,T1,T2) → Horner's syndrome, shoulder pain, rib destruction, atrophy of hand muscles
  superior vena cava syndrome: central tumor → SVC compression → dyspnea, headache, facial swelling, venous distention of neck and chest wall
- **Extrathoracic metastases**: brain, bone, liver, adrenal, skin
- **Paraneoplastic syndromes**
  Endocrine
  ACTH (SCLC) → **Cushing's syndrome**; ADH (SCLC) → **SIADH**
  PTH-rP (squamous cell) → **hypercalcemia**
  Skeletal: digital clubbing (non-small cell), **hypertrophic pulmonary osteoarthropathy** (adenocarcinoma) = symmetric polyarthritis and proliferative periostitis of long bones
  Neurologic (usually small cell): **Eaton-Lambert**, periph. neuropathy, cerebellar degen.
  Cutaneous: acanthosis nigricans, dermatomyositis
  Hematologic: hypercoagulable state (adenocarcinoma), DIC, marantic endocarditis

Screening (*NEJM* 2005;352:2714)
- No proven survival benefit to screening CXR or sputum cytology, even in high-risk Pts
- Survival benefit of screening chest CT in observational studies controversial (*NEJM* 2006;355:1763; *JAMA* 2007;297:953); await RCTs

Diagnostic and staging evaluation
- **Imaging**: CXR, chest CT (include liver and adrenal glands)
- **Tissue**
  bronchoscopy (for central lesions) or **CT-guided needle biopsy** (for peripheral lesions or accessible sites of suspected metastasis)
  mediastinoscopy (lymph node bx), VATS (eval. of pleura peripheral lesions), thoracentesis (cell block for cytology), or sputum cytology (for central lesions)
- **Staging**
  Intrathoracic: mediastinoscopy or VATS; thoracentesis if pleural effusion
  Extrathoracic:
  PET scan or integrated PET-CT more Se than CT alone for detecting mediastinal and distant mets as well as bone mets (*NEJM* 2000;343:254 & 2003;348:2500)
  brain MRI for all Pts and bone scan for those w/ localizing sx or lab abnormalities
- PFTs with quantitative V/Q if planned treatment includes surgical resection

TNM Staging System for NSCLC					
	N stage	N0	N1	N2	N3
T stage	**Definition**	no ⊕ nodes	ipsilat. hilar	ipsilat. mediast.	contralat. or supraclav.
T1	Tumor ≤3 cm	IA	IIA		
T2	Tumor >3 cm	IB	IIB		
T3	Direct invasion of chest wall, diaphragm, mediast. pleura, pericard.	IIB		IIIA	
T4	Malig. pleural effusion; invasion of mediast., heart, great vessels, trachea, carina, esophagus, vertebral body				IIIB

NSCLC treatment

- **Stages I & II**: surgical resection + **adjuvant chemo** for stage IB-II (NEJM 2004;350:351 & 2005;352:2589); gene expression data identifies early NSCLC w/ ↑ risk of recurrence that may benefit from more aggressive chemo (NEJM 2006;355:570)
- **Stage III**: optimal **combo/sequence of chemo, radiation, & surgery** unknown IIIA has been viewed as potentially resectable and IIIB as unresectable neoadjuvant chemoradiation may convert unresectable → resectable
- **Stage IV**: **chemotherapy** ↑ survival c/w best supportive care standard is a platinum-based doublet (eg, carboplatin + paclitaxel) *no single regimen proven superior* (NEJM 2002;346:92) palliative radiation used to control local symptoms caused by tumor or metastasis solitary brain metastasis: surgical resection + whole brain irradiation may ↑ survival
- **Biologic therapy** (for stage IIIB/IV) erlotinib (EGFR inhibitor) if progress after chemo → ↑ median survival by 2 mos c/w supportive care (NEJM 2005;353:123); consider targeting to Pts w/ EGFR mutations (more common in Asians, females, nonsmokers, bronchioalveolar histology) bevacizumab (anti-VEGF mAb) added to chemo → ↑ median survival by 2 mos; ↑ risk of bleeding, ∴ exclude if brain mets or squamous cell CA (hemoptysis) (NEJM 2006;355:2542)

NSCLC Simplified Staging Schema, Treatment, and 5-y survival				
Stage	**at dx**	**Definition**	**Treatment**	**5-y**
I	10%	Isolated lesion	Surgery + chemo	>60%
II	20%	Hilar node spread	Surgery ± radiation ± chemo	40-50%
IIIA	15%	Mediast. spread, but resectable	Neoadjuvant chemotherapy ± radiation → surgical resection	25-30%
IIIB	15%	Unresectable	Chemotherapy ± radiation ± biologic ± surgery (selected cases)	10-20%
IV	40%	Metastatic	Chemo ± biologic and/or supportive care Palliative radiation	1%

NSCLC prognosis

- ERCC1 (excision repair cross-complementation group 1) expression may identify Pts who do not respond to cisplatin-based chemo (NEJM 2006;355:983)
- Gene expression data may aid in prognosis (NEJM 2006;355:570 & 2007;356:11)

SCLC Treatment

- SCLC usually disseminated at presentation, but can be **very** responsive to chemoradiation
- **Chemotherapy** (platinum + etoposide) is primary treatment modality
- **Thoracic radiation** added to chemotherapy improves survival in limited stage disease
- **Prophylactic cranial irradiation** (PCI) improves survival for limited stage disease in complete remission (NEJM 1999;341:476)

SCLC Staging Schema and Treatment				
Stage	**% at dx**	**Definition**	**Treatment**	**Median survival**
Limited	30-40%	Confined to ipsilat. hemithorax w/in one radiation port	Radiation + chemotherapy ± PCI	1-2 y
Extensive	60-70%	Beyond one radiation port	Chemotherapy	~1 y

BREAST CANCER

Epidemiology and risk factors (Risk assessment tool: www.cancer.gov/bcrisktool/)
- Most common cancer in U.S. women; 2nd most common cause of cancer death in women
- **Age**: incidence rates ↑ with age, with decrease in slope at age of menopause
- **Genetics** (NEJM 2003;348:2339): 15-20% have ⊕ FHx
    Risk depends on # of affected 1st-degree relatives and their age at dx
    ~45% of cases of familial cases are associated with known germline mutations
    BRCA1/2: 50-85% lifetime risk of breast cancer & ↑ risk of **ovarian cancer**; ? ↑ colon & prostate cancer; BRCA2: also w/ ↑ *male* breast cancer and ? ↑ pancreatic cancer
- Endogenous or exogenous **estrogen**: ↑ risk with early menarche, late menopause, late parity, or nulliparity (NEJM 2006;354:270); ↑ risk with prolonged HRT (RR = 1.24 after 5.6 y, JAMA 2003;289:3243); no ↑ risk shown with OCP use (NEJM 2002;346:2025)
- Benign breast conditions: ↑ risk w/ atypia (atypical ductal or lobular hyperplasia) & proliferative (ductal hyperplasia, papilloma, radial scar, or sclerosing adenosis) features; no ↑ risk w/ cysts, fibroadenoma, or columnar changes (NEJM 2005;352:229)
- Radiation

Clinical manifestations
- Breast mass (hard, irregular, fixed, nontender; nipple discharge (higher risk if unilateral, limited to one duct, bloody, associated with mass)
- Special types: **Paget's** disease → unilateral nipple eczema + nipple discharge; **inflammatory** breast cancer → skin erythema and edema (peau d'orange)
- Metastases: lymph nodes, bone, liver, lung, brain

Screening
- **Self breast exam** (SBE): no proven mortality benefit (JNCI 2002;94:1445)
- **Clinical breast exam** (CBE): benefit independent of mammography not established
- **Mammography**: ~20-30% ↓ in breast cancer mortality (smaller absolute benefit in women <50) (Lancet 2001;358:1340 & 2002;359:909; Annals 2002;137:347; Lancet 2006;368:2053)
    suspicious lesions: clustered **microcalcifications**, **spiculated** or **enlarging** masses
- Most U.S. groups recommend annual mammography + CBE beginning at age 40
    Women at ↑ risk: screen earlier (age 25 in BRCA1/2 carrier, 5-10 y before earliest ⊕ FHx index case, 8-10 y after thoracic irradiation, upon dx of ↑ risk benign conditions)
    MRI superior to mammo in high-risk Pts (NEJM 2004;351:427; Lancet 2005;365:1769)
    Women with strong FHx should be evaluated for possible genetic testing
- **MRI**: consider if >20-25% lifetime risk (eg, ⊕⊕ FHx, BRCA 1 or 2, prior chest XRT) (JAMA 2006;295:2375; CA 2007;57:75)

Diagnostic evaluation
- **Palpable breast mass**:
    Age <30 y → observe for resolution over 1-2 menstrual cycles
    Age <30 y, unchanging mass → **U/S** → aspiration if mass not simple cyst
    Age >30 y or solid mass on U/S or bloody aspirate or recurrence after aspiration → **mammo** (detect other lesions) *and* either **fine-needle aspir.** or **core-needle bx**
    Clearly cancerous on exam or indeter. read/atypia on needle bx → **excisional bx**
- **Suspicious mammogram** with normal exam: stereotactically-guided bx
- **MRI**: detects contralateral cancer in 3% of women w/ recently dx breast cancer & negative contralateral mammogram (but PPV only 21%) (NEJM 2007;356:1295); whether to use routinely remains unclear

Staging
- **Anatomic**: tumor size, chest wall invasion, axillary LN mets (*strongest prognostic factor*)
- **Histopathologic**: type (little prognostic relevance) & grade; lymphatic/vascular invasion
    In situ carcinoma: no invasion of surrounding stroma
        Ductal (DCIS): ↑ risk of invasive cancer in *ipsilateral* breast (~30%/10 y)
        Lobular (LCIS): marker of ↑ risk of invasive cancer in *either* breast (~1%/y)
    Invasive carcinoma: infiltrating ductal (70-80%); invasive lobular (5-10%); tubular, medullary, and mucinous (10%, better prognosis); papillary (1-2%); other (1-2%)
    Inflammatory breast cancer (see above): not a histologic type but a clinical reflection of tumor invasion of dermal lymphatics; very poor prognosis
    Paget disease: ductal cancer invading nipple epidermis ± associated mass
- **Biologic**: estrogen and progesterone receptor (ER/PR) status; HER2/neu overexpression
    4 basic subtypes include: luminal A (ER⊕ HER2⊖), luminal B (ER⊕ HER2⊕), basal-like or "triple negative" (ER⊖PR⊖Her2⊖), and ER⊖HER2⊕
- Bone marrow micrometastases associated w/ ~2× ↑ risk of death (NEJM 2005;353:793)
- Recurrence score (multigene RT-PCR assay) may be sent to help predict recurrence risk in node ⊖, ER⊕ Pts (NEJM 2004;351:2817 & 2006;355:560)

Simplified Staging System for Breast Cancer			
Stage	Characteristics	Description	5-y surv
I	Tumor ≤2 cm	Operable locoregional	90%
IIA	Tumor >2 cm or *mobile* axillary nodes		80%
IIB	Tumor >5 cm		65%
IIIA	Internal mammary or *fixed* axillary nodes	Locally advanced	50%
IIIB	Direct extension to chest wall or skin	Inoperable locoregional	45%
IIIC	Infraclavicular or supraclavicular nodes		40%
IV	Distant metastases	Metastatic	15%

Treatment

- **Local control: surgery and radiation therapy (RT)**
    Breast-conserving = lumpectomy + breast RT + axillary node dissection (ALND) is
    equivalent to *mastectomy* + ALND (NEJM 2002;347:1227, 1233); contraindications:
    multicentric disease, diffuse microcalcifications, prior RT, pregnancy, ? tumor >5 cm
    Radiation therapy (RT) after mastectomy for ≥4 ⊕ LN, tumor >5 cm or ⊕ surgical
    margins → ↓ locoregional recurrence and ↑ survival (Lancet 2005;366:2087)
- **Systemic therapy: chemotherapy and other adjuvant therapy**
    Chemotherapy: **anthracycline**-based AC (adriamycin + cyclophosphamide) + **taxanes**
    (paclitaxel or docetaxel) for advanced disease, node ⊕ tumors (Lancet 2005;352:2302), or
    high-risk node ⊖ tumors (eg, HER2⊕). Little benefit of adding taxanes in ER⊕ tumors.
    Biologic
       trastuzumab (Herceptin; anti-HER2/*neu* mAb) ↑ survival in HER2⊕ tumors (15-20%),
       but ↑ cardotoxicity w/ anthracyclines (NEJM 2005;353:1659, 1673; Lancet 2007;369:29)
       lapatinib (tyrosine kinase inhib. of HER2 & EGFR): delays progression in Pts who have
       failed trastuzumab (NEJM 2006;355:2733)
    Hormonal (in ER/PR ⊕ or unknown status)
       tamoxifen: 41% ↓ recurrence and 34% ↓ breast cancer mortality in *postmenopausal*
       Pts (Lancet 2005;365:1687)
       aromatase inhibitors (AI) (anastrozole, letrozole, exemestane): ~18% ↓ recurrence
       c/w tamoxifen in *postmenopausal* Pts (Lancet 2005;365:60; NEJM 2005;353:2747)
       options include upfront AI or tamoxifen × 2-3 y followed by AI (Lancet 2007;369:559)
       2nd-line: ovarian ablation with LHRH agonists (goserelin) or oophorectomy if
       premenopausal; pure antiestrogens (fulvestrant) if *postmenopausal*
       ovarian ablation + AI or tamoxifen for *premenopausal* women is under study

Treatment of Carcinoma *in situ* and Invasive Carcinoma of the Breast	
LCIS	Close surveillance ± chemoprevention; ? prophylactic bilat. mastectomy
DCIS	Mastectomy or lumpectomy + RT; ALND *not* indicated; ± chemoprevention (NEJM 2004;350:1430)
I II	Surgery + RT + Adjuvant chemo if ↑ risk: tumor >1 cm or ⊕ LN or ER/PR ⊖ (Lancet 1998;352:930) + Hormonal therapy for ER/PR ⊕ (or unknown status) tumors + Trastuzumab if HER2⊕ and tumor ≥1 cm or ⊕ LN
III	Neoadjuvant chemo → surgery + RT ± adjuvant chemotherapy + Hormonal therapy for ER/PR ⊕ (or unknown status) tumors + Trastuzumab if HER2⊕
IV	ER/PR ⊕: hormonal therapy ± chemotherapy ER/PR ⊖, HER2⊕: chemo + trastuzumab ER/PR ⊖, HER2⊖: chemotherapy Bony mets: bisphosphonates ↓ skeletal complic. (NEJM 1998;339:357)

Prevention

- **Selective estrogen receptor modulators (SERMs)**
    Tamoxifen: ↓ risk of contralateral breast cancer in adjuvant setting;
       risk-benefit unclear when given as 1° prevention in Pts at ↑ risk: ↓ invasive breast
       cancer, but ↑ DVT & uterine CA risk, and ? ↑ in all-cause mortality (Lancet 2002;360:817)
    Raloxifene: ↓ risk of invasive breast cancer & vertebral fx, ↑ risk of stroke & DVT/PE
       (RUTH, NEJM 2006;355:125); ≈ tamoxifen in prevention of breast cancer w/ ↓ risk of
       DVT/PE & cataracts, trend towards ↓ uterine cancer (STAR, JAMA 2006;295:2727)
    Aromatase inhibitors under study
- BRCA1/2 carriers: several options, including intensified surveillance as described above
    Prophylactic bilateral mastectomy (NEJM 2001;345:159) and bilateral salpingo-oophorectomy
    (↓ risk of ovarian *and* breast cancer; NEJM 2002;346:1609; JAMA 2006;296:185) are effective.
    Chemoprevention: limited data supports use of tamoxifen for risk reduction

PROSTATE CANCER

Epidemiology and risk factors (NEJM 2003;349:366)
- Most common cancer in U.S. men; 2nd most common cause of cancer death in men
- Lifetime risk of prostate cancer dx ~16%; lifetime risk of dying of prostate cancer ~3%
- More common with ↑ age (rare if <45 y), in African Americans, and if ⊕ FHx

Clinical manifestations (usually asymptomatic at presentation)
- **Obstructive sx** (more common with BPH): hesitancy, ↓ stream, retention, nocturia
- **Irritative sx** (also seen with prostatitis): frequency, dysuria, urgency
- Periprostatic spread: hematuria, hematospermia, new-onset erectile dysfunction
- Metastatic disease: bone pain, spinal cord compression, cytopenias

Screening (NEJM 2001;344:1373)
- Mortality benefit from screening has not been established (Annals 2002;137:915, 917)
- **Digital rectal exam** (DRE): size, consistency, lesions
- **PSA**: 4 ng/ml cutpoint neither Se nor Sp; can ↑ with BPH, prostatitis, acute retention, after bx or TURP, and ejaculation (no affect ↑ after DRE, cystoscopy); ↓ free PSA %,
  ↑ PSA velocity, ↑ PSA density, & age-adjusted PSA reference ranges may ↑ test utility
  15% of men >62 y w/ PSA <4 & nl DRE have bx-proven T1 cancer (NEJM 2004;350:2239)
- Offer DRE + PSA screening to men age ≥50 (≥45 if high risk) with life expectancy ≥10 y

Diagnostic and staging evaluation
- **Transrectal ultrasound** (TRUS) **guided biopsy**, with 6-12 core specimens
- **Histology**: **Gleason grade** (2-10; low grade ≤6) = sum of the differentiation score (1 = best, 5 = worst) of the two most prevalent patterns in the bx; correlates with prognosis
- **Imaging**: to evaluate extraprostatic spread
  bone scan: for PSA >10 ng/ml, high Gleason grade, or clinically advanced tumor
  abdomen-pelvis CT: inaccurate for detecting extracapsular spread and lymph node mets
  endorectal coil MRI: improves assessment of extracapsular spread

			TNM Staging & Treatment of Prostate Cancer
Stage	**Tumor**	**Nodes, Mets**	**Treatment**
I	T1a = non-palp., not visible on imaging	N0, M0, Gleason 2-4	**Watchful waiting** (consider if limited life expect.) **Radiation** (external beam or brachytherapy; NEJM 2006;355:1583) **Radical prostatectomy** (± radiation and/or hormonal Rx if high-risk features found at surgery)
II	T1/T2 = w/ in prostate	N0, M0	
III	T3 = extends thru capsule	N0, M0	**Radiation** + androgen ablation (see below)
IV	T4 = invades adjacent structures	N0, M0	**Radiation** (for M0 disease) **Androgen deprivation** (JAMA 2005;294:238) orchiectomy
	Any T	N1, M0	**GnRH analogues** (leuprolide, goserelin) antiandrogens (flutamide, bicalutamide) 2nd-line: antiandrogen withdrawal, different antiandrogen, androgen synthesis inhib. (ketoconazole, aminoglutethimide), estrogens
	Any T	Any N, M1*	**Chemo** (docetaxel) if hormone-refractory (NEJM 2004;351:1502, 1513)

*Bisphosphonates (alendronate, zolendronate) & palliative radiation for bone mets

Prognosis
- PSA level, Gleason grade, and age are predictors of metastatic disease
- In surgically treated Pts, 5-y relapse-free survival >90% if disease confined to organ, ~75% if extension through capsule, and ~40% if seminal vesicle invasion
- Compared to watchful waiting, surgery ↓ prostate cancer mortality & overall mortality in patients <75 (NEJM 2005;352:1977); comparisons of surgery and radiation are underway
- PSA doubling time, Gleason, & time to biochemical recurrence predict mortality following recurrence. For local recurrence following RP, salvage RT may be beneficial if low PSA.
- Metastatic disease: median survival ~24-30 mos; all progress to androgen independence

Prevention
- Finasteride ↓ total prostate cancers detected by bx, but ↑ number of high Gleason grade tumors (NEJM 2003;349:215)

COLORECTAL CANCER (CRC)

Epidemiology and risk factors
- 3rd most common cancer in U.S men and women; 2nd leading cause of cancer death overall
- Age: rare before 40, 90% of cases occurring after age 50
- **Genetics:** up to 25% of patients have ⊕ FHx: risk depends on number of 1st-degree relatives (with CRC or polyp) and age at dx; ~5% have an identifiable germline mutation
  - **Familial adenomatous polyposis (FAP):** mutation of APC tumor suppressor → 1000s of polyps at young age → ~100% lifetime risk; ↑ risk of thyroid, stomach, SI cancers
  - **Hereditary nonpolyposis colorectal cancer (HNPCC):** mutations in DNA mismatch repair genes → ↑ tumor progression → ~80% lifetime risk; predom. **right-sided** tumors; ↑ risk of **endometrial**, ovarian, stomach, small bowel cancers
- **Inflammatory bowel disease:** ↑ risk with ↑ extent and duration of disease
- ↓ risk of adenomas w/ ASA & NSAIDs, incl. COX-2 (NEJM 2006;355:873, 885), but ↑ bleeding and ↑ CV events w/ COX-2; ↓ COX-2-expressing colorectal cancer after prolonged ASA (NEJM 2007;356:2131; Lancet 2007;369:1603); currently not recommended (Annals 2007;146:361)

Pathology
- **Adenoma → carcinoma sequence** reflects accumulation of multiple genetic mutations
  ↑ risk of malignancy with large (>2.5 cm), villous, sessile adenomatous polyps
- ~50% of colon tumors are proximal to splenic flexure

Clinical manifestations
- Distal colon: Δ **bowel habits**, **obstruction**, colicky abdominal pain, **hematochezia**
- Proximal colon: **iron defic. anemia**, dull vague abd pain; obstruction atypical due to larger lumen, liquid stool, and polypoid tumors (vs. annular distal tumors)
- Metastases: nodes, **liver**, lung, peritoneum → RUQ tenderness, ascites, supraclavicular LN
- Associated with Streptococcus bovis bacteremia and Clostridium septicum sepsis

Screening (NEJM 2002;346:40)
- **Average risk** & age >50: q5y flex sig + q1y FOBT or q10y colonoscopy
- **↑ risk:** earlier (age 40 if ⊕ FHx) and/or more frequent screening based on risk factor(s)
- **Endoscopy: colonoscopy** test of choice as examines entire colon; ~1/2 of Pts w/ advanced proximal neoplasms have no distal polyps (NEJM 2000;343:162, 169) flexible sigmoidoscopy vs. ∅ endo. shown to ↓ distal CRC mortality (NEJM 1992;326:653)
- **Fecal occult blood test (FOBT):** ↓ mortality (NEJM 1993;328:1365 & 2000;343:1603), 6-sample (3 cards) home testing much more Se (24% vs. 5%) than single physician DRE/FOBT at identifying advanced neoplasia (Annals 2005;142:81)
- **Fecal DNA:** ↑ Se, ≈ Sp c/w FOBT, but less Se than colonoscopy (NEJM 2004;351:2704)
- Imaging: air-contrast barium enema (ACBE) and CT colonography are both less Se than colonoscopy (Lancet 2005;365:305), especially for lesions <1 cm

Staging
- **Colonoscopy** + biopsy/polypectomy
- Abdomen/pelvis CT (but inaccurate for assessing depth of invasion & malignant LN)
- **Intraoperative staging** is essential for evaluating extracolonic spread
- Tumor markers: baseline **CEA** in Pt with known CRC has prognostic significance and is useful to follow response to therapy and detect recurrence; not a screening tool

Treatment Based on TNM and Modified Dukes Staging of Colorectal Cancer				
TNM	**Dukes**	**Criteria**	**5-y surv.**	**Treatment**
I	A	Into submucosa	95%	Surgery alone
	B1	Into muscularis	90%	
IIA	B2	Into serosa	80%	Surgery; no established role for adjuvant chemotherapy*
IIB	B2	Direct invasion	70%	
IIIA/B	C	≤4 ⊕ LNs	65%	Surgery + chemotherapy*
IIIC	C	≥4 ⊕ LNs	35%	**5-FU + leucovorin + oxaliplatin =** FOLFOX
IV	D	Distant metastases	5%	Chemotherapy 1st line: FOLFOX or irinotecan (FOLFIRI) + bevacizumab 2nd line: irinotecan + cetuximab ± palliative surgery†

*Consider adjuvant chemo for high-risk stage II (obstruct./perf., adherence to adj. structures, inadeq. nodal sampling, lymphovasc. invasion, poorly differentiated). For stage II or III **rectal cancer**: combined chemoradiation → surgery → chemo. † Surgical resection of isolated liver or lung metastases associated with ~30% 5-y survival. (NEJM 2004;350:2343 & 2004: 351:337 & 2005;352:476 & 2006;355:1114)

PANCREATIC CANCER

Epidemiology and risk factors (*Lancet* 2004;363:1049)
- 4th leading cause of cancer death in U.S. men and women
- Acquired risk factors: **smoking**, obesity, chronic pancreatitis, ? diabetes
- Hereditary risk factors: genetic susceptibility may play a role in 5-10% of cases
  Hereditary chronic pancreatitis: mutation in cationic trypsinogen gene
  Familial cancer syndromes and gene mutations with ↑ risk: Peutz-Jeghers (LKB1), familial
    atypical multiple mole melanoma syndrome (p16), and ataxia-telangiectasia (ATM);
    hereditary colorectal cancer and BRCA2 mutations may also ↑ risk

Pathology
- ≥95% of malignant pancreatic neoplasms arise from **exocrine** (ductal or acinar) cells
- ~60% arise in head, 15% in body, 5% in tail; in 20% tumor diffusely involves whole gland

Clinical manifestations
- **Painless jaundice** (w/ pancreatic head mass), **pain** (radiating to back), **weight loss**
- New-onset atypical diabetes mellitus; unexplained malabsorption; unexplained pancreatitis
- Migratory thrombophlebitis (Trousseau's sign)
- Exam: abdominal mass; nontender, palpable gallbladder (Courvoisier's sign, but more often
    seen with biliary tract cancers); hepatomegaly; ascites; left supraclavicular (Virchow's)
    node & palpable rectal shelf (both nonspecific signs of carcinomatosis)
- Laboratory tests may show ↑ bilirubin, ↑ Aϕ, anemia

Diagnostic and staging evaluation
- **Pancreatic protocol CT scan** (I$^+$ w/ arterial & venous phase imaging)
- If no lesion seen → EUS, ERCP, MRI/MRCP may reveal mass or malignant ductal strictures
- Biopsy pancreatic lesion via EUS-guided FNA (preferred in potential surgical candidates) or
    CT-guided (potential risk of seeding) or biopsy metastasis
- Tumor markers: ↑ CA 19-9; may be useful to follow disease postoperatively

Clinical (Radiologic) Staging & Prognosis of Pancreatic Adenocarcinoma		
Stage & % at dx	**Criteria**	**Median Survival**
Resectable 15-20%	No extrapancreatic disease Patent SMV & portal vein; celiac axis & SMA not involved No bulky nodes	10-20 mo (favorable: tumor <3 cm, ⊖ marg., well-differen.) 5-y survival ~30% if node ⊖ vs. ~10% if node ⊕
Locally advanced (unresectable) 40%	Extensive PV, SMV, celiac axis, or SMA involvement No distant mets	8-12 mo
Metastatic 40%	Typically liver & peritoneum; occasionally lung	3-6 mo

Treatment
- Resectable: surgery ± adjuvant (neoadjuvant or postoperative) therapy
    pancreaticoduodenectomy = **Whipple procedure** = resection of pancreatic head,
    duodenum, CBD and gallbladder ± partial gastrectomy
    adjuvant therapy: ↑ survival w/ **chemoradiation** (eg, postoperative 5-FU/radiation +
    gemcitabine) (*NEJM* 2004;350:2713; *JCO* 2005;23:4532; *JAMA* 2007;297:267)
- Locally advanced: **5-FU chemorad** ↑ survival over chemo or XRT alone; ? followed by
    gemcitabine (*JCO* 2005;23:4538)
- Metastatic: **gemcitabine** improves survival over 5-FU (*JCO* 1997;15:2403), adding erlotinib
    to gemcitabine provides slight additional benefit (*JCO* 2005;23:16S,1)
- Palliative and supportive care
    obstructive jaundice or gastric outlet obstruction: endoscopic stenting or surgical bypass
    pain: opiates, celiac plexus neurolysis, radiation therapy
    weight loss: pancreatic enzyme replacement for suspected fat malabsorption
    nutrition consult

FEVER AND NEUTROPENIA (FN)

Definition
- Fever: single oral temp ≥38.3°C (101°F) or ≥38°C (100.4°F) for ≥1 h
- **Neutropenia**: ANC <500 cells/μl or <1000 cells/μl with predicted nadir <500 cells/μl

Pathophysiology and microbiology
- Predisposing factors: catheters, skin breakdown, mucositis throughout GI tract, obstruction (lymphatics, biliary tract, GI, urinary tract), immune defect associated with malignancy
- Majority of episodes thought to result from seeding of bloodstream by GI flora
- GNRs (especially *P. aeruginosa*) were historically most common
- Gram ⊕ infections have recently become more common (60–70% of identified organisms)
- Fungal superinfection often results from prolonged neutropenia & antibiotic use
- Infection with atypical organisms and bacterial meningitis is rare

Prevention
- Levofloxacin (500 mg qd) ↓ febrile episodes & bacterial infections in chemo-related high-risk neutropenic patients; no difference in mortality (*NEJM* 2005;353:977, 988)

Diagnostic evaluation
- Exam: skin, oropharynx, lung, perirectal area, surgical & catheter sites; avoid DRE
- Labs: CBC with differential, electrolytes, BUN/Cr, LFTs, U/A
- Micro: blood (peripheral & through each indwelling catheter port), urine, & sputum cx; for localizing s/s → ✓ stool, peritoneal, CSF or skin biopsy cultures
- Imaging: CXR; for localizing s/s → CNS, sinus, chest, or abdomen/pelvis imaging
- Caveats: neutropenia → impaired inflammatory response → *exam and radiographic findings may be subtle*; absence of neutrophils by Gram stain does *not* r/o infection

Risk stratification (factors that predict lower risk)
- History: age <60, no symptoms, no major comorbidities, cancer in remission, solid tumor, no h/o fungal infection or recent antifungal Rx
- Exam: temp <39 °C, no tachypnea, no hypotension, no Δ MS, no dehydration
- Studies: ANC >100 cells/μl, anticipated duration of neutropenia <10 d, normal CXR

Initial antibiotic therapy
- Empiric regimens should include a drug with **antipseudomonal activity**
- PO abx can be used in low-risk Pts: cipro + amoxicillin-clavulanate (*NEJM* 1999;341:305, 312)
- IV antibiotics: no clearly superior regimen; monotherapy or 2-drug regimens can be used
  Monotherapy: ceftazidime, cefepime, imipenem-cilastatin, or meropenem
  2-drug therapy: aminoglycoside + antipseudomonal β-lactam
  PCN-allergic: levofloxacin + aztreonam or aminoglycoside
- **Vancomycin** added in select cases (hypotension, indwelling catheter, severe mucositis, MRSA colonization, h/o quinolone prophylaxis), discontinue when cultures ⊖ × 48 h

Modification to initial antibiotic regimen
- Low-risk Pts who become afebrile w/in 3–5 d can be switched to PO antibiotics
- Empiric antibiotics are changed for fever >3–5 d with progressive disease
- Antifungal therapy is added for neutropenic fever >5 d
  liposomal amphotericin B, caspofungin, micafungin, anidulafungin, voriconazole, posaconazole all options (*NEJM* 2002;346:225 & 2007;356:348)

Duration of therapy
- Known source: complete standard course (eg, 14 d for bacteremia)
- Unknown source: continue antibiotics until afebrile *and* ANC >500 cells/μl
- Less clear when to d/c abx when Pt is afebrile but prolonged neutropenia

Role of hematopoietic growth factors (*JCO* 2000;18:3558)
- Granulocyte (G-CSF) and granulocyte-macrophage (GM-CSF) colony-stimulating factors can be used as 1° prophylaxis when expected FN incidence >40% or as 2° prophylaxis after FN has occurred in a previous cycle (to maintain dose-intensity for curable tumors)
- Colony-stimulating factors can be considered as adjuvant therapy in high-risk FN Pts

---

SPINAL CORD COMPRESSION

Clinical manifestations
- Metastases located in vertebral body extend and cause epidural spinal cord compression
- **Prostate**, **breast**, and **lung** cancer are the most common causes, followed by renal cell carcinoma, NHL, and myeloma

- **Site of involvement: thoracic** (70%), **lumbar** (20%), **cervical** (10%)
- Signs and symptoms: **pain** (96%), **weakness, autonomic dysfunction** (urinary retention, ↓ anal sphincter tone), **sensory loss**

Diagnostic evaluation
- Always take back pain in Pts with solid tumors very seriously
- Do *not* wait for neurologic signs to develop before initiating evaluation b/c duration & severity of neurologic dysfunction before Rx are best predictors of neurologic outcome
- Urgent **whole spine MRI** is study of choice

Treatment
- **Dexamethasone** (10 mg IV → 4 mg IV or PO q6h)
  initiate immediately while awaiting imaging if back pain + neurologic deficits
- Emergent XRT or surgical decompression if confirmed compression / neuro deficits
- Neurosurgery superior to XRT in regaining neuro fxn for solid tumors *(Lancet 2005;366:643)*
- If pathologic fracture causing compression → surgery; if not surgical candidate → XRT

TUMOR LYSIS SYNDROME

Clinical manifestations
- Large tumor burden or a rapidly proliferating tumor → spontaneous or chemotherapy-induced release of intracellular electrolytes and nucleic acids
- Most common w/Rx of high-grade lymphomas (**Burkitt's**) and leukemias (**ALL, AML, CML in blast crisis**); rare with solid tumors; rarely due to spontaneous necrosis
- Electrolyte abnormalities: ↑ K, ↑ uric acid, ↑ PO_4 → ↓ Ca
- **Renal failure** (urate nephropathy)

Prophylaxis
- Allopurinol 300 mg qd to bid PO or 200–400 mg/m^2 IV (adjusted for renal fxn) & aggressive hydration prior to beginning chemotherapy or XRT
- Rasburicase (recombinant urate oxidase) 0.15 mg/kg or 6 mg fixed dose (except in obese Pts) & aggressive hydration prior to beginning chemotherapy or XRT (see below)

Treatment
- *Avoid IV contrast and NSAIDs*
- Allopurinol + IV hydration ± diuretics to ↑ UOP
- Alkalinization of urine w/ isotonic $NaHCO_3$ ↑ UA solubility & ↓ risk of urate nephropathy
- Rasburicase (recombinant urate oxidase, 0.15–0.2 mg/kg/d × 3–7 d) for severe hyperuricemia, especially in aggressive malignancy; uric acid levels must be drawn on ice to quench *ex vivo* enzyme activity *(JCO 2003;21:4402; Acta Haematol 2006;115:35)*
- Treat hyperkalemia, hyperphosphatemia, and symptomatic hypocalcemia
- Hemodialysis may be necessary; early renal consultation for Pts w/ renal insuffic. or ARF

CANCER OF UNKNOWN PRIMARY SITE

Evaluation of Cancer of Unknown Primary				
Path	Possible Sources	Markers	Imaging	Additional Path
Adeno.	Colon, Upper GI, Panc.	CEA, CA19-9	Endoscopy/EUS	CDX1, CK7/20
	HCC	AFP	Abd/Pelvic CT	
	Breast	CA-15-3	Mammography	ER/PR, GCDFP
	Ovarian, Prostate	CA125, PSA	Pelvic U/S	CA-125, PSAP
	Lung		Chest CT	TTF1, CK7
Squam.	Lung	None	Chest CT	TTF1, CK7
	Head & Neck		Laryngoscopy	
	Esophageal		Endoscopy	
	Cervix, Anus			
Poorly Differen.	Germ cell	hCG, AFP	Testicular U/S	PLAP, isochrom 12p
	Lymphoma	LDH	PET	LCA, flow, cytogenetics
	Thyroid	Thyroglob.	Thyroid U/S	Thyroglobulin
	GIST, Sarcoma		Abd/Pelvic CT	c-KIT, desmin, vimentin
	Neuroendocrine			NSE, chromogranin
				Consider EM for all

Additional studies for each possible source listed in same row. May also need tests for adeno/squam for poorly-diff.

Microbiology of Pneumonia	
Clinical Setting	**Etiologies**
Community-acquired (NEJM 2002;347:2039)	*S. pneumoniae* *Mycoplasma, Chlamydia,* viral (espec. in young & healthy) *H. influenzae, M. catarrhalis* (espec. in COPD'ers) *Legionella* (espec. in elderly, smokers, ↓ immunity) *Klebsiella* & other GNR (especially in alcoholics & aspirators) *S. aureus* (espec. postviral infection) Influenza A & B (espec. in elderly and pulm. disease) (no organism identified in 40-60% cases)
Hospital-acquired	GNR including *Pseudomonas, Klebsiella, E. coli, Enterobacter, Serratia, Acinetobacter,* & *S. aureus* (MRSA)
Immuno-compromised	All of the above + PCP, fungi, *Nocardia,* atypical mycobacteria, CMV, HSV

Aspiration (NEJM 2001;334:665)	*Chemical pneumonitis* due to aspiration of sterile gastric contents
	 Bacterial pneumonia due to inhalation of oropharyngeal microbes
	     outpatients: typical oral flora (*Strep, Staph,* anaerobes)
	     inpatients or chronically ill: GNR and *S. aureus*

Clinical manifestations
- "Typical": acute onset of fever, cough productive of purulent sputum, dyspnea, consolidation on CXR
- "Atypical" (originally described as culture ⊖): insidious onset of dry cough, extrapulmonary sx (N/V, diarrhea, headache, myalgias, sore throat), patchy interstitial pattern on CXR
- Symptoms do not reliably distinguish between "typical" (*S. pneumoniae, H. influenzae*) and "atypical" (*Mycoplasma, Chlamydia, Legionella*) pathogens
- Influenza: fever, chills, sweats, malaise, headache, myalgias, nonproductive cough serious illness, espec. in elderly and in those w/ cardiopulmonary disease can lead to 2° bacterial pneumonia

Diagnostic studies
- **Sputum Gram stain**: utility debated
  Is it a good sample (ie, sputum or spit)? → should be <10 squamous cells/lpf
  Is it a purulent sample? → should be >25 PMNs/lpf
- **Sputum culture**: sample should be transported to lab w/in 1-2 h of collection
- Blood cultures (*before antibiotics!*): ⊕ in ~10% of inPts, depending on pathogen
- **CXR** (PA & lateral); effusions >1 cm should be tapped
- **S$_a$O$_2$** or **P$_a$O$_2$**
- Other laboratory evaluation: CBC w/ differential, electrolytes, BUN/Cr, glucose, LFTs
- Special microbiologic studies:
  Mycoplasma: PCR of throat or sputum/BAL
  Legionella: urine Ag (detects *L. pneumophilia* L1 serotype, 70% of clinical disease)
  S. pneumoniae urinary Ag
  Rapid influenza assay (Se ~70%)
  MTb: induced sputum for acid-fast stain and mycobacterial cx (*empiric respiratory isolation while results pending*); request rapid DNA probe if stain ⊕
  Induced sputum for PCP if HIV ⊕ or known decreased cell-mediated immunity
  Viruses: nasal washings or swabs for EIA or DFA
  HIV test if Pt 15-54 y
- Bronchoscopy: consider if Pt immunosuppressed, critically ill, failing to respond, or has chronic pneumonia. Also in suspected MTb if no adequate sputum and in suspected PCP if induced sputum unavailable or ⊖.
- CT scan: consider if failing to respond to appropriate therapy

P.O.R.T. Score, Prognosis, and Recommended Triage			
Class	Score	Mortality	Suggested Triage
I	age <50, no comorbidities	<1%	Outpatient
II	≤70	<1%	Outpatient
III	71-90	2.8%	? Brief inpatient
IV	91-130	8.2%	Inpatient
V	>130	29.2%	ICU
Variables	Points		
Demograph.	Men (age in y), women (age - 10), nursing home resident (+10)		
Coexist. probs	Neoplasm (+30), liver disease (+20), CHF (+10), CVA (+10), renal disease (+10)		
Exam	ΔMS (+20), RR >30 (+20), SBP <90 (+20), Temp <35° or >40° (+15), HR >125 (+10)		
Laboratory	pH <7.35 (+30), BUN >30 (+20), Na <130 (+20), glc >250 (+10), Hct <30 (+10), P_aO_2 <60 or S_aO_2 <90 (+10), pleural effusion (+10)		

(NEJM 1997;336:243)

Treatment	
Clinical scenario	Empiric treatment guidelines*
Outpatient	No recent abx: macrolide or doxycycline Recent abx: [macrolide + (high-dose amoxicillin or amoxicillin/clavulanate or 2nd generation ceph.)] or respiratory FQ
Community-acquired, hospitalized	[3rd gen. ceph. + macrolide] or respiratory FQ
Community-acquired, hospitalized, ICU	[3rd gen. ceph. + macrolide] or respiratory FQ (assuming no risk for Pseudomonas)
Hospital-acquired with risk factors for MDR pathogens	[Antipseudomonal PCN or 3rd gen. ceph. or FQ or carbapenem] and vancomycin use FQ or add azithromycin if suspect Legionella
Immunocompromised	As above ± TMP-SMX ± steroids to cover PCP
Aspiration	[3rd gen. ceph. or FQ] ± [clindamycin or metronidazole]
Influenza A & B	M2 inhib. (amantidine, rimantidine) effective against A only Neuraminidase inhib. (oseltamivir, zanamivir) effective against A & B Drugs ↓ duration of illness only if started <48 h from onset
Route of therapy	Inpatients should initially be treated with IV antibiotics Δ to PO when clinically responding and able to take POs

*When possible, organism-directed therapy, guided by in vitro susceptibilities or local patterns of drug resistance should be utilized. For ventilator-associated pneumonia, 8 ≈ 15 d of Rx, except for Pseudomonas and other non-fermenting GNR (JAMA 2003;290:2588). (CID 2003;37:1405; AJRCCM 2005;171:388; MMWR 2005;54:1)

Prognosis (also see PORT score above)
- Pneumonia and influenza are the 8th leading cause of death in the USA
- Pts usually stabilize in 2-3 d (JAMA 1998;279:1452)
- For low-risk Pts, can discharge immediately after switching to PO abx (Chest 1998;113:142)
- CXR resolves in most by 6 wks; important to document complete resolution to r/o underlying malignancy

Prevention
- Inactivated influenza vaccine: persons >50 y of age, at risk for complications of influenza, health care workers, caretakers of high-risk persons
- Pneumococcal polysaccharide vaccine: persons >65 y of age and those with high-risk medical illness

Candida species
- **Microbiology**: C. albicans and nonalbicans species (consider imidazole resistance if prior treatment or nonalbicans species)
- **Risk factors**: neutropenia, immunosuppression, broad-spectrum abx, intravascular catheters (especially if TPN), IVDA, abdominal surgery, renal failure
- **Clinical manifestations**

  Mucocutaneous: cutaneous (eg, red, macerated lesions in intertriginous zones); oral thrush (if unexplained, r/o HIV); esophageal (odynophagia; ± oral thrush); vulvovaginal

  Candiduria: typically colonization due to broad-spectrum abx and/or indwelling catheter; failure to clear raises possibility of upper UTI

  Candidemia (4th or 5th leading cause of nosocomial blood stream infection): typically due to intravascular catheter; r/o retinal involvement; endocarditis rare (but more common w/ nonalbicans and if prosthetic valve)

  Hepatosplenic: intestinal seeding of portal & venous circulation; seen in acute leukemics

  Hematogenous dissemination → lung, brain, meninges

Empiric Treatment	
Mucocutaneous	Clotrimazole, nystatin, fluconazole, itraconazole
Candidemia w/o neutropenia	Ampho B or fluconazole or caspofungin or [fluc + ampho B]
Febrile neutropenia	Ampho B or caspofungin

Remove intravascular catheters (CID 2004;38:161)

Histoplasmosis
- **Epidemiology**: hyperendemic in central & SE U.S. (especially in areas w/ bird & bat droppings), present in river banks including northeast
- **Clinical manifestations**

  Acute pulmonary: often subclinical

  Chronic pulmonary: ↑ productive cough, wt loss, night sweats, infiltrates, cavitation

  Disseminated (immunocompromised): fever, wt loss, HSM, LAN, oral ulcers, skin lesion
- **Treatment**: itraconazole; amphotericin if severe or disseminated (CID 2000;30:688)

Coccidioidomycosis
- **Epidemiology**: SW U.S. (San Joaquin or "Valley" fever)
- **Clinical manifestations**

  Acute pulmonary: often subclinical; chest pain, cough, fever, arthralgias

  Chronic pulmonary: cough, hemoptysis, fever, night sweats, wt loss

  Chronic disseminated (in immunocompromised, pregnant, & diabetics): fever, malaise, diffuse pulmonary process, bone, skin, & meningeal involvement
- **Treatment** for disseminated or high-risk 1° pulmonary: fluconazole or itraconazole, or amphotericin if severe (CID 2005;41:1217)

Blastomycosis
- **Epidemiology**: south central, SE, and midwest U.S.
- **Clinical manifestations**

  Often asymptomatic, acute pneumonia, chronic pneumonia

  Extrapulmonary: verrucous & ulcerated skin lesions, bone & GU involvement

  Disseminated: can involve CNS
- **Treatment**: itraconazole; amphotericin if severe (CID 2000;30:679)

Aspergillus (Chest 2002;121:1988)
- **ABPA**: see "Interstitial Lung Disease"
- **Hypersensitivity pneumonitis**: see "Interstitial Lung Disease"
- **Aspergilloma**: usually in pre-existing cavity (from TB, etc.); most asx, but can lead to hemoptysis; sputum cx ⊕ in <50%; CT → mobile intracavitary mass with air crescent Rx: antifungals w/o benefit; embolization or surgery for persistent hemoptysis
- **Necrotizing tracheitis**: white necrotic pseudomembranes in Pts w/ AIDS or lung tx
- **Chronic necrotizing (semi-invasive)**: seen in COPD or mild immunosuppression; p/w sputum, fever, wt loss over months; CT shows infiltrate ± nodule ± pleural thickening; lung bx → invasion; Rx = amphotericin or voriconazole
- **Invasive/disseminated**: seen if immunocompromised (neutropenia, s/p transplant, glucocorticoid Rx, AIDS); clinical: s/s pneumonia including chest pain and hemoptysis; CT shows nodules, halo sign, air crescent sign, lung bx if prior testing inconclusive Rx: amphotericin B or voriconazole

Definitions
- **Anatomic**
  lower: urethritis, cystitis (superficial infection of bladder)
  upper: pyelonephritis (inflammatory process of the renal parenchyma), renal or
    perinephric abscess, prostatitis
- **Clinical**
  uncomplicated: cystitis in nonpregnant women w/o underlying structural or
    neurological disease
  complicated: upper tract infection in women or UTI in men or pregnant women or
    UTI with underlying structural disease or immunosuppression

Microbiology
- Uncomplicated UTI: **E. coli** (80%), Proteus, Klebsiella, S. saprophyticus (CID 2004;39:75)
- Complicated UTI: E. coli (30%), enterococci (20%), Pseudomonas (20%), S. epidermidis
  (15%), other GNR
- Catheter-associated UTI: **yeast** (30%), E. coli (25%), other GNR, enterococci, S. epi
- Urethritis: Chlamydia trachomatis, Neisseria gonorrhoeae, Ureaplasma urealyticum,
  Trichomonas vaginalis, Mycoplasma genitalium, HSV

Clinical manifestations
- **Cystitis**: dysuria, **urgency**, **frequency**, Δ in urine color/odor, suprapubic pain;
  fever generally *absent*
- **Urethritis**: may be identical to cystitis except *urethral discharge is present*
- **Prostatitis**
  chronic: similar to cystitis except *symptoms of obstruction* (hesitancy, weak stream)
  acute: perineal pain, fever, tenderness on prostate exam
- **Pyelonephritis**: fever, shaking chills, flank or back pain, nausea, vomiting, diarrhea
- **Renal abscess** (intrarenal or perinephric): identical to pyelonephritis except *persistent
  fever despite appropriate antibiotics*

Diagnostic studies
- **Urinalysis: pyuria** + **bacteriuria** ± hematuria
  significant bacterial counts: $\geq 10^5$ CFU/ml in asx women, $\geq 10^3$ CFU/ml in men,
    $\geq 10^2$ CFU/ml in sx or catheterized Pts
  sterile pyuria → urethritis, renal tuberculosis, foreign body
- **Urine Gram stain and cx** (from clean-catch midstream or straight-cath specimen)
- Pregnant women & those undergoing urologic surgery *screen for asymptomatic bacteriuria*
- Blood cultures: in febrile and possibly complicated UTIs
- DNA detection/cx for *C. trachomatis/N. gonorrhoeae* in sexually active Pts or sterile pyuria
- First-void and midstream urine specimens, prostatic expressate, and post-prostatic
  massage urine specimens in cases of suspected prostatitis
- Abdominal CT to r/o abscess in Pts with pyelo who fail to defervesce after 72 h
- Urologic workup (renal U/S, abd CT, voiding cystography) if recurrent UTIs in men

Treatment of UTIs	
Clinical scenario	**Empiric treatment guidelines***
Cystitis	FQ or TMP-SMX PO × 3 d (uncompl.) or × 10-14 d (complicated) Asx bacteriuria in pregnant women or prior to urologic surgery → abx × 3 d
Urethritis	Treat for both Neisseria and Chlamydia Neisseria: ceftriaxone 125 mg IM × 1 or levofloxacin 250 mg PO × 1 Chlamydia: doxy 100 mg PO bid × 7 d or azithromycin 1 g PO × 1
Prostatitis	FQ or TMP-SMX PO × 14-28 d (acute) or 6-12 wks (chronic)
Pyelonephritis	Outpatient: FQ or amoxicillin/clav or oral ceph. PO × 14 d Inpatient: ceftriaxone IV or FQ PO or [amp IV + gent] or ampicillin/sulbactam × 14 d (Δ IV → PO when Pt improved clinically and afebrile × 24-48 h and then complete 14 d course)
Renal abscess	Drainage + antibiotics as for pyelonephritis

*When possible, organism-directed therapy, guided by *in vitro* susceptibilities or local patterns of drug
resistance should be utilized.

SOFT TISSUE AND BONE INFECTIONS

CELLULITIS

Infection of superficial and deep dermis and subcutaneous fat

Microbiology (NEJM 2004;350:904)
- Streptococcus and *Staphylococcus* including MRSA (15-74% of purulent skin and soft tissue infections; high-risk groups include athletic teams, military, prison, MSM, communities or families w/ MRSA infections; NEJM 2005;355:666)
- Cat bite: *P. multocida*; dog bite: *P. multocida* & *C. canimorsus*
- Penetrating injury: *Pseudomonas*
- Fish spine: *E. rhusiopathiae*, *V. vulnificus*

Clinical manifestations
- Erythema, edema, warmth, pain (rubor, tumor, calor, dolor)
- ± Lymphadenitis (proximal red streaking) and regional lymphadenopathy
- *P. multocida* → rapid onset; *C. canimorsus* → sepsis w/ symmetric, peripheral gangrene in splenectomized and other immunocompromised Pts

Diagnosis
- Largely clinical diagnosis; blood cx low yield but useful if ⊕
- Aspirate of bulla or pus from furuncle or pustule may provide dx

Treatment
- **Antibiotics**: penicillinase-resistant PCN or 1st gen. ceph.; if MRSA suspected → vanco if hospitalized, TMP-SMX if outPt
- **Limb elevation** (erythema may get *worse* after initiation of abx b/c bacterial killing → release of inflammatory enzymes)

"DIABETIC FOOT"

Infected neuropathic foot ulcer

Microbiology
- **Mild** (superficial, no bone or joint involvement): usually *S. aureus* or aerobic streptococci
- **Limb or life-threatening** = deep, bone/joint involvement, systemic tox., limb ischemia monomicrobial or polymicrobial with aerobes + anaerobes
  aerobes = staphylococci, streptococci, enterococci, and GNR (including *Pseudomonas*)
  anaerobes = anaerobic streptococci, *Bacteroides*, *Clostridium* (rare)

Clinical manifestations
- Ulcer with surrounding erythema and warmth ± purulent drainage
- Tenderness may be absent due to neuropathy
- ± Crepitus (indicating gas and ∴ mixed infection w/ GNR & anaerobes or *Clostridium*)
- ± Underlying osteomyelitis
- ± Systemic toxicity (fever, chills, leukocytosis, hyperglycemia)

Diagnostic studies
- Superficial swabs from ulcers *not* helpful (only yield superficial colonizing organisms)
- Wound cx (eg, curettage at base of ulcer after débridement) has ↑ Se
- Blood cx should be obtained in all Pts, ⊕ in 10-15%
- **Osteomyelitis should always be ruled out** (see below for specific imaging tests) probing to bone (ability to reach bone via ulcer/tract) has high Sp but low Se bone bx most reliable

Treatment (NEJM 1994;331:854)
- Bedrest, elevation, non-weight-bearing status
- Antibiotics

Severity of infection	Empiric antibiotics
Mild	penicillinase-resistant PCN or 1st gen. ceph. (TMP-SMX if MRSA suspected)
Chronic non-limb/life-threatening	[FQ + clindamycin] *or* ampicillin-sulbactam *or* ticarcillin-clavulanate
Life-threatening	[Imipenem + vanco] *or* [vanco + aztreonam + metronidazole] *or* [ampicillin-sulbactam + AG]

- **Surgery**: early, aggressive, and repeated surgical débridement; revascularization or amputation may be necessary

Definition
- Infection and necrosis of superficial fascia, subcutaneous fat, and deep fascia (necrosis of arteries and nerves in subcutaneous fat → gangrene)
- Fournier's gangrene: necrotizing fasciitis of the male genitalia (used by some to describe involvement of male or female perineum)

Epidemiology
- ↑ risk in diabetes, PVD, alcohol abuse, IVDA, immunosuppression, cirrhosis
- Can also affect healthy individuals

Microbiology
- Group I (often after abd/perineal surgery): polymicrobial (anaerobe + facultative anaerobe + GNR); often with DM, PVD and other comorbidities.
- Group II (extremities): Strep pyogenes ± Staph; often healthy w/o obvious portal of entry; up to half have toxic shock syndrome (TSS)
- Group III: marine Vibrio infection

Clinical manifestations
- Most common sites: extremities, abdominal wall, and perineum, but can occur anywhere
- **Cellulitic skin ∆s with poorly defined margins + rapid spread + systemic toxicity**
- **Pain out of proportion** to degree of apparent cellulitis; skin hyperesthetic and later anesthetic
- **Bullae formation** (serous → hemorrhagic); darkening of skin to bluish-gray → **cutaneous gangrene ± crepitus** or radiographically visible gas

Diagnostic signs
- Need high degree of clinical suspicion because of nonspecific physical exam
- Aspiration of necrotic center; blood cultures; Gram stain; ✓ CK for tissue necrosis
- Imaging studies: plain radiographs → soft tissue gas; CT → extent of infection, soft tissue gas; MRI → best tissue contrast
- Clinical diagnosis enough to initiate **urgent surgical exploration**

Treatment
- Definitive treatment is **surgical débridement** of necrotic tissue and fasciotomy
- Type I: breadth of GNR coverage determined by host, prev hosp, prev Rx and initial Gram stain; eg, carbapenem or [3rd gen ceph + amp + (clinda or metranidazole)]
- Type II: PCN + clindamycin. If community-acquired MRSA a consideration, + vanco. If TSS, add high dose IVIG.
- **Hyperbaric oxygen**: useful adjunct, but should not delay definitive surgical treatment

Prognosis
- Generally fatal if untreated; reported mortality 20-50%

CLOSTRIDIAL MYONECROSIS (GAS GANGRENE)

Definition
- Life-threatening, fulminant clostridial infection of skeletal muscle
- Usually **muscle trauma + wound contamination** with clostridial spores
- Most commonly C. perfringens or septicum + malignancy (heme or GI)

Clinical manifestations
- Incubation period 6 h to 2-3 d
- Acute onset with sense of heaviness or pain, often at site of trauma or surg, that rapidly ↑'s with marked systemic toxicity
- Bronze discoloration of skin, tense bullae, serosanguineous or dark fluid and necrotic areas
- **Crepitus** present but not prominent (gas is in muscle) may be obscured by edema

Diagnostic studies
- Gram stain of discharge: **large, Gram ⊕ bacilli with blunt ends,** very few polys
- Clostridial bacteremia in ~15%
- Plain radiographs: gas dissecting into muscle

Treatment
- **Surgical exploration with débridement,** fasciotomies, and amputation if necessary
- **Antibiotics**: high-dose **penicillin G** 24 MU IV divided q2-3h + **clinda** 900 mg IV q8h
- ? Hyperbaric oxygen

OSTEOMYELITIS

Infection of bone due to hematogenous seeding or direct spread from contiguous focus

Microbiology (NEJM 1997;336:999)
- **Hematogenous**: *S. aureus*; mycobacterial infection of vertebral body = Pott's disease
- **Contiguous focus** (may be acute or chronic)
  open fracture, orthopedic surgery, etc.: *S. aureus* and *S. epi*
  + vasc. insuffic. (eg, diabetic foot): **polymicrobial** (aerobic + anaerobic GPC & GNR)

Clinical manifestations
- Surrounding soft-tissue compromise ± fistula to superficial skin
- Vertebral osteomyelitis (common manifestation in adults over 50 y): unremitting, focal back pain and usually fever
- ± Fever, malaise, and night sweats (more common in hematogenous than contiguous)

Diagnostic studies
- Identification of the causative organism is key
- **Culture data from tissue** (surgical sampling/needle bx) *not* swabs of ulcers/fistulae
- **Blood cultures** (more often ⊕ with acute hematogenous osteomyelitis)
- Imaging
  plain radiographs: normal early in disease; lytic lesions seen after 2-6 wks
  CT: can demonstrate periosteal reaction and cortical and medullary destruction
  MRI: can detect very early changes
  CT & MRI very Se but not completely Sp; false ⊕ if contiguous focus w/ periosteal reaction, Charcot changes
  radionuclide imaging: very Se but non-Sp (false ⊕ if soft-tissue inflammation)

Treatment
- **Antibiotics** (based on cx data) × 4-6 wks
- **Surgery** should be considered for any of the following:
  acute osteo that fails to respond to medical therapy
  chronic osteo
  complications of pyogenic vertebral osteo (eg, early signs of cord compression, spinal instability, epidural abscess)
  infected prosthesis

EPIDURAL ABSCESS

Etiology
- Hematogenous spread (2/3): skin infection, soft tissue (dental abscess), or endocarditis
- Direct extension (1/3): vertebral osteomyelitis, sacral decubitus ulcer, spinal anesthesia or surgery, lumbar puncture
- Risk factors: diabetes, renal failure, alcoholism, IVDA, immunosuppression
- *S. aureus* most common pathogen

Clinical manifestations
- **Back pain** (unremitting midline) + usually **fever** ± nerve root or cord signs

Diagnostic studies
- **MRI**
- Blood cx (frequently ⊖)

Treatment
- **Antibiotics** + **surgery** (decompressive laminectomy and débridement) for failure to improve on medical therapy or early signs or symptoms of cord compression (with vertebral osteo and epidural abscess, may see paraplegia 48-72 h after first signs)

ACUTE BACTERIAL MENINGITIS

Definition
- Bacterial infection of the subarachnoid space

Microbiology in Adult Meningitis	
Etiology	**Comments**
S. pneumoniae (30-60%)	Most common cause in adults. Look for distant infection (eg, Osler's triad = meningitis, pneumonia, endocarditis). Drug-resistant *S. pneumoniae* (DRSP): ~40% PCN-resistant (20% intermed.; 15-20% high) ~<10% 3rd gen. ceph.-resistant (5% intermed.; <5% high) *even intermed. resistance problematic for Rx of meningitis*
N. meningitidis (10-35%)	Primarily in children and young adults; may be associated with petechiae or purpura. Deficiencies in terminal complement predispose to recurrent meningococcemia & rarely, meningitis.
H. influenzae (<5%)	↓ incidence in children because of *H. influenzae* type b vaccine. Look for predisposing factors in adults (eg, CSF leak, recent neurosurgical procedure, trauma, mastoiditis).
L. monocytogenes (5-10%)	Seen in elderly, alcoholics, or patients with malignancy, immunosuppression, or iron overload. Outbreaks associated with contaminated milk, cheese, coleslaw, raw vegetables. Despite name, often associated with *poly-predominant* pleocytosis.
GNRs (1-10%)	Usually nosocomial or postprocedure or in elderly or immunosuppressed.
Staphylococci (5%)	Seen with indwelling CSF shunt (*S. epidermidis*) or following neurosurgery or head trauma (*S. aureus*).
Mixed infection	Suspect parameningeal focus or CSF leak.

Clinical manifestations (NEJM 2006;354:14)
- **Fever** (77%)
- **Headache** (87%), **stiff neck** (83%), and **photosensitivity**
- Δ **MS** (69%) (defined as GCS < 14), **seizures** (5%)
- 2 of 4 (fever, HA, stiff neck, Δ MS) present in 95%
- Presentation may be *atypical* in elderly and immunocompromised, with primarily lethargy and confusion, and no fever

Physical exam
- **Nuchal rigidity** (Se 30%), **Kernig's sign** (Pt supine, hip flexed at 90°, knee flexed at 90°; ⊕ if passive extension of knee results in resistance), **Brudzinski's sign** (Pt supine and limbs supine; ⊕ if passive neck flexion → involuntary hip and/or knee flexion) nb, Kernig's and Brudzinski's signs ⊕ in only ~5% of Pts (CID 2002;35:46)
- ± Focal neuro findings (~30%; hemiparesis, aphasia, visual field cuts, CN palsies)
- ± Funduscopic findings: papilledema, absent venous pulsations
- ± Rash: maculopapular, petechial, or purpuric

Diagnostic studies
- **Blood cultures**
- *Consider* **head CT** to r/o mass effect before LP *if* presence of high-risk feature (age >60 y, immunocompromised, h/o CNS disease, new onset seizure, Δ MS, focal neuro findings); absence of all these has NPV 97%; however, should be noted that in Pts w/ mass effect, herniation may occur even w/o LP and may not occur even w/ LP (NEJM 2001;345:1727)
- **Lumbar puncture** (NEJM 2006;355:e12): CSF Gram stain has 60-90% Se; cx has 70-85% Se

CSF Findings in Meningitis					
Condition	Appearance	Pressure (cm)	WBC/mm³ _Predom type_	Glc (mg/dl)	TP (mg/dl)
Normal	Clear	9-18	0-5 _lymphs_	50-75	15-40
Bacterial	Cloudy	18-30	100-10,000 _polys_	<45	100-1000
TB	Cloudy	18-30	<500 _lymphs_	<45	100-200
Fungal	Cloudy	18-30	<300 _lymphs_	<45	40-300
Aseptic	Clear	9-18	<300 _polys → lymphs_	50-100	50-100

- Additional CSF studies depending on clinical suspicion: acid-fast smear and cx, India ink preparation, cryptococcal antigen, fungal cx, PCR (eg, of HSV, VZV, enteroviral), cytology

Treatment of Meningitis	
Clinical scenario	Empiric treatment guidelines*
Normal adult	**Ceftriaxone 2 g IV q12h + Vancomycin 1 g IV q12h** (nb, Cftx in case PCN-resistant _S. pneumo_; Vanco, which has poorer CSF penetration, in case Cftx-resistant _S. Pneumo_) If >50 y old: + Ampicillin 2 g IV q4h for _Listeria_ TMP/SMX + vancomycin if β-lactam allergic
Immuno-compromised	Ampicillin + ceftazidime ± vancomycin + acyclovir
CSF shunts, recent neurosurgery, or head trauma	Vancomycin + ceftazidime
Empiric antibiotics should be started as soon as possible. If concerned about ↑ ICP, obtain BCx → start empiric abx → obtain head CT → LP (if not contraindicated); yield of CSF fluid unlikely to be changed if obtained w/in ~ 4h of initiation of abx.	
Corticosteroids: Dexamethasone 10 mg IV q6h × 4 d → ↓ neuro disability & mort. by ~50% w/ _S. pneumo_ & GCS 8-11. Must start before or w/ 1st dose of abx (_NEJM_ 2002;347:1549).	
Prophylaxis: rifampin (600 mg PO bid × 2 d) or ciprofloxacin (500 mg PO × 1) or ceftriaxone (250 mg IM × 1) for close contacts of Pt w/ meningococcal meningitis.	

*When possible, organism-directed Rx, guided by suscept. or local patterns of drug resistance should be used.

Prognosis
- For community-acquired _S. pneumo_ mort. 19-37%; 30% have long-term neuro sequelae

ASEPTIC MENINGITIS

Definition
- **Negative bacterial microbiologic data**, CSF pleocytosis with ⊖ appropriate blood and CSF cultures (aseptic meningitis can be neutrophilic, though less common)
- Misnomer, as "aseptic" only in sense that less likely to be acute bacterial meningitis, but can be due to both infectious and noninfectious etiologies

Etiologies (_Neurology_ 2006;66:75)
- **Viral**: enteroviruses (most common), HIV, HSV (type 2 > 1), VZV, mumps, lymphocytic choriomeningitis virus, encephalitis viruses, adenovirus, polio, CMV, EBV
- **Parameningeal focus of infection** (eg, brain abscess, epidural abscess, septic thrombophlebitis of dural venous sinuses, or subdural empyema)
- **Tuberculosis**, **fungal**, **spirochetal** (Lyme disease, syphilis, leptospirosis), **rickettsial**, _Coxiella_, _Ehrlichia_
- Partially treated bacterial meningitis
- **Medications**: TMP/SMX, NSAIDs, penicillin, isoniazid
- **Systemic illness**: SLE, sarcoidosis, Behçet's, Sjögren's syndrome, rheumatoid arthritis
- **Neoplasms**: intracranial tumors (or cysts), lymphomatous or carcinomatous meningitis

Empiric treatment
- No abx if suspect viral (cell count <500 w/ >50% lymphs, TP <80-100 mg/dl, normal glc, ⊖ Gram stain, not elderly/immunocompromised); o/w start empiric abx, wait for cx data
- MTb: antimyobacterial Rx + dexamethasone (_NEJM_ 2004;351:1741)

VIRAL ENCEPHALITIS

Definition
• Viral infection of the brain parenchyma

Etiologies (Lancet 2002;359:507; Neurology 2006;66:75)
• **HSV-1** (~9%)
• **Arboviruses** (~9%): Eastern equine, Western equine, West Nile, St. Louis
• **Enteroviruses**: Coxsackie, echo
• Others: VZV (~9%), CMV, EBV, HIV, rabies, adenoviruses
• Nonviral etiologies that mimic: bacterial endocarditis, abscess, toxoplasmosis, TB, toxins, vasculitis, subdural hematoma

Clinical manifestations
• Fever, HA, Δ MS, ± seizures and focal neuro findings (latter atypical for viral *meningitis*)

Diagnostic studies
• **Lumbar puncture**: lymphocytic pleocytosis; PCRs available for HSV, VZV, CMV, adeno, enterovirus in right setting; ELISA or DFA of nasal or resp swabs for adenovirus or flu Ags serologies
• **MRI**
• Etiologic dx in only about 25% of cases

Treatment
• HSV: acyclovir 10 mg/kg IV q8h (recovery related to promptness of Rx) + good hydration

Definition
- Infection of endothelium of heart (including but not limited to the valves)
- Acute (ABE): infection of normal valves with a virulent organism (eg, *S. aureus*)
- Subacute (SBE): indolent infection of abnormal valves with a less virulent organism (eg, *S. viridans*)

Predisposing conditions
- **Abnormal valve**
  high-risk: prior endocarditis, rheumatic valvular disease, AoV disease, complex cyanotic lesions, prosthesis (1.5-3% at 12 mos, 3-6% at 5 y), HCMP
  medium-risk: MV disease (including MVP w/ MR or leaflet thickening), HCMP
- **Abnormal risk of bacteremia**: IVDA, indwelling venous catheters (20% of bacteremic Pts develop endocarditis), poor dentition, hemodialysis, diabetes mellitus

Modified Duke Criteria	
Major	**Minor**

• **Sustained bacteremia** by an organism known to cause endocarditis (or 1 BCx or ⊕ serology for *Coxiella*)
• **Endocardial involvement** document by *either*
  ⊕ echocardiogram (vegetation, abscess, prosthetic dehiscence)
  or
  new valvular regurgitation
	• Predisposing condition (see above)
	• Fever
	• **Vascular phenomena**: septic arterial or pulmonary emboli, mycotic aneurysms, ICH, Janeway lesions
	• **Immune phenomena**: ⊕ RF, GN, Osler's nodes, Roth spots
	• ⊕ **blood cx** not meeting major criteria

Definitive (ie, highly probable): 2 major *or* 1 major + 3 minor *or* 5 minor criteria	
Possible: 1 major + 1 minor *or* 3 minor criteria	

(CID 2000;30:633)

Microbiology of Endocarditis				
	Native valve endocarditis (NVE)		**Prosthetic valve endocarditis (PVE)**	
Etiology	**Non-IVDA**	**IVDA**	**early** (<6 mo post)	**late** (>6 mo post)
S. viridans et al.	40%	10%	<10%	35%
Enterococcus	10%	10%	<5%	10%
S. aureus	30%	60%	25%	20%
S. epidermidis	5%	<5%	40%	20%
GNR	5%	10%	10%	<5%
Other	<5%	<5%	10%	10%
Culture ⊖	5%	<5%	<5%	5%
Culture ⊖ = nutritionally-deficient streptococci, HACEK (*Haemophilus parainfluenzae & aphrophilus, Actinobacillus, Cardiobacterium, Eikenella,* and *Kingella*), *Bartonella, Coxiella, Chlamydia, Legionella, Brucella*				

(Adapted from Braunwald, E, ed., Heart Disease, 5th ed., 1997; W. B. Saunders, Phila.)

Clinical manifestations *(NEJM 2001;345:1318)*
- **Persistent bacteremia**: fever (80-90%), anorexia, weight loss, night sweats, fatigue
- **Valvular or perivalvular infection**: new murmur, CHF, conduction abnormalities
- **Septic emboli**: systemic emboli (eg, to periphery, CNS, kidneys, spleen, or joints), pulmonary emboli (if right-sided), mycotic aneurysm, MI (coronary artery embolism)
- **Immune complex phenomena**: arthritis, glomerulonephritis, ⊕ RF, ↑ ESR

Physical exam
- HEENT: **Roth spots** (retinal hemorrhage + pale center), **petechiae** (conjunctivae, palate)
- Cardiac: **valvular regurgitation** ± thrill (fenestrated valve or ruptured chordae), muffled prosthetic valve sounds, pericardial rub. *Frequent examinations* for changing murmurs.
- Abdomen: tender splenomegaly
- Musculoskeletal: arthritis, vertebral tenderness
- Extremities *(typically seen in SBE not ABE)*
  Janeway lesions (septic emboli → nontender, hemorrhagic macules on palms or soles)
  Osler's nodes (immune complexes → tender nodules on pads of digits)
  proximal nailbed splinter hemorrhages; clubbing
- Neuro: Δ MS or focal deficits

Diagnostic studies
- **Blood cultures** (*before antibiotics*): at least 3 sets (aerobic & anaerobic bottles) from different sites, ideally spaced ≥1 h apart. ✓ BCx (at least 2 sets) after appropriate antibiotics have been initiated to document clearance; repeat q24-48h until ⊖.
- CBC with differential, ESR, rheumatoid factor, BUN, Cr, U/A & UCx
- **ECG** (on admission and at regular intervals): to assess for new conduction abnormalities
- **Echocardiogram**: obtain TTE; TEE if (1) intermediate pretest probability (4-60%), (2) prosthetic valve, (3) TTE nondiagnostic, (4) TTE ⊖ but endocarditis strongly suspected, or (5) suspect progressive or invasive infection (eg, persistent bacteremia or fever, new conduction abnormality, intracardiac shunt, etc.) (*NEJM* 2001;345:1318)

Method	Sensitivity		
	NVE	**PVE**	**Abscess**
Transthoracic (TTE)	~65%	~25%	28%
Transesophageal (TEE)	>90%	~90%	87%

(*Chest* 1991;100:351; *NEJM* 1991;324:795; *JACC* 1991;18:391; *AJC* 1993;71:201)

Treatment
- Obtain culture data first

  ABE → antibiotics should be started promptly after culture data obtained

  SBE → if Pt hemodynamically stable, antibiotics may be delayed in order to properly obtain adequate blood culture data, especially in the case of prior antibiotic treatment
- **Suggested empiric therapy**

  native valve ABE: [naf + gent] or [vanco + gent] if high prev. of MRSA

  native valve SBE: penicillin/ampicillin + gentamicin

  prosthetic valve: vancomycin + gentamicin + rifampin
- Adjust antibiotic regimen based on organism and sensitivities
- Repeat BCx qd until Pt defervesces and BCx ⊖; usually 2-3 d
- Fever may persist up to 1 wk after appropriate antibiotic therapy instituted or in setting of metastatic sites of infection
- Systemic anticoagulation relatively *contraindicated* given risk of hemorrhagic transformation of cerebral embolic strokes (however, in absence of cerebral emboli, can continue anticoagulation for preexisting indication)
- Duration of therapy is usually **4-6 wks**, except in cases of uncomplicated right-sided endocarditis, in which 2 wks of therapy may have comparable outcomes

Indications for surgery
- In general, try to deliver as many days of abx as possible, in hopes of ↓ incidence of recurrent infection in prosthesis, as well as to improve structural integrity of tissue that will receive prosthesis
- Cerebral septic embolism historically considered a relative *contraindication* to immediate surgery as risk of hemorrhagic conversion during cardiopulmonary bypass high during the first 10-14 d; recent studies suggest in modern bypass area, risk lower (*Stroke* 2006;37:2094)
- Indications for surgery

  refractory CHF (ie, despite maximal, ICU-level medical therapy)

  persistent or refractory infection (eg, ⊕ BCx after 1 wk of appropriate IV abx and no drainable metastatic focus)

  invasive infection (ring abscess, worsening conduction; seen in 15% native, 60% prosthetic)

  prosthetic valve, especially with valve malfunction or dehiscence or S. aureus infection

  hard-to-eradicate infections (eg, fungi)

  high risk for embolic complications

Prognosis
- Non-IVDA ABE w/ *S. aureus* → 55-70% survival
- IVDA ABE w/ *S. aureus* → 85-90% survival
- SBE → 85-90% survival

Endocarditis Prophylaxis	
Cardiac conditions	**Prosthetic valve; previous endocarditis; congenital heart disease** (CHD) including unrepaired or incompletely repaired cyanotic CHD (palliative shunts or conduits), 1st 6 mos after completely repaired CHD using prosthetic material; **cardiac transplant recipients w/ valvulopathy** (Nb, prophylaxis no longer rec. in Pts w/ acquired valvular dysfxn, bicuspid AoV, MVP with leaflet thickening or regurgitation, HCMP)
Procedures	**Dental:** that involve manipulation of gingival tissue or periapical region of teeth or perforation of oral mucosa (eg, extractions, periodontal procedures, implants, root canal, cleanings) **Respiratory:** incision or biopsy of respiratory mucosa (Nb, prophylaxis no longer rec. for GI or GU procedures)
Regimens	Oral: **amoxicillin 2 g 30-60 min before** Unable to take PO: amp 2 g IM/IV or cefazolin or Cftx 1 g IM/IV PCN-allergic: clindamycin 600 mg PO/IM/IV

(Circ 2007;115:epub)

BACTEREMIA

Etiologies
- 1° infxn due to direct inoculation of the blood, frequently assoc. w/ intravascular catheters
- 2° infxn due to infection in another site (eg, UTI, lung, skin) spreading to blood

Microbiology
- 1° infxn/indwelling catheters (CID 2004;39:309)
  Coagulase-neg staphylococci (includes S. epidermidis and others) 31%
  Staphylococcus aureus 20%
  Enterococci 9%
  Candida species 9%
  E. coli 6%
  Klebsiella species 5%
- 2° infxn: dependent upon the source

Risk factors for true bacteremia (JAMA 1992;267:1962)
- **Pt**: fever, shaking chills, IVDA, major comorbidities
- **Organism**
  higher risk: S. aureus, β-hemolytic Strep, enterococci, GNR, S. pneumonia, Neisseria
  lower risk: coag-neg staph (~10%), diptheroids & *Propionibacterium* (~0%)
- **Time to growth**: <24 h → higher risk, >72 h → lower risk (except for slow-growing organisms such as HACEK group)
- **Confirmatory cultures**

Treatment
- **1° infxn**: antibiotics based upon culture results
  empiric initial vanco to cover coag-neg staph and MRSA while awaiting sensi.
  also Rx line tip w/ >15 colonies (in clinical setting suggestive of infxn; NEJM 1985; 312:1142)
- S. aureus: d/c catheter, echo to r/o endocarditis; if echo ⊖, Rx × 2 wks from first ⊖ BCx
- Coag-neg staph: may consider leaving catheter in place, Rx × 2 wks
  Cleared 80% of time w/ line left in unless tunnel infxn or clot (c/w 10% if S. aureus)
  If catheter left in place, re✓ BCx >1 wk after completion of abx regimen
- **2° infxn**: assess for primary source of infection and treat underlying infection
- **Persistently ⊕ BCx**: d/c indwelling catheters, consider metastatic infxn, consider infected thrombosis

TUBERCULOSIS

Epidemiology
- U.S. prevalence of infection: 10-15 million people; worldwide prevalence: ~2 billion people
- ↑ incidence in U.S. from 1984-1992 due to HIV, poverty, homelessness, immigration
- **Pt is more likely to develop TB disease if:**
  High-prevalence populations (more likely to be exposed to and infected with bacillus):
    immigrant from high-prevalence areas, homeless or medically underserved, resident
    or worker in jail or long-term care facility, HCW at facility w/ TB, close contact
    to Pt w/ active TB
  High-risk populations (more likely to progress from infection → active disease):
    HIV ⊕ or other immunodeficiencies, chronic renal failure, diabetes mellitus, IVDA,
    alcoholics, malnourished, malignancy, s/p gastrectomy

Microbiology and natural history
- Transmission of *Mycobacterium tuberculosis* via small-particle aerosols (ie, droplet nuclei)
- 90% of infected normal hosts will never develop clinically evident disease, 10% will
- Localized disease: healing & calcification *or* progressive 1° TB
- Hematogenous spread: latent infection ± reactivation TB *or* progressive disseminated TB
- Two-thirds of clinically evident disease due to reactivation in U.S.; risk ~2%/y for first
  2-3 y after infection

Screening for prior infection
- **Whom to screen**: high-prevalence and high-risk populations (HIV ⊕ Pts should
  have PPD testing as part of initial evaluation and annually thereafter)
- **How to screen**: Mantoux tuberculin test (ie, purified protein derivative or PPD)
  inject 5-TU (0.1 ml) intermed. strength PPD intradermally → wheal; examine 48-72 h
- **How to interpret**: determine maximum diameter of induration by palpation

Size of reaction	Persons considered to have ⊕ test
>5 mm	HIV ⊕ or immunosuppressed (eg, prednisone 15 mg/d × >1 mo) Close contacts with Pt w/ active TB CXR c/w prior TB
>10 mm	All other high-risk populations Recent conversion (↑ in induration by >10 mm in last 2 y)
>15 mm	Everyone else
False ⊖	Faulty application, anergy, acute TB (2-10 wk to convert), acute non-TB infections, malignancy
False ⊕	Improper reading, cross-reaction with atypicals, BCG vaccination (although usually <10 mm by adulthood)
Booster effect	↑ induration b/c immunologic boost provided by prior skin test in previously sensitized (ie, infected) individual. Test goes from ⊖ → ⊕, but does *not* represent true conversion due to *recent* infection. 2nd test is Pt's true baseline. Can be seen 1 y after initial skin test.

(NEJM 2002;347:1860)

- IFN-γ assays may be superior for screening purposes b/c of ↑ Sp (Lancet 2001;357:2017; JAMA
  2001;286:1740; Lancet 2006;367:1328, MMWR Dec. 16, 2005)

Clinical manifestations
- **Primary tuberculous pneumonia**: middle or lower lobe **consolidation**,
  ± effusion, ± cavitation
- **Tuberculous pleurisy**: can occur with primary or reactivation. Due to breakdown of
  granuloma with spilling of contents into pleural cavity and local inflammation.
  Pulmonary effusion ± pericardial and peritoneal effusions (tuberculous polyserositis).
- **Reactivation tuberculous pulmonary dis.**: apical infiltrate ± volume loss ± cavitation
- **Miliary tuberculosis**: acute or insidious; wide dissemination 2° hematogenous spread;
  usually in immunocompromised, diabetic, alcoholic, elderly or malnourished Pts.
  Constitutional symptoms (fever, night sweats, weight loss) prominent.
  Pulmonary disease w/ small millet seed-like lesions (2-4 mm) on CXR or chest CT
  (latter more Se, but not present in everyone with miliary TB).
- **Extrapulmonary tuberculosis**: lymphadenitis, pericarditis, peritonitis, meningitis,
  nephritis, osteomyelitis (vertebral = Pott's disease), hepatitis, cutaneous
- **Tuberculosis and HIV infection**: HIV-infected and other immunosuppressed Pts at
  ↑ risk for reactivation and progressive primary infection. Risk of progression from
  infection to disease 8-10%/y.

Diagnostic studies for active TB *(high index of suspicion is key!)*
- **Acid-fast smear** (rapid diagnosis) and **culture** (more Se and allows susceptibility testing) of sputum, bronchoscopic alveolar lavage, pleura, or other clinical specimens
- PCR: 94-97% Se c/w smear; 40-77% Se c/w culture
- CXR: classically fibrocavitary apical disease in reactivation vs. middle & lower lobe consolidation in 1° TB, but distinction imperfect and HIV ⊕ strongly assoc. with non-apical disease, regardless of timing *(JAMA 2005;293:2740)*

Preventive therapy *(JAMA 2005;293:2776)*
- Appropriate prophylaxis reduces incidence of subsequent disease by 65-75%
- Treat Pts who are ⊕ based on screening guidelines listed above
- **Rule out active disease** in any Pt w/ suggestive s/s before starting INH

Scenario	Regimen
Likely INH-sensitive	INH 300 mg PO qd + pyridoxine 25 mg PO qd × 6-9 mo
HIV ⊕	INH 300 mg PO qd + pyridoxine 25 mg PO qd × 9 mo
Contact case INH-resistant	RIF × 4 mo
Contact case known or suspected to have multi-drug resistant TB	No proven regimen: ? PZA + ETB, ? PZA + FQ

(INH = isoniazid, RIF = rifampin, PZA = pyrazinamide, ETB = ethambutol, FQ = fluoroquinolone)

- **Monitor for hepatitis:** if aminotransferases 5× normal (risk ↑ w/ age; *Chest 2005;128:116*) or symptomatic → d/c current anti-TB medications and reevaluate

Treatment of active tuberculosis *(Lancet 2003;362:887; JAMA 2005;293:2776)*
- Isolate Pt
- Use regimens containing multiple drugs to which the organism is susceptible
- Promote adherence to therapy; directly observed therapy (DOT) cost effective for Pts at high risk for nonadherence
- Screen for HIV in all Pts in whom initiating anti-TB Rx

Antituberculous Medications		
Drug	Dose	Adverse effects
Isoniazid (INH)	300 mg PO qd	Hepatitis, peripheral neuropathy (prevented by concomitant pyridoxine), lupus-like syndrome
Rifampin (RIF)	600 mg PO qd	Orange discoloration of urine/tears, hepatitis, GI upset, hypersensitivity, fever
Pyrazinamide (PZA)	25 mg/kg PO qd	Hepatitis, hyperuricemia, arthritis
Ethambutol (EMB)	15-25 mg/kg PO qd	Optic neuritis
Streptomycin (SM)	15 mg/kg IM qd	Ototoxicity, nephrotoxicity
Amikacin (AMK)	15 mg/kg IM qd	Ototoxicity, nephrotoxicity
Quinolone Moxifloxacin	400 mg PO qd	GI upset

Antituberculous Regimens*	
Scenario	Regimen
Pulmonary TB **≥4% INH-resist. in community** (includes most of U.S.)	INH + RIF + PZA + (EMB) until suscept. known If *sensitive* to INH & RIF → INH + RIF + PZA × 2 mos, then → INH + RIF × 4 mos If *resistant*, see next row
Drug-resistant TB (INH-, RIF-, or multidrug-resistant)	Consult ID specialist
Extrapulmonary TB	Consult ID specialist
TB in HIV ⊕ patient	Consult ID specialist

*Individualize duration based on host, disease form, and rate of clinical/microbiologic improvement.

Definition
- AIDS: HIV + CD4 count <200/mm³ or opportunistic infection (OI) or malignancy

Epidemiology
- ~1 million Americans infected w/ HIV; 6th leading cause of death in 25-44 y-old age group
- ~40 million individuals infected worldwide
- Routes: sexual (risk is 0.3% for male-to-male, 0.2% for male-to-female, 0.1% for female-to-male transmission), IVDA, transfusions, needle sticks (0.3%), vertical (15-40%)

Acute retroviral syndrome (ARS)
- Occurs in ~40-70% of HIV ⊕ Pts ~4 wks after infection; ⊕ ELISA, ⊕ viral load
- Manifestations: mononucleosis-like syndrome (↑ incidence of mucocutaneous and neurologic manifestations c/w EBV or CMV)

Diagnostic studies
- **ELISA** for HIV-1 Ab: ⊕ 1-12 wks after acute infection; >99% Se; 1° screen test
- **Western blot**: ⊕ if ≥2 bands from diff regions of HIV genome; >99% Sp; confirmatory after ⊕ ELISA
- **Rapid preliminary tests**: 4 Ab tests; use saliva, plasma, blood, or serum; 99% Se & Sp
- **PCR (viral load)**: detects HIV-1 RNA in plasma; standard (limit 200-400 copies per ml) and ultrasensitive assays (limit 20-75 copies per ml). ~2-4% false ⊕ rate, but usually low # of copies; in contrast, should be very high (>750k) in primary infection.
- When testing, obtain informed consent for ELISA, Western, and PCR
- HIV screening is recommended for all Pts in all health care settings *(MMWR Sept 22, 2006)*
- **CD4 count**: not a dx test *per se*, as may be HIV ⊕ and have a normal CD4 count or may have a low CD4 count and *not* be HIV ⊕; many other illnesses impact CD4 count

Initial approach to HIV ⊕ Pt
- **Document** HIV infection (if adequate documentation is not available, repeat dx studies)
- **H & P** (evidence of OIs, malignancies, STDs); review all meds
- **Laboratory evaluation**: CD4 count, viral load, genotype test, CBC with diff., Cr, lytes, LFTs, fasting glc, PPD, syphilis, toxoplasmosis, CMV, fasting lipids, hepatitis serologies, baseline CXR, Pap smear in women

Antiretrovirals	
Drugs	**Side Effects**
NRTI zidovudine (AZT; Retrovir) stavudine (d4T; Zerit) didanosine (ddI; Videx) zalcitabine (ddC; Hivid) abacavir (ABC; Ziagen) lamivudine (3TC; Epivir) tenofovir (TDF; Virend) emtricitabine (FTC; Emtriva)	class: GI intol. common (less w/ 3TC, ABC, TDF) facial/peripheral lipoatrophy (less w/ 3TC, FTC, ABC, TDF) lactic acidosis (less w/ 3TC/FTC, ABC, TDF) ddI & d4T → peripheral neuropathy & pancreatitis AZT → BM suppression ABC → hypersensitivity (3%)
NNRTI nevirapine (NVP; Viramune) efavirenz (EFV; Sustiva) delaverdine (DLV; Rescriptor)	class: rash, induce or inhibit CYP₄₅₀ EFV → CNS effects
PI amprenavir (APV; Agenerase) atazanavir (ATV; Reyataz) indinavir (IDV; Crixivan) fosamprenavir (FPV; Lexiva) lopinavir/riton. (LPV/r; Kaletra) ritonavir (RTV; Norvir) nelfinavir (NFV; Viracept) saquinavir (SQV; Fortavase) tipranavir (TPV; Aptivus) darunavir (DRV; Prezista)	class: GI intolerance inhibit CYP₄₅₀ type II DM truncal obesity hyperlipidemia (less w/ ATV) IDV → nephrolithiasis
FI enfurvitide (T20; Fuzeon)	injection site reaction

NRTI = nucleoside/tide reverse transcriptase inhibitor; NNRTI = nonnucleoside RTI; PI = protease inhibitor; FI = fusion inhibitor

- **Use of antiretrovirals should be done in consultation with an HIV specialist** as recommendations continue to be in flux and drug resistance and adverse reactions can be complicated to manage. Below are some guidelines for initiation *(JAMA 2006;296:827)*.

- Indications for initiation of therapy (HAART)
  AIDS or **symptomatic HIV** (eg, thrush, unexplained fevers)
  asymptomatic + **high viral load** (>35-50,000 copies/ml) or **low CD4** (consider at 200-350/mm^3, definite at <200/mm^3)
- Resistance testing recommended for all Pts in US starting therapy
- Regimens *(JAMA 2006;296:827)*
  [NNRTI + 2 NRTI] or [PI (± low-dose ritonavir) + 2 NRTI]
  NNRTI (EFV) + 2 NRTI better tolerated and achieved greater virologic suppression c/w PI (NFV) + 2 NRTI or 4-drug regimen *(Lancet 2006;368:287)*
  EFV + TDF + FTC reasonable regimen (superior to EFV + AZT + 3TC; *NEJM 2006;354:251*)
  ? NRTI + [NNRTI or PI] better tolerated and as effective as 3 drugs *(Lancet 2006;368:2125)*
  Integrase inhibitors under study *(Lancet 2007;369:1261)*
- Viral load should ↓ 1 log copies/ml per month
- Initiation of antiretrovirals may *transiently worsen* existing OIs for several wks b/c ↑ immune response ("Immune Reconstitution Syndrome" or IRS)
- If Rx needs to be interrupted, *stop all antiretrovirals* to minimize development of resistance
- Failing regimen = unable to achieve undetectable viral load (? perhaps okay if <10k; *Lancet 2004;364:51*), ↑ viral load, ↓ CD4 count, or clinical deterioration (with detectable viral load consider genotypic or phenotypic assay)

OI Prophylaxis		
OI	**Indication**	**1° Prophylaxis**
Tuberculosis	⊕ PPD (≥5 mm) or High-risk exposure	INH + vitamin B$_6$ × 9 mo
Pneumocystis jiroveci	CD4 count <200/mm^3 or CD4% <14% or thrush	TMP-SMX DS or SS qd or DS tiw or dapsone 100 mg qd or atovaquone 1500 mg qd or pentamidine 300 mg inh q4wk
Toxoplasmosis	CD4 count <100/mm^3 and ⊕ Toxoplasma serology	TMP-SMX DS qd or dapsone 200 mg qd + pyrimethamine 75 mg qd + leucovorin 25 qwk
MAC	CD4 count <50/mm^3	azithro 1200 mg qwk or clarithro 500 mg bid
Stop 1° prophylaxis if CD4 > initiation threshold >3-6 mo on HAART		
Stop 2° prophylaxis (maintenance therapy of existing OI; drugs and doses differ for different OIs) if there has been clinical resolution or stabilization and CD4 thresholds have been exceeded × 3-6 mo		

(MMWR June 14, 2002)

COMPLICATIONS OF HIV/AIDS

CD4 count	Complications
<500	Constitutional symptoms Seborrheic dermatitis, oral hairy leukoplakia, Kaposi's sarcoma, lymphoma Oral, esophageal, and recurrent vaginal candidiasis Recurrent bacterial infections Pulmonary and extrapulmonary tuberculosis HSV, VZV
<200	*Pneumocystis jiroveci* pneumonia ("PCP"), *Toxoplasma, Bartonella Cryptococcus, Histoplasma, Coccidioides*
<50-100	CMV, MAC Invasive aspergillosis, bacillary angiomatosis (disseminated *Bartonella*) CNS lymphoma, PML

Fever
- Etiologies *(CID 1999;28:341)*
  infxn (88%): MAC, CMV, early PCP, TB, histoplasmosis, sinusitis, endocarditis
  lymphoma
  drug reaction
- Workup: guided by CD4 count, s/s, epi & exposures
  CBC, extended chemistries, LFTs, BCx, CXR, UA, ✓ medications, ? ✓ abd CT
  CD4 <100-200 → serum cryptococcal Ag, LP, urinary Histo Ag, mycobacterial and fungal isolators, CMV

pulmonary s/s → CXR; ABG; sputum for bacterial culture, PCP, AFB; bronchoscopy
diarrhea → stool for fecal leukocytes, culture, O&P, AFB; endoscopy
abnormal LFTs → abdominal CT, liver biopsy
cytopenias → bone marrow biopsy (include aspirate for culture)

Cutaneous
- Seborrheic dermatitis; eosinophilic folliculitis; HSV and VZV infections; prurigo nodularis; scabies; cutaneous candidiasis; eczema; psoriasis; cutaneous drug eruptions
- Dermatophyte infections: proximal subungual onychomycosis (onychomycosis starting at nailbed) virtually pathognomonic for HIV
- **Molluscum contagiosum** (poxvirus): 2-5 mm pearly papules with central umbilication
- **Kaposi's sarcoma** (KSHV or HHV8): red-purple nonblanching nodular lesions
- **Bacillary angiomatosis** (disseminated *Bartonella*): friable violaceous vascular papules
- **Warts** (HPV infection)

Ophthalmologic
- **CMV retinitis** (CD4 count usually <50); Rx: ganciclovir, valganciclovir, ganciclovir ocular insert, foscarnet, or cidofovir (also HZV, VZV)

Oral
- **Aphthous ulcers**
- **Thrush** (oral candidiasis): typically associated with burning or pain. Types: exudative (curdlike patches that reveal raw surface when scraped off), erythematous (erythema without exudates), atrophic
- **Oral hairy leukoplakia**: painless proliferation of papillae. Caused by EBV but not precancerous; *adherent* white coating usually on *lateral* tongue.
- **Kaposi's sarcoma**

Cardiac
- Dilated CMP; PHT; PI → ↑ risk of MI (but absolute risk small; *NEJM* 2007;356:1723)

Pulmonary

Radiographic pattern	Common causes
Normal	Early *P. jiroveci* (PCP)
Diffuse interstitial infiltrates	*P. jiroveci*, TB, viral or disseminated fungal PNA
Focal consolidation or masses	Bacterial or fungal PNA, TB, Kaposi's sarcoma
Cavitary lesions	TB, aspergillosis and other fungal PNA Bacterial PNA (including *Nocardia* and *Rhodococcus*)
Pleural effusion	TB, bacterial or fungal PNA Kaposi's sarcoma, lymphoma

- *Pneumocystis jioveci* ("PCP") pneumonia (CD4 <200)
  constitutional sx, fever, night sweats, dyspnea on exertion, nonproductive cough
  CXR w/ interstitial pattern, ↓ P$_a$O$_2$, ↑ A-a ∇, ↑ LDH, ⊕ PCP sputum stain
  Rx if P$_a$O$_2$ >70: **TMP-SMX DS 2 tabs PO q8h** or [TMP 5 mg/kg PO tid + dapsone 100 mg PO qd] or [clindamycin + primaquine] or atovaquone
  Rx if P$_a$O$_2$ <70: **prednisone** (40 mg PO bid then ↓ after 5 d; start *before* TMP/SMX; *NEJM* 1990;323:1444, 1451); **TMP-SMX 15 mg of TMP/kg IV divided q6-8h** or [clindamycin + primaquine] or pentamidine or trimetrexate

Gastrointestinal
- **Esophagitis**: *Candida*, CMV, HSV, aphthous ulcers, pill-induced
  upper endoscopy if no thrush or unresponsive to empiric antifungal therapy
- **Enterocolitis**
  bacterial (usually acute): *Salmonella*, *Shigella*, *Campylobacter*, *Yersinia*, *C. difficile*
  protozoal (usually chronic): *Giardia*, *Entamoeba*, *Cryptosporidium*, *Isospora*, *Microsporidium*, *Cyclospora*
  viral (CMV, adenovirus); fungal (histoplasmosis); MAC; AIDS enteropathy
- **GI bleeding**: CMV, Kaposi's sarcoma, lymphoma, histo
- **Proctitis**: HSV, CMV, *Chlamydia*, gonococcal

Hepatobiliary
- **Hepatitis**: HBV, HCV, CMV, MAC, drug-induced
- **AIDS cholangiopathy**: often in assoc. w/ CMV or *Cryptosporidium* or *Microsporidium*

Renal
- **HIV-associated** nephropathy (collapsing FGS); nephrotoxic drugs

Hematologic

- **Anemia**: ACD, BM infiltration by infxn or tumor, drug toxicity, hemolysis
- **Leukopenia**
- **Thrombocytopenia**: bone marrow involvement, ITP
- **↑ globulin**

Oncologic

- **Non-Hodgkin's lymphoma**: ↑ frequency regardless of CD4 count, but incidence ↑ as CD4 count ↓
- **CNS lymphoma**: CD4 count <50, EBV-associated
- **Kaposi's sarcoma** (HHV-8): can occur at any CD4 count, but incidence ↑ as CD4 count ↓ usually occurs in MSM
  mucocutaneous: red-purple nodular lesions
  pulmonary: nodules, infiltrates, effusions, LAN
  GI: GI bleeding, obstruction, obstructive jaundice
  Rx: limited disease → alitretinoin gel, XRT, cryo, or intralesional vinblastine; systemic → chemotherapy
- **Cervical cancer**

Endocrine/metabolic

- **Hypogonadism**
- **Adrenal insufficiency**, CMV adrenalitis
- **Wasting syndrome**
- **Lipodystrophy and metabolic syndrome**: central obesity, lipoatrophy of extremities, dyslipidemia, hyperglycemia (insulin resistance)
- **Lactic acidosis**: N/V, abdominal pain; ? mitochondrial toxicity of AZT, d4T, ddI, and, less commonly, other NRTI

Neurologic

- **Meningitis**: *Cryptococcus*, bacterial (incl. *Listeria*), viral (HSV, CMV, HIV seroconversion), tuberculosis, lymphomatous, histoplasmosis, cocci
- **Neurosyphilis**: meningitis, cranial nerve palsies, dementia
- **Space-occupying lesions**: may present as headache, focal deficits, or Δ MS
  workup: MRI, stereotactic brain bx if suspect non-*Toxoplasma* etiology (toxoplasma sero⊖) or if Pt fails to respond to 2-wk trial of empiric toxoplasmosis Rx (of those who ultimately respond, 50% do so by d 3, 86% by d 7, 91% by d 14, *NEJM* 1993;329:995)

Etiology	Imaging Appearance	Diagnostic studies
Toxoplasmosis	enhancing lesions (can be multiple)	⊕ *Toxoplasma* serology
CNS lymphoma	enhancing lesion (usually single)	⊕ CSF PCR for EBV ⊕ SPECT or PET scan
Progressive multifocal leukencephalopathy (PML)	Multiple nonenhancing lesions in white matter	⊕ CSF PCR for JC virus
Other: bacterial abscess, nocardiosis, cryptococcoma, tuberculoma, CMV, HIV	Variable	Biopsy

- **AIDS dementia complex**: memory loss, gait disorder, spasticity
- **Myelopathy**: **infection** (CMV, HSV), **cord compression** (epidural abscess, lymphoma), **vacuolar** (HIV)
- **Peripheral neuropathy**: meds, HIV, CMV, demyelinating

Mycobacterium avium complex (MAC)

- Clinical manifestations: fever, night sweats, wt loss, hepatosplenomegaly, diarrhea, pancytopenia. May see enteritis and mesenteric lymphadenitis with CD4 <100-150, bacteremia usually when CD4 <50.
- Treatment: clarithromycin + ethambutol ± rifabutin

Cytomegalovirus (CMV)

- Clinical manifestations: retinitis, esophagitis, colitis, hepatitis, neuropathies, encephalitis
- Treatment: valganciclovir, ganciclovir, foscarnet, or cidofovir

LYME DISEASE

Microbiology
- Infection with **spirochete** *Borrelia burgdorferi* (consider coinfection w/ *Ehrlichia*, *Babesia*)
- Transmitted by **ticks** (*Ixodes*); animal hosts include deer and mice
- Infection usually requires **tick attachment >36-48 h**

Epidemiology
- Lyme disease most common vector-borne illness
- Peak incidence is in the summer months (May-Aug)
- Majority of cases in NY, NJ, CT, RI, WI, PA, MA, ME, NH, MI, MD, DE
- Humans contact ticks usually in fields with low brush near wooded areas

Clinical Manifestations	
Stage	**Manifestations**
Stage 1 (early localized) wks after infection	Due to local effects of spirochete *General*: **flu-like illness** *Dermatologic* (~80%): **erythema chronicum migrans** (ECM) = macular, erythematous lesion with central clearing, ranging in size from 6-38 cm; lymphocytomas; regional LAN
Stage 2 (early dissem.) wks to mos after infection	Due to spirochetemia and immune response *General*: fatigue, malaise, LAN, HA; fever uncommon *Derm*: **multiple (1-100) annular lesions ≈ ECM** *Rheumatologic* (~10%): **migratory arthralgias** (knee & hip) **& myalgias**, oligoarthritis *Neurologic* (~15%): **Bell's palsy** (or other cranial neuropathies); aseptic meningitis, mononeuritis multiplex (may be painful), transverse myelitis *Cardiac* (~8%): **heart block**, myocarditis
Stage 3 (late persistent) mos to y after infection	Due to chronic infection *or* autoimmune response *Derm*: **acrodermatitis chronica atrophicans**, panniculitis *Rheumatologic* (~60%): joint pain, **recurrent mono- or oligoarthritis of large joints**, synovitis *Neurologic*: subacute encephalomyelitis, polyneuropathy, dementia

(NEJM 2001;345:115; Lancet 2003;362:1639)

Diagnostic studies
- In general, a *clinical* diagnosis
- **Serology** (in right clinical setting)
  screen with **ELISA**, but
    false ⊕ due to other spirochetal diseases, SLE, RA, EBV, HIV, etc.
    false ⊖ due to early antibiotic therapy
  confirm ⊕ ELISA results with **Western blot** (↑ Sp)
- CSF examination in Pts with suspected neurologic disease
    ⊕ intrathecal Ab production if (CSF IgG/serum IgG)/(CSF albumin/serum albumin) >1

Treatment *(NEJM 2006;354:2794)*
- Prophylaxis
    protective clothing, tick ✓ q24h, DEET (all help prevent tick-borne diseases)
    doxycycline 200 mg po × 1 w/in 72 h of finding partially engorged, nymphal *Ixodes* tick attached ↓ risk of Lyme from 3.2 to 0.4%. Even in hyperendemic area, would need to treat 40-150 people to prevent 1 case of Lyme *(NEJM 2001;345:79)*.
- Antibiotics: *if* clin. manifestations *and* ⊕ serology (? *and* h/o tick bite if nonendemic area)
    local or early dissem. w/o neuro or cardiac involvement: **doxycycline** 100 mg PO bid (standard duration rec. has been 3-4 wks, but recent studies suggest 10 d to 3 wks may be just as effective) *(NEJM 1997;337:289)*
    neuro (other than Bell's palsy), cardiac, chronic arthritis, pregnancy: **ceftriaxone** 2 g IV qd × 2-4 wks *(NEJM 1997;337:289)*
- Vaccine: 78% ↓ in occurrence of Lyme disease in Pts in endemic areas at risk for exposure *(NEJM 1998;339:209)*; currently unavailable because of concerns re: joint & neuro toxicity

Rocky Mountain Spotted Fever (RMSF)

Microbiology
- Infection with *Rickettsia rickettsii* (Gram ⊖ obligate intracellular bacterium)
- Transmitted by *Dermacentor variabilis*, *Dermacentor andersoni*

Epidemiology
- Coastal mid-Atlantic, New England, midwest, northwest, southeast, Canada, Mexico, Central America, and in parts of South America
- Peak incidence spring and early summer

Clinical manifestations
- **Fever, headache**
- **Rash** (2-3 d after onset): starts on ankles and wrists → trunk, palms & soles
- Myalgias, N/V, occasionally abdominal pain

Diagnosis
- Usually a clinical diagnosis
- During acute illness can dx by examining skin bx for rickettsiae (Se ~70%)
- 7-10 d after onset of sx, serology (indirect fluorescent antibody test) turns ⊕

Treatment
- Doxycycline 100 mg PO bid

Ehrlichiosis

Microbiology
- Infection with an obligate Gram-negative intracellular bacteria
- **Human monocytic ehrlichiosis** (*Ehrlichiosis chaffeensis*) (HME)
- **Human granulocytic anaplasmosis** (*Anaplama phagocytophilum*) (HGA)
- Transmission: HME by *Amblyomma americanum*, *Dermacentor variabilis*; HGA by *Ixodes*

Epidemiology
- Majority of HGA cases found in RI, MN, CT, NY, MD
- Majority of cases of HME found in SE, southcentral, and mid-Atlantic regions of U.S.
- Peak incidence spring and early summer

Clinical manifestations
- Fever, myalgia, malaise, headache, occasional cough, dyspnea, renal dysfunction
- Laboratory: leukopenia or neutropenia, thrombocytopenia, ↑ aminotransferases, LDH, A\φ

Diagnosis
- Usually a clinical diagnosis
- Acute illness: intraleukocytic morulae on peripheral blood smear (rare); PCR; later: serology

Treatment
- Doxycycline 100 mg PO bid

Babesiosis

Microbiology
- Infection with parasite *Babesia microti* (U.S.), *Babesia divergens* (Europe)
- Transmitted by *Ixodes*

Epidemiology
- Europe & U.S. (more commonly coastal areas & islands off of MA, NY, RI, CT)
- Peak incidence spring and summer

Clinical manifestations
- Range from asx to fevers, sweats, myalgias, & headache to severe hemolytic anemia, hemoglobinurea, & death
- Risk factors for severe disease include asplenia, depressed cellular immunity, ↑ age

Diagnosis
- Blood smear with intraerythrocytic parasites; PCR; serology (late)

Treatment
- [Atovaquone + azithromycin] or [clindamycin + quinine]
- Exchange transfusion if parasitemia >10%, severe hemolysis, or SIRS

Definition
- **Fever >101°F** or **>38.5°C** on more than one occasion
- Duration ≥3 weeks
- **No diagnosis** despite 1 wk of intensive evaluation

Etiologies
- Differential extensive, but following are some of the more common causes
- More likely to be *subtle manifestation of common disease* than an uncommon disease
- In Pts with HIV: 75% infectious, *rarely due to HIV itself*
- Up to 30% of cases undiagnosed, most spontaneously defervesce

Category	Etiologies of Classic FUO
Infection ~30%	**Tuberculosis**: disseminated or extrapulmonary disease can have normal CXR, PPD, sputum AFB; biopsy (lung, liver, bone marrow) for granulomas has 80-90% yield in miliary disease **Endocarditis**: consider HACEK organisms, *Bartonella, Legionella,* and *Coxiella* **Intra-abdominal abscess**: hepatic, splenic, subphrenic, pancreatic, perinephric, pelvic, prostatic, appendicitis **Osteomyelitis**, dental abscess, sinusitis, paraspinal abscess CMV, EBV, Lyme disease, malaria, babesiosis, amebiasis, fungal infxn
Connective tissue disease ~30%	**Giant cell arteritis**: headache, scalp pain, jaw claudication, visual disturbances, PMR, ↑ ESR **Adult onset Still's disease** (juvenile rheumatoid arthritis): fevers with evanescent, salmon-colored macular truncal rash during fevers may precede arthritis **Polyarteritis nodosa, other vasculitides** RA, SLE
Neoplasm ~20%	**Lymphoma**: LAN, HSM, ↓ Hct or plt, ↑ LDH **Renal cell carcinoma**: microscopic hematuria, ↑ Hct **Hepatocellular carcinoma, pancreatic cancer, colon cancer** Atrial myxomas: obstruction, embolism, constitutional symptoms Leukemia, myelodysplasia
Miscellaneous ~20%	Drugs, factitious DVT, PE, hematoma Thyroid, adrenal insufficiency, pheochromocytoma Granulomatous hepatitis, sarcoidosis Familial Mediterranean fever (mutation in pyrin in myeloid cells; episodic fever, peritonitis, pleuritis; ↑ WBC & ESR during attacks)

(*Lancet* 1997;350:575; *Archives* 2003;163:545, 1033)

Workup
- History: fever curve, infectious contacts, travel, pets, occupation, medications, thorough ROS, PMHx and PSHx, TB history
- Discontinue unnecessary medications (only 20% w/ med-induced FUO will have eosinophilia or rash); reassess 1-3 wks after meds d/c'd
- Careful physical exam with attention to skin findings, LAN, murmurs, HSM, arthritis
- Laboratory evaluation
  CBC with diff, lytes, BUN, Cr, LFTs, ESR, CRP, ANA, RF, cryoglobulin, LDH
  BCx × 3 sets (off abx; hold for HACEK, RMSF, Q fever, Brucella), U/A, UCx, PPD, heterophile Ab, CMV antigenemia test, HIV Ab test (PCR if 1° infxn suspected)
- Imaging studies: CXR, chest & abdominal CT (oral & IV contrast), ? tagged WBC or gallium scan, ? FDG PET, ? echocardiogram
- Consider temporal artery bx if ↑ ESR and age >60, particularly if other s/sx
- ? Bone marrow aspirate and bx (esp if signs of marrow infiltration) or liver bx (especially if ↑ Aφ): even w/o localizing signs or symptoms, yield may be up to 15%

Treatment
- Empiric antibiotics are *not* indicated (unless Pt neutropenic)

HYPOPITUITARY SYNDROMES

Panhypopituitarism
* Etiologies
  Primary: surgery, radiation, tumors (primary or metastatic), infection, infiltration (sarcoid, hemochromatosis), autoimmune, ischemia (including Sheehan's syndrome caused by pituitary infarction intrapartum), carotid aneurysms, cavernous sinus thrombosis, trauma
  Secondary (hypothalamic dysfunction or stalk interruption): tumors (including craniopharyngioma), infection, infiltration, radiation, surgery, trauma
* Clinical manifestations
  Hormonal: weakness, easy fatigability, hypotension, bradycardia, sexual dysfunction, loss of axillary & pubic hair, hypotension, polyuria, & polydipsia
  Mass effect: headache, visual field Δs, cranial nerve palsies, galactorrhea
  Apoplexy (pituitary hemorrhage or infarction, usually w/ underlying pituitary adenoma): sudden headache, N/V, visual field Δs, cranial nerve palsies, meningismus, Δ MS, hypoglycemia, hypotension
* Diagnostic studies
  Hormonal studies
  chronic: ↓ target gland hormone + ↓ or normal trophic pituitary hormone
  acute: target gland hormonal studies may be *normal*
  partial hypopituitarism is more common than panhypopituitarism
  Pituitary MRI
* Treatment
  Replace deficient target gland hormones
  Most important deficiencies to recognize and treat in inpatients are *adrenal insufficiency* and *hypothyroidism*; if both present, treat with glucocorticoids first, then replace thyroid hormone so as not to precipitate adrenal crisis

↓ACTH
* Adrenal insufficiency similar to 1° (see "Adrenal Disorders") *except*:
  no salt cravings or hypokalemia (b/c aldo preserved)
  no hyperpigmentation (b/c ACTH/MSH is not ↑)

↓TSH
* Central hypothyroidism similar to 1° (see "Thyroid Disorders") *except* absence of goiter
* Free T_4 in addition to TSH must be ✓'d as TSH may be low or *inappropriately normal*

↓PRL
* Inability to lactate

↓GH
* ↑ risk for osteoporosis, fatigue
* Dx with failure to ↑ GH w/ appropriate stimulus (eg, GHRH/arginine stimulation or insulin tolerance test)
* GH replacement in adults controversial

↓FSH & LH
* Clinical manifestations: ↓ libido, impotence, oligo- or amenorrhea, infertility
* Physical examination: loss of axillary, pubic, and body hair
* Diagnostic studies: ↓ testosterone or estradiol with ↓ or normal FSH/LH (all levels ↓ in acute illness, ∴ don't measure in hospitalized Pts)
* Treatment: testosterone or estrogen replacement *vs.* correction of the underlying cause

↓ADH (hypothalamic or stalk disease): diabetes insipidus
* Clinical manifestations: *severe* polyuria, *mild* hypernatremia (*severe* if ↓ access to H_2O)
* Diagnostic studies: see "Disorders of Sodium Homeostasis"

Pituitary tumors
- Pathophysiology: adenoma → excess of ≥1 trophic hormones (if tumor fxnal, but 30-40% are not) and potentially *deficiencies* in other trophic hormones due to compression; cosecretion of PRL and growth hormone in 10% of prolactinoma
- Clinical manifestations: syndromes due to oversecretion of hormones (see below)
  Anatomic consequences: headache, visual Δs, diplopia, cranial neuropathies
- Workup: MRI, hormone levels, consider MEN1 (see below)

Hyperprolactinemia (NEJM 2003;349:2035)
- Etiology
  prolactinoma (50% of pituitary adenomas)
  stalk compression due to nonprolactinoma → ↓ inhibitory dopamine → ↑ PRL (mild)
- Physiology: PRL induces lactation and inhibits GnRH → ↓ FSH & LH
- Clinical manifestations: **amenorrhea, galactorrhea, infertility,** ↓ libido, impotence
- Diagnostic studies
  ↑ **PRL**, but elevated in many situations, ∴ r/o pregnancy, hypothyroidism, psychotropic meds, antiemetics, renal failure (↓ clearance), cirrhosis, stress, ↑ carb diet
  MRI to evaluate for tumor, visual field testing if MRI shows compression of optic chiasm
- Treatment
  If asx (no H/A or hypogonadal sx) and microadenoma (<**10 mm**) → follow with MRI
  If sx or macroadenoma (≥**10 mm**) options include:
    medical with dopamine agonist such as bromocriptine (70-100% success rate) or cabergoline (better tolerated); side effects include N/V, orthostasis, nasal congestion
    surgical: transsphenoidal surgery (main indications failed medical Rx, GH cosecretion, or neurologic sx not improving); 10-20% recurrence rate
    radiation: if medical or surgical therapy have failed or are not tolerated

Acromegaly (↑ GH; 10% of adenomas)
- Physiology: stimulates secretion of insulin-like growth factor 1 (IGF-1)
- Clinical manifestations: ↑ soft tissue, arthralgias, jaw enlargement, headache, carpal tunnel syndrome, macroglossia, hoarseness, sleep apnea, amenorrhea, impotence, diabetes mellitus, acanthosis/skin tags, ↑ sweating, HTN/CMP, colonic polyps
- Diagnostic studies: *no utility in checking random GH levels because of pulsatile secretion*
  ↑ **IGF-1** (somatomedin C); ± ↑ PRL
  oral glucose tolerance test → GH *not* suppressed to <2 ng/ml by 2 h
  pituitary MRI to evaluate for tumor
- Treatment: surgery, octreotide (long- and short-acting preparations), dopamine agonists, pegvisomant (GH receptor antagonist), radiation
- Prognosis: w/o Rx there is 2-3× ↑ mortality, risk of pituitary insufficiency, colon cancer

Cushing's disease (↑ACTH): 10-15% of adenomas; see "Adrenal Disorders"

Central hyperthyroidism (↑TSH, ↑ alpha subunit): very rare; see "Thyroid Disorders"

↑ **FSH & LH:** usually non-fxn, presents as *hypopituitarism* b/c of compression effects

DISORDERS OF MULTIPLE ENDOCRINE SYSTEMS

Multiple Endocrine Neoplasia (MEN) Syndromes	
Type	Features
1 (*MENIN* inactiv.)	Parathyroid hyperplasia/adenomas → hypercalcemia (~100% penetrance) Pancreatic islet cell neoplasia (gastrin, VIP, insulin, glucagon) Pituitary adenomas
2A (*RET* proto-oncogene)	Medullary thyroid carcinoma (MTC) Pheochromocytoma (~50%) Parathyroid hyperplasia → hypercalcemia (15-20%)
2B (*RET* proto-oncogene)	Medullary thyroid carcinoma (MTC) Pheochromocytoma (~50%) Mucosal and gastrointestinal neuromas

Polyglandular Autoimmune (PGA) Syndromes	
Type	Features
I (children)	Mucocutaneous candidiasis, hypoparathyroidism, adrenal insufficiency
II (adults)	Adrenal insufficiency, autoimmune thyroid disease, diabetes mellitus type 1

Diagnostic Studies in Thyroid Disorders	
Test	**Comments**
Thyroid-stimulating hormone (TSH)	*Most sensitive test* to detect 1° hypo- and hyperthyroidism May be inappropriately normal in central etiologies ↓'d by dopamine, steroids, severe illness
T_3 and T_4 immunoassays	Measure *total* serum concentrations (∴ influenced by TBG)
Free T_4 immunoassay (FT$_4$)	Free T_4, not influenced by TBG, increasingly popular
Thyroxine-binding globulin (TBG)	↑TBG (∴ ↑T_4): estrogens, OCP, pregnancy, hepatitis ↓TBG (∴ ↓T_4): androgens, glucocorticoids, nephrotic syndrome, cirrhosis, acromegaly, phenytoin
Reverse T_3	Inactive, ↑'d in sick euthyroid syndrome
Thyroid antibodies	Antithyroid peroxidase (TPO) → Hashimoto's Thyroid-stimulating Ig (TSI) → Graves' disease
Thyroglobulin	↑'d in thyroid injury, inflammation, and cancer (∴ useful marker of *recurrence* of papillary and follicular cancer)

Radioactive iodine uptake (RAIU) scan	Useful to differentiate causes of hyperthyroidism
	↑ **uptake**
	  homogeneous = Graves' disease
	  heterogeneous = multinodular goiter
	  1 focus of uptake w/ suppression of rest of gland = hot nodule
	no uptake = subacute painful or silent thyroiditis, exogenous thyroid hormone, struma ovarii, recent iodine load, or antithyroid drugs

Figure 7-1 Approach to thyroid disorders

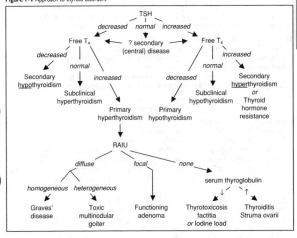

HYPOTHYROIDISM

Etiologies
- Primary (>90% of cases of hypothyroidism; ↓ **free T₄**, ↑TSH)
  Goitrous: **Hashimoto's thyroiditis**, recovery phase after thyroiditis, iodine deficiency
  Nongoitrous: surgical destruction, s/p radioactive iodine or XRT, amiodarone, lithium
- Secondary (↓ free T₄, variable TSH): hypothalamic or pituitary failure (TSH levels ↓ or "normal," can be slightly ↑ although functionally inactive due to abnormal glycosylation)

Hashimoto's thyroiditis
- Autoimmune destruction with patchy lymphocytic infiltration
- Usually seen in women 20-60 y old; may be part of PGA syndrome type II
  (hypothyroidism, Addison's, diabetes mellitus); associated w/ ↑ incidence of Sjögren's syndrome, pernicious anemia, & primary biliary cirrhosis
- ⊕ antithyroid peroxidase (anti-TPO) and antithyroglobulin (anti-Tg) abs in >90%

Clinical manifestations (Lancet 2004;363:793)
- **Early**: weakness, fatigue, arthralgias, myalgias, headache, depression, cold intolerance, weight gain, constipation, menorrhagia, dry skin, coarse brittle hair, brittle nails, carpal tunnel syndrome, delayed DTRs ("hung up" reflexes), diastolic HTN, hyperlipidemia
- **Late**: slow speech, hoarseness, loss of outer third of eyebrows, **myxedema** (nonpitting skin thickening due to ↑ glycosaminoglycans), periorbital puffiness, bradycardia, pleural, pericardial, & peritoneal effusions, atherosclerosis
- **Myxedema coma**: hypothermia, hypotension, hypoventilation, Δ MS

Diagnostic studies
- ↓ **FT₄**; ↑**TSH** in primary hypothyroidism; ⊕ antithyroid Ab in Hashimoto's thyroiditis
- May see hyponatremia, hypoglycemia, anemia, ↑ LDL, ↓ HDL, and ↑ CK
- Screening recommended for pregnant women

Treatment of overt hypothyroidism
- Levothyroxine (1.5-1.7 µg/kg/d), re✓ TSH q5-6wks and titrate until euthyroid; sx can take mos to resolve; **lower starting dose** (0.3-0.5 ug/kg/d) if at risk for ischemic heart disease; advise Pts to keep same formulation of levothyroxine
- Myxedema coma: load 5-8 µg/kg T₄ IV, then 50-100 µg IV qd; b/c peripheral conversion is impaired, may also give 5-10 µg T₃ IV q8h (T₃ more arrhythmogenic); must give empiric *adrenal replacement therapy* as ↓ adrenal reserves in myxedema coma

Subclinical hypothyroidism (NEJM 2001;345:260)
- Mild ↑TSH and **normal free T₄** with only subtle or no sx
- If ↑ titers of antithyroid Abs, progression to overt hypothyroidism is ~4%/y
- Rx controversial: follow expectantly or treat to improve ? mild sx or dyslipidemia
  most initiate Rx if TSH >10 mU/L, goiter, pregnancy, or infertility
  risk of precipitating atrial fibrillation & angina and accelerating osteoporosis

HYPERTHYROIDISM

Etiologies (Lancet 2003;362:459)
- **Graves' disease** (60-80% of thyrotoxicosis)
- **Thyroiditis**: thyrotoxic phase of subacute thyroiditis
- **Toxic adenomas** (single or multinodular goiter) or, rarely, functioning thyroid carcinoma
- TSH-secreting pituitary tumor or pituitary resistance to thyroid hormone (↑TSH, ↑ free T₄)
- Misc: amiodarone, iodine-induced, thyrotoxicosis factitia, struma ovarii (3% of ovarian dermoid tumors and teratomas), hCG-secreting tumors (eg, choriocarcinoma)

Graves' disease
- Female:male ratio is 5-10:1, most Pts between 40-60 y at dx
- ⊕ **thyroid antibodies**: TSI (⊕ in 80%), antimicrosomal, antithyroglobulin; ANA
- Clinical manifestations in addition to those of hyperthyroidism (see below):
  goiter: diffuse, nontender, w/ thyroid bruit
  ophthalmopathy (50%; up to 90% if formally tested): periorbital edema, proptosis (✓ if sclera visible between lower iris and lower lid), conjunctivitis, diplopia (EOM infiltration); associated w/ smoking
  pretibial myxedema (3%): infiltrative dermopathy

Clinical manifestations of hyperthyroidism
- Restlessness, sweating, tremor, moist warm skin, fine hair, tachycardia, AF, weight loss, ↑ frequency of stools, menstrual irregularities, hyperreflexia, osteoporosis, stare and lid lag (due sympathetic overactivity)
- **Subclinical** (↓TSH, **normal FT_4 and T_3**): ↑ risk of atrial fibrillation and osteoporosis, may account for 10% of new-onset AF (*NEJM 2001;345:512*)
- **Apathetic thyrotoxicosis**: seen in elderly who can present with lethargy as only sx
- **Thyroid storm** (extremely rare): delirium, fever, tachycardia, systolic hypertension but wide pulse pressure and ↓ MAP, GI symptoms; 20-50% mortality

Laboratory testing
- ↑ FT_4 and FT_3; ↓TSH (except in TSH-secreting tumors)
- **RAIU scan** is very useful study to differentiate causes (see table on page 7-3)
- Rarely need to ✓ for autoantibodies except in pregnancy (to assess risk of fetal Graves')
- May see hypercalciuria ± hypercalcemia, ↑ AΦ, anemia

Treatment
- β-blockers: control tachycardia (propranolol also ↓ $T_4 \rightarrow T_3$ conversion)
- Graves' disease: either antithyroid drugs or radioactive iodine (*NEJM 2005;352:905*)
  propylthiouracil (PTU) or **methimazole**: 50% chance of recurrence after 1 y; side effects include pruritus, rash, arthralgia, fever, N/V, and *agranulocytosis* in 0.5%
  radioactive iodine (RAI): preRx w/ antithyroid drugs to prevent ↑ thyrotoxicosis, stop > 5 d before to allow RAI uptake; > 75% of treated Pts become hypothyroid
  surgery: rarely chosen for Graves', usually for Pts w/ obstructive goiter
- Toxic adenoma or toxic multinodular goiter: RAI or surgery (± PTU or methimazole preRx)
- Thyroid storm: β-blocker, PTU, iopanoic acid or iodide (for "Wolff-Chaikoff" effect) >1 h after PTU, ± steroids (↓ $T_4 \rightarrow T_3$)
- Ophthalmopathy: can worsen after RAI, sometimes responds to prednisone; can be treated w/ radiation and/or surgical decompression of the orbits

THYROIDITIS (*NEJM 2003;348:2646*)
- **Acute:** bacterial infection (fever, ↑ ESR, normal TFTs), radiation, amiodarone, trauma
- **Subacute:** transient thyrotoxicosis → transient hypothyroidism → normal thyroid fxn
  painful (= viral, granulomatous, or de Quervain's): fever, ↑ ESR; Rx = NSAIDs, steroids
  silent (= postpartum, autoimmune, or lymphocytic): painless; ⊕ TPO Abs
- **Chronic:** Hashimoto's (hypothyroidism), Riedel's (idiopathic fibrosis, normal TFTs)

NONTHYROIDAL ILLNESS (SICK EUTHYROID SYNDROME)
- TFT abnormalities in Pts w/ severe nonthyroidal illness (∴in acute illness, ✓ TFTs only if ↑ concern for thyroid disease); *may* have acquired transient central hypothyroidism
- If thyroid dysfxn suspected in critically ill Pt, TSH alone not reliable; must measure total T_4, FT_4, & T_3
- Mild illness: ↓$T_4 \rightarrow T_3$ conversion, ↑ rT_3 ⇒ ↓ T_3; in severe illness: ↓ TBG & albumin, ↑↑ rT_3 ⇒ ↓↓T_3, ↑ degradation of T_4, central ↓TSH ⇒ ↓↓T_3, ↓↓ T_4, ↓ FT_4 ↓ TSH
- Recovery phase: ↑ TSH followed by recovery of T_4 and then T_3
- Replacement thyroxine **not** helpful or recommended for critically ill Pts w/ ↓ T_3 and T_4 unless other s/s of hypothyroidism

AMIODARONE AND THYROID DISEASE
Risk of thyroid dysfunction is lower with lower doses
✓ TSH prior to therapy, at 4-mo intervals on amio, and for 1 y after if amio d/c'd

Hypothyroidism (occurs in ~10%; more common in iodine-replete areas)
- Pathophysiology
  (1) "Wolff-Chaikoff" effect: iodine load ↓ I^- uptake, organification, and release of T_4 & T_3
  (2) inhibits $T_4 \rightarrow T_3$ conversion
  (3) ? direct/immune-mediated thyroid destruction
- Normal individuals: ↓T_4; then escape Wolff-Chaikoff effect and have ↑ T_4, ↓ T_3, ↑ TSH; then TSH normalizes (after 1-3 mos)
- Susceptible individuals (eg, subclinical Hashimoto's, ∴ ✓ anti-TPO) do *not* escape effects
- Treatment: thyroxine to normalize TSH; may need larger than usual dose

Hyperthyroidism (3% of Pts on amio; ~10-20% of Pts in iodine-*deficient* areas)
- Type 1 = underlying multinodular goiter or autonomous thyroid tissue
  pathophysiology: Jodbasedow effect (iodine load → ↑ synthesis of T_4 and T_3 in
  autonomous tissue)
  diagnostic studies: ↑ thyroid blood flow on Doppler U/S; treatment: methimazole
- Type 2 = destructive thyroiditis
  pathophysiology: ↑ **release** of preformed T4 & T3 → hyperthyroidism
  → hypothyroidism → recovery
  diagnostic studies: ↑ ESR, ↓ flow on Doppler U/S; treatment: steroids
- Type 1 vs. 2 often difficult to distinguish and Rx for both initiated (*JCEM* 2001;86:3)

THYROID NODULES

- Prevalence 5-10% (20-60% if screen with U/S), ~5% malignant
- Features associated w/ ↑ risk of malignancy: age < 20 or >70, male sex, h/o neck XRT,
  fixed lesion, "cold nodule" on RAIU, large size, worrisome U/S findings (hypoechoic, solid,
  irregular borders, microcalcifications, central blood flow), cervical LAN
- Features associated w/ benign dx: FHx of autoimmune thyroid disease or goiter, presence
  of hypo- or hyperthyroidism, nodule tenderness
- Screening U/S recommended for those with FHx of MEN2 or medullary thyroid cancer,
  personal h/o neck XRT, palpable nodules or multinodular goiter
- FNA should be performed for nodules >10 mm with irregular borders, microcalcifications,
  or chaotic intranodular vascular spots; FNA any nodules in Pts with h/o neck XRT or
  FHx of MEN2 or MTC

Figure 7-2 Approach to thyroid nodules (*Endocr Pract* 2006;12:63)

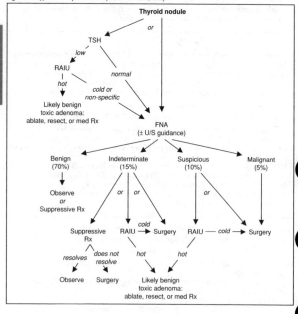

CUSHING'S SYNDROME (HYPERCORTISOLISM)

Definitions
- Cushing's syndrome = cortisol excess
- Cushing's disease = Cushing's syndrome 2° to pituitary ACTH hypersecretion

Etiologies of hypercortisolism
- Most common cause is iatrogenic Cushing's syndrome caused by exogenous glucocorticoids
- **Cushing's disease** (60-70%): pituitary adenoma (usually microadenoma) or hyperplasia
- **Adrenal tumor** (15-25%): adenoma or carcinoma
- **Ectopic ACTH** (5-10%): SCLC, carcinoid, islet cell tumors, medullary thyroid cancer, pheo

Clinical manifestations
- Glucose intolerance or DM, HTN, obesity, and oligomenorrhea (all nonspecific)
- Central obesity, buffalo hump, moon facies, wasting of extremities, proximal myopathy, spontaneous bruising, wide striae, osteoporosis, and hypokalemia (all more specific)
- Other: depression, insomnia, psychosis, impaired cognition, facial plethora, acne, hirsutism, hyperpigmentation (if ↑ ACTH), fungal skin infxns, nephrolithiasis, polyuria

Figure 7-3 Approach to suspected Cushing's syndrome

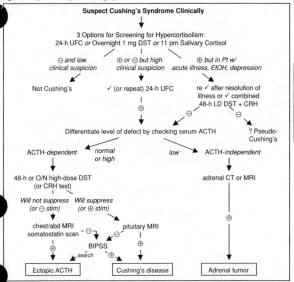

CRH = corticotropin-releasing hormone; DST = dexamethasone suppression test; UFC = urinary free cortisol
Overnight 1 mg DST = give 1 mg at 11 pm; ✓ 8 am serum cortisol (suppression if <5 μg/dl); 1-2% false ⊕
   (primarily used to evaluate subclinical Cushing's in Pts w/ adrenal "incidentaloma")
11 pm salivary cortisol = abnl if level ↑; 24-h UFC = abnl if level ↑, > 4 × ULN virtually diagnostic
48-h LD DST + CRH = 0.5 mg q6h × 2 d, then IV CRH 2 h later; ✓ serum cortisol 15 min later (⊕ = > 1.4 μg/dl)
48-h LD DST = 0.5 mg q6h × 2 d; ✓ 24-h UFC at base. & during last 24 h of dex (suppress if <10% of base)
48-h HD DST = 2 mg q6h × 2 d; ✓ 24-h UFC as per LD DST
O/N HD DST = 8 mg at 11 pm; ✓ 9 am serum cortisol (suppression if <32% of baseline)
CRH test = 1 μg/kg IV; ✓ cortisol and ACTH (⊕ stim if > 35% ↑ in ACTH or >20% ↑ in cortisol above baseline)
BIPSS = bilat. inferior petrosal sinus vein sampling; ✓ petrosal:peripheral ACTH ratio (⊕ = >2 basal, >3 after CRH)
(Endo & Metab Clin North Am 2005;34:385)

Treatment of Cushing's syndrome

- Surgical resection of pituitary adenoma, adrenal tumor, or ectopic ACTH-secreting tumor
- If transsphenoidal surgery (TSS) not successful → pituitary XRT, medical adrenalectomy w/ mitotane, or bilat surgical adrenalectomy; ketoconazole (± metyrapone) to ↓ cortisol
- Glucocorticoid replacement therapy × 6-36 mos after TSS (lifelong glucocorticoid + mineralocorticoid replacement if medical or surgical adrenalectomy)

HYPERALDOSTERONISM

Etiologies

- **Primary** (adrenal disorders, ↑ aldosterone is renin independent)
  adrenal hyperplasia (70%), adenoma (**Conn's syndrome,** 25%), carcinoma (5%)
  glucocorticoid-remediable aldosteronism (GRA; ACTH-dep. promoter rearrangement)
- **Secondary** (extra-adrenal disorders, ↑ aldosterone is renin dependent)
  Primary reninism: renin-secreting tumor
  Secondary reninism
  renovascular disease: RAS, malignant hypertension
  edematous states w/ ↓ effective arterial volume: CHF, cirrhosis, nephrotic syndrome
  hypovolemia, diuretics, Bartter's (defective Na/K/2Cl transporter ≈ receiving loop diuretic), Gitelman's (defective renal Na/Cl transporter ≈ receiving thiazide diuretic)
- **Nonaldosterone mineralocorticoid excess** mimics hyperaldosteronism
  Cushing's syndrome, CAH (some enzyme defects → shunting to mineralocorticoids)
  11β-OHSD deficiency (buildup of cortisol, which binds to mineralocorticoid receptor)
  Licorice (glycyrrhizinic acid inhibits 11β-OHSD), exogenous mineralocorticoids
  Liddle's syndrome (constitutively activated/overexpressed distal tubular renal Na channel)

Clinical manifestations

- **Mild to moderate diastolic HTN**, headache, muscle weakness, polyuria, polydipsia; no peripheral edema because of "escape" from Na retention; malignant HTN is rare
- Classically **hypokalemia** (but often normal), metabolic alkalosis, mild hypernatremia

Diagnostic studies

- 5-10% of Pts w/ HTN; ∴ screen if HTN + hypokalemia, adrenal mass, or refractory HTN
- **Aldosterone** (>15-20 ng/dl) and **plasma aldosterone:renin ratio** (>20 if 1°)
  obtain 8 a.m. paired values (off spironolactone & eplerenone for 6 wks); Se & Sp >85%
- ACEI/ARB, diuretics, CCB can ↑ renin activity → ↓ PAC/PRA ratio and β-blockers may ↑ PAC/PRA ratio; ∴ avoid. α-blockers generally best to control HTN during dx testing.
- Confirm with sodium suppression test (fail to suppress aldo after sodium load)
  oral salt load (+ KCl) × 3 d, ✓ 24-h urine (⊕ if aldo >12 μg/d while Na >200 mEq/d)
  or 2L NS over 4 h, measure aldo at end of infusion (⊕ if aldo >5 ng/dl)

Figure 7-4 Approach to suspected hyperaldosteronism

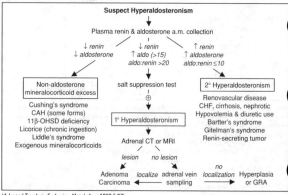

(Adapted *Trends in Endocrine Metabolism* 1999;5:97)

Treatment
- Adenoma or carcinoma → surgery
- Hyperplasia → spironolactone or eplerenone; GRA → glucocorticoids ± spironolactone

---

ADRENAL INSUFFICIENCY

Etiologies
- **Primary** = adrenocortical disease = **Addison's disease**
  autoimmune: isolated or in assoc w/ PGA syndromes (see table on page 7-2)
  infection: tuberculosis, CMV, histoplasmosis
  vascular: hemorrhage (usually in setting of sepsis), thrombosis, and trauma
  metastatic disease: (90% of adrenals must be destroyed to cause insufficiency)
  deposition diseases: hemochromatosis, amyloidosis, sarcoidosis
  drugs: ketoconazole, etomidate (even after single dose), rifampin, anticonvulsants
- **Secondary** = pituitary failure of ACTH secretion (but aldosterone **intact** b/c RAA axis)
  any cause of primary or secondary hypopituitarism (see "Pituitary Disorders")
  glucocorticoid therapy (occurs after ≥2 wks of "suppressive doses," which are
     extremely variable; even 7.5 mg/d of prednisone can be suppressive)
  megestrol (a progestin with some glucocorticoid activity)

Clinical manifestations (NEJM 1996;335:1206)
- **Primary** or **secondary**: weakness and fatigability (99%), **anorexia** (99%),
  orthostatic hypotension (90%), nausea (86%), vomiting (75%), hyponatremia (88%)
- **Primary only** (extra s/s due to lack of aldosterone and ↑ ACTH): marked orthostatic
  hypotension (because volume-depleted), **hyperpigmentation** (seen in creases, mucous
  membranes, pressure areas, nipples), **hyperkalemia**
- **Secondary only**: ± other manifestations of hypopituitarism (see "Pituitary Disorders")

Diagnostic studies
- Early a.m. serum cortisol: <3 μg/dl virtually diagnostic; >18 μg/dl rules it out (except in
  critical illness—see below)
- ↑ dose (250 μg) **cosyntropin stimulation test** (testing ability of ACTH → ↑ cortisol)
  normal = 60-min post-ACTH cortisol ≥18 μg/dl
  abnormal in *primary* b/c adrenal gland diseased and unable to give adequate output
  abnormal in *chronic secondary* b/c adrenals atrophied and unable to respond
  may be *normal* in *acute secondary* b/c adrenals still able to respond
- ↓ dose (1 μg) cort stim: ? more sensitive than high-dose test (controversial)
- Other tests to evaluate HPA axis (w/ guidance by endocrinologist): insulin-induced
  hypoglycemia (measure serum cortisol response); metyrapone (blocks cortisol synthesis
  and therefore stimulates ACTH, measure plasma 11-deoxycortisol and urinary 17-
  hydroxycorticosteroid levels)
- Other lab abnormalities: hypoglycemia, eosinophilia, lymphocytosis, ± neutropenia
- ACTH: ↑ in 1°, ↓ or low-normal in 2°
- Imaging studies to consider
  pituitary MRI to detect pituitary abnormalities
  adrenal CT: small, noncalcified adrenals in autoimmune, enlarged in metastatic disease,
    hemorrhage, infection, and deposition (although may be normal-appearing)

Adrenal insufficiency and critical illness (NEJM 2003;348:727)
- Controversial; no consensus exists on diagnosing *relative* adrenal insufficiency
- Serum free cortisol may be more useful in critically ill Pt (NEJM 2004;350:1629)
- Perform ACTH stim as soon as possible in critically ill Pt suspected to have adrenal insuffic.
  → insufficiency if baseline cortisol < 15 μg/dl or if Δ ≤9 μg/dl
  poor prognosis also associated with elevated baseline cortisol >34 μg/dl
- Initiate corticosteroids early if adrenal insufficiency suspected:
  hydrocortisone 50-100 mg IV q6-8h
  use dexamethasone 2-4 mg IV q6h + fludrocortisone 50 μg daily prior to ACTH stim,
  but change to hydrocortisone once test performed

Treatment
- *Acute* adrenal insufficiency
  Hydrocortisone IV as above + volume resuscitation with normal saline
- *Chronic* adrenal insufficiency
  Hydrocortisone: 20-30 mg PO qd (2/3 in am, 1/3 in pm) or prednisone ~5 mg PO qd
  Fludrocortisone (*not* needed in 2° adrenal insufficiency): 0.05-0.1 mg PO qam
  back-up dexamethasone 4 mg IM prefilled syringe given to Pt for emergency situations

PHEOCHROMOCYTOMA

Clinical manifestations (five Ps)
- **Pressure** (hypertension, paroxysmal in 50%, severe and resistant to therapy)
- **Pain** (headache, chest pain)
- **Palpitations** (tachycardia, tremor, wt loss, fever)
- **Perspiration** (profuse)
- **Pallor** (vasoconstrictive spell)
- "Rule of 10": 10% extra-adrenal (known as paraganglioma), 10% in children, 10% multiple or bilateral, 10% recur (↑ in paraganglioma), 10% malignant (↑ in paraganglioma), 10% familial, 10% incidentaloma
- Emotional stress does not trigger paroxysms, but abdominal manipulation can trigger catecholamine release; some reports of IV contrast causing paroxysms
- Associated with MEN 2A/2B, Von Hippel Lindau, neurofibromatosis type 1, familial paraganglioma (mutations in succinate dehydrogenase gene B and D)

Diagnostic studies
- 24° urinary fractionated metanephrines and catecholamines: 90% Se, 98% Sp screening test of choice if low-risk (⊕ with severe illness, renal failure, OSA, labetalol due to assay interference, TCAs, medications containing sympathomimetics)
- Plasma free metanephrines: 99% Se, 89% Sp (JAMA 2002;287:1427) screening test of choice if high-risk, but ↑ rate of false ⊕ in low-preval. population
- Adrenal CT or MRI; consider MIBG scintigraphy if CT/MRI ⊖, PET can be used to localize nonadrenal mass, but usually easy to find

Treatment
- α-blockade first (usually phenoxybenzamine) ± β-blockade (often propranolol) → surgery

ADRENAL INCIDENTALOMAS

Epidemiology
- 4% of Pts undergoing abdominal CT scan have incidentally discovered adrenal mass; prevalence ↑ with age

Differential diagnosis
- **Nonfunctioning mass**: adenoma, cysts, abscesses, granuloma, hemorrhage, lipoma, myelolipoma, primary or metastatic malignancy
- **Functioning mass**: pheochromocytoma, adenoma (cortisol, aldosterone, sex hormones), nonclassical CAH, other endocrine tumor, carcinoma
- **Nonadrenal mass**: renal, pancreatic, gastric, artifact

Workup (NEJM 2007;356:601)
- **Rule out subclinical Cushing's syndrome** in all Pts using 1 mg overnight DST (Sp 91%). Abnormal results require confirmatory testing.
- **Rule out hyperaldosteronism** if hypertensive w/ plasma aldo & renin (see above).
- **Rule out pheochromocytoma** in all Pts (b/c of morbidity un Rx'd pheo) using 24-h urine fractionated metanephrines and catecholamines or plasma free metanephrines.
- Rule out metastatic cancer and infection by history or CT-guided biopsy if suspicious
- CT and MRI characteristics may suggest adenoma vs. carcinoma
  Benign features: size <4 cm; smooth margins, homogenous and hypodense appearance; unenhanced CT <10 Hounsfield units or CT contrast-medium washout >50% at 10 min. Can follow such incidentalomas w/ periodic scans.
  Suspicious features: size >4 cm or ↑ size on repeat scan; irregular margins, heterogeneous, dense, or vascular appearance; unenhanced CT >10 Hounsfield units or CT contrast-medium washout < 50% at 10 min; h/o malignancy or young age (incidentaloma less common). Such incidentalomas warrant FNA biopsy, repeat scan in 3 mos, or resection.

CALCIUM DISORDERS

Laboratory Findings in Calcium Disorders			
Ca	PTH	Disease	PO$_4$
↑	↑↑	Hyperparathyroidism (1° and 3°)	↓
	↑ or nl	Familial hypocalciuric hypercalcemia	↓
	↓	Malignancy	var.
		Vitamin D excess	↑
		Milk-alkali syndrome, thiazides	↓
		↑ Bone turnover	↑
↓	↑↑	Pseudohypoparathyroidism	↑
	↑	Vitamin D deficiency	↓
		Chronic renal failure (2° hyperpara)	↑
	var.	Acute calcium sequestration	var.
	↓	Hypoparathyroidism	↑

Pitfalls in measuring calcium
- Physiologically active Ca is free or ionized (ICa). Serum Ca reflects total calcium (bound + unbound) and ∴ influenced by albumin (main Ca-binding protein).
- Corrected Ca (mg/dl) = measured Ca (mg/dl) + [0.8 × (4 - albumin (gm/dl))]
- Alkalosis will cause more Ca to be bound to albumin (∴ total Ca may be normal but ↓ ICa)
- Best to measure **ionized Ca** directly

HYPERCALCEMIA

Etiologies of Hypercalcemia	
Category	Etiologies
Hyperparathyroidism	**1°**: adenoma (85%), hyperplasia (15-20%; spont. vs. MEN 1/2A), carcinoma (<1%) **3°**: after long-standing 2° hyperparathyroidism (as in renal failure) → autonomous nodule develops, requires surgery Lithium → ↑ PTH
Familial hypocalciuric hypercalcemia (FHH)	Mutation in Ca-sensing receptor in parathyroid and kidney → ↑ Ca set point; ± ↑ PTH (and less ↑ than in 1° hyperpara.) Acquired form due to autoAb vs. Ca-sensing receptor (rare)
Malignancy	PTH-related peptide (PTHrP) → humoral ↑ Ca of malignancy (eg, squamous cell cancers, renal, breast, bladder) Cytokines & ↑ 1,25-(OH)$_2$D$_3$ (eg, hematologic malignancies) Local osteolysis (eg, breast cancer, myeloma)
Vitamin D excess	Granulomas (sarcoid, TB, histo, Wegener's) → ↑ 1-OH → ↑ 1,25-(OH)$_2$D Vitamin D intoxication
↑ bone turnover	Hyperthyroidism, immobilization + Paget's disease, vitamin A
Miscellaneous	Thiazides; Ca-based antacids or massive dairy consumption (milk-alkali syndrome); adrenal insufficiency

(JCEM 2005;90:6316)

Clinical manifestations ("bones, stones, abdominal groans, and psychic moans")
- **Hypercalcemic crisis** (usually when Ca 13-15): polyuria, dehydration, mental status Δs
  Ca toxic to renal tubules → blocks ADH activity, causes vasoconstriction, and ↓ GFR → polyuria but ↑ Ca reabsorption → ↑ serum Ca → ↑ nephrotoxicity and CNS sx
- Osteopenia, fractures, and osteitis fibrosa cystica (latter seen in severe hyperpara only → ↑ osteoclast activity → cysts, fibrous nodules, salt & pepper appearance on X-ray)
- Nephrolithiasis, nephrocalcinosis, nephrogenic DI
- Abdominal pain, anorexia, nausea, vomiting, constipation, pancreatitis, PUD
- Fatigue, weakness, depression, confusion, coma, ↓ DTRs, short QT interval
- **Calciphylaxis** (calcific uremic arteriolopathy): calcification of media of small- to medium-sized blood vessels of dermis & SC fat → ischemia and skin necrosis
  (NEJM 2007;356:1049).
  Associated w/ uremia, ↑ PTH, ↑ Ca, ↑ PO$_4$, and ↑ (Ca × PO$_4$) product. Dx by biopsy.
  Rx: aggressive wound care, keep Ca & PO$_4$ nl (goal < 55), avoid vitamin D & Ca suppl.
  IV Na thiosulfate & parathyroidectomy controversial.
  Overall portends a poor prognosis.

Diagnostic studies
- Hyperparathyroidism and malignancy account for 90% of cases of hypercalcemia
  hyperparathyroidism more likely if asx or chronic hypercalcemia
  malignancy more likely if acute or sx; malignancy usually overt or becomes so in mos
- Ca, alb, ICa, PTH (may be inappropriately normal in 1° hyperparathyroidism & FHH), PO_4;
  based on results consider checking PTHrP, 25-(OH)D, 1,25-(OH)$_2$D, Aϕ, U_{Ca}

Acute Treatment of Hypercalcemia			
Treatment	Onset	Duration	Comments
Normal saline (4-6 L/d)	h	during Rx	natriuresis → ↑ renal Ca excretion
Furosemide (IV q6h)	h	during Rx	Start only *after* intravascularly replete. Promotes natriuresis and ∴ ↑ Ca excretion.
Bisphosphonates	1-2 d	var.	Inhibit osteoclasts, useful in malignancy; caution in renal failure; risk of jaw osteonecrosis
Calcitonin	h	2-3 d	Quickly develop tachyphylaxis
Glucocorticoids	days	days	? Useful in some malig. & vitamin D intox.

(NEJM 2005;352:373)

HYPOCALCEMIA

Etiologies of Hypocalcemia	
Category	Etiologies
Hypoparathyroidism	Isolated; familial (PGA 1, activating Ca-sensing receptor mutations; see 7-2); iatrogenic (s/p thyroid, cancer surgery, neck irradiation); Wilson's; hemochromatosis; hypoMg (↓ secretion and effect); activating Ca-sensing receptor autoAb
Pseudo-hypoparathyroidism	Ia and Ib: PTH end-organ resistance (∴ ↑ serum PTH) Ia: + skeletal abnormalities, short stature, & retardation Pseudopseudohypoparathyroidism = Ia syndrome but *nl* Ca & PTH
Vitamin D deficiency or resistance	Nutritional/sunlight deprivation; GI disease/fat malabs.; drugs (anticonvulsants, rifampin, ketoconazole, 5-FU/leucovorin); genetic (1α-hydroxylase, VDR mutations)
Chronic renal failure	↓ 1,25-(OH)$_2$D production, ↑ PO_4 from ↓ clearance
Accelerated net bone formation	Post-parathyroidectomy, Rx of severe vit D deficiency or Paget's disease, osteoblastic metastases
Calcium sequestration	Pancreatitis, citrate excess (eg, after blood transfusions), acute ↑↑ PO_4 (ARF, rhabdomyolysis, tumor lysis)

Clinical manifestations
- **Neuromuscular irritability**: perioral paresthesias, cramps, ⊕ **Chvostek's** (tapping facial nerve → contraction of facial muscles), ⊕ **Trousseau's** (inflation of BP cuff → carpal spasm), laryngospasm; irritability, depression, psychosis, ↑ ICP, seizures, ↑ QT
- **Rickets** and/or **osteomalacia**: chronic ↓ vit D → ↓ Ca, ↓ PO_4 → ↓ bone/cartilage mineralization, growth failure, bone pain, muscle weakness
- **Renal osteodystrophy** (↓ vit D & ↑ PTH in renal failure): osteomalacia (↓ mineralization of bone due to ↓ Ca and 1,25-(OH)$_2$D) & osteitis fibrosa cystica (due to ↑ PTH)

Diagnostic studies
- Ca, alb, ICa, PTH, 25-(OH)D, 1,25-(OH)$_2$D (if renal failure or rickets), Cr, Mg, PO_4, Aϕ, U_{Ca}

Treatment (also treat concomitant vitamin D deficiency)
- Symptomatic: intravenous Ca gluconate (1-2 g IV over 20 mins) + vitamin D (calcitriol most effective in acute hypocalcemia, but takes h to work) ± Mg (50-100 mEq/d)
- Asymptomatic and/or chronic: **oral Ca** (1-3 g/d) & vitamin D (eg, ergocalciferol 50,000 IU PO q wk × 8-10 wks). In chronic hypopara, calcitriol is needed, consider also thiazide.
- Chronic renal failure: phosphate binder(s), oral Ca, calcitriol or analog (calcimimetic may be needed later to prevent hypercalcemia)

DIABETES MELLITUS

Definition (Diabetes Care 2003;26:S33)
- Fasting glc >126 mg/dl or rand. glc >200 mg/dl × 2 or 75 g OGTT w/ 2-h glc >200 mg/dl
- Blood glc higher than normal, but not frank diabetes:
  Impaired fasting glc (IFG) = 100-125 mg/dl
  Impaired glc tolerance (IGT): 2-h after 75 g OGTT 140-199 mg/dl
- ? ↑ Hb_{A1C} (no accepted criterion yet)

Categories
- **Type 1**: islet cell destruction; absolute insulin deficiency; ketosis in absence of insulin
  prevalence 0.4%; usual onset in childhood; ↑ risk if ⊕ FHx; HLA associations
  anti-GAD, anti-islet cell & anti-insulin autoantibodies
- **Type 2**: insulin resistance + relative insulin deficiency (prevent ketosis but not ↑ glc)
  insulin resistance → ↑ glc → ↑ insulin secretion →→→ pancreatic failure → overt diabetes
  prevalence 8%; onset in later life; ↑↑ risk if ⊕ FHx; no HLA associations
  risk factors: age, race, FHx, obesity, sedentary lifestyle, metabolic abnormalities
- **Type 2 DM p/w DKA** ("Flatbush Diabetes"): most often seen in young blacks, anti-GAD
  neg, often do not require insulin following Rx of DKA (Diabetes 1994;43:741)
- **M**ature-**O**nset **D**iabetes of the **Y**oung (**MODY**): autosomal dominant inherited form
  of DM due to defects in insulin secretion genes; occurs in lean young adults who do
  not normally require insulin (NEJM 2001;345:971)
- **Secondary causes of diabetes**: exogenous or endogenous glucocorticoids, glucagonoma
  (3 D's = DM, DVT, diarrhea), pancreatic (pancreatitis, hemochromatosis, CF, resection)

Clinical manifestations
- Polyuria, polydipsia, polyphagia with unexplained weight loss; can also be asymptomatic

Diabetes Treatment Options	
Diet	Type 1: ADA diet; Type 2: wt reduction diet + exercise
Metformin	↓ hepatic gluconeogenesis, ↓ Hb_{A1C} 1.5% Wt neutral, N/V & rare lactic acidosis Contraindic. in renal or liver failure Consider first-line Rx w/ lifestyle mod. for all DM2 w/ Hb_{A1C} ≥7%
Sulfonylureas (SU)	↑ insulin secretion, ↓ Hb_{A1C} 1.5% Hypoglycemia, wt gain
Thiazolidinediones (TZD)	↑ insulin Se in adipose & muscle (PPAR-γ agonist) ↓ Hb_{A1C} 0.5-1.4% Wt gain, hepatotoxicity, fluid retention & CHF, ? ↑ MI Contraindic. in liver disease and NYHA III-IV, monitor LFTs
Glinides	↑ insulin secretion, ↓ Hb_{A1C} 1.5% Hypoglycemia (but less than w/ SU), wt gain
Exenitide	↑ glc-depend insulin secretion (GLP-1 agonist), ↓ Hb_{A1C} 0.5% Wt loss, N/V & diarrhea (30-45%) To be used in combination with an oral agent
α-glucosidase inhibitor	↓ intestinal CHO absorption, ↓ Hb_{A1C} 0.5-0.8%. GI distress (gas).
Pramlintide	Delays gastric emptying & ↓ glucagon, ↓ Hb_{A1C} 0.5% To be used as adjunctive Rx w/ insulin in DM1 or DM2
DPP-4 inhibitor	Blocks degrad. of GLP-1 & GIP → ↑ insulin. ↓ Hb_{A1C} 0.5%
Insulin (Additional DM1 options: insulin pump, pancreatic or islet cell transplant)	↓ Hb_{A1C} 1.5-2.5%; hypoglycemia, wt gain Generally combine intermed./long-acting (NPH or glargine) and short/rapid-acting (regular or lispro) insulin. Consider starting if mono oral Rx not adequate (espec if ↑ Hb_{A1C} high) and definitely start if combo oral Rx not adequate.

(JAMA 2002;287:360, 373; Diabetologia 2006;49:1711)

Insulin Preparations				
Preparation	Onset	Peak	Duration	Side effects/Comments
Lispro, aspart	5-15 min	60-90 min	2-4 h	Give immediately before meal
Regular	30-60 min	2-4 h	5-8 h	Give ~30 min before meal
NPH	1-2 h	4-8 h	12-18 h	Can cause protamine Ab prod
Glargine	2 h	No peak	20-24 h	Once daily (AM or PM)
Inhaled	5-15 min	~2-4 h	~6-8 h	Causes cough, variable absorp

(NEJM 2005;352:174)

Complications

- **Retinopathy**
  non-proliferative: "dot & blot" and retinal hemorrhages, cotton wool/protein exudates
  proliferative: neovascularization, vitreous hemorrhage, retinal detachment, blindness
  treatment: photocoagulation
- **Nephropathy**: microalbuminuria → proteinuria ± nephrotic syndrome → renal failure
  diffuse glomerular basement membrane thickening/nodular pattern (Kimmelstiel-Wilson)
  usually accompanied by retinopathy; lack of retinopathy suggests another cause
  treatment: strict BP control, ACE inhibitors (*NEJM* 1993;329:1456; *Lancet* 1997;349:1787) &
    ARBs (*NEJM* 2001;345:851, 861), low-protein diet, dialysis, or transplant
- **Neuropathy**
  symmetric peripheral: symmetric distal sensory loss, paresthesias, ± motor loss
  autonomic: gastroparesis, neurogenic bladder, impotence, orthostatic hypotension
  mononeuropathy: sudden onset peripheral or CN deficit (footdrop, CN III > VI > IV)
- **Accelerated atherosclerosis**: coronary, cerebral, and peripheral arterial beds
- **Infections**: candidiasis, mucormycosis, necrotizing external otitis
- **Dermatologic**: necrobiosis lipoidica diabeticorum, lipodystrophy, acanthosis nigricans

Outpatient screening and treatment goals (*Diabetes Care* 2006;29:S4)

- ✓ Hb$_{A1C}$ q3-6mos, goal <7%; microvascular & macrovascular complications ↓ by strict glycemic control, in DM1 (DCCT, *NEJM* 1993;329:997 & 2005;353:2643) & DM2 (UKPDS, *Lancet* 1998;352:837)
- Microalbuminuria yearly with spot microalbumin/Cr ratio, goal <30 mg/g
- BP <130/80; LDL <100, TG <150, HDL >40; benefit of statins in all diabetics even w/o overt CAD (*Lancet* 2003;361:2005 & 2004;364:685); ASA if age ≥40 or other cardiac risk factors
- Dilated retinal exam yearly; podiatrist yearly at a minimum

DIABETIC KETOACIDOSIS (DKA)

Precipitants (the I's)

- **Insulin deficiency** (ie, failure to take enough insulin)
- **Infection** (pneumonia, UTI) or **Inflammation** (pancreatitis, cholecystitis)
- **Ischemia** or **Infarction** (myocardial, cerebral, gut)
- **Intoxication** (alcohol, drugs)
- **Iatrogenesis** glucocorticoids, thiazides

Pathophysiology

- Occurs in **type 1 diabetics** (and *rarely* in type 2 diabetics)
- ↑ glucagon & ↓ insulin
- Hyperglycemia due to: ↑ gluconeogenesis, ↑ glycogenolysis, ↓ glucose uptake into cells
- Ketosis due to: inability to utilize glucose → mobilization and oxidation of fatty acids,
  ↑ substrate for ketogenesis, ↑ ketogenic state of the liver, ↓ ketone clearance
- Mortality ~1% when Pts cared for in tertiary care centers

Clinical manifestations (*Diabetes Care* 2003;26:S109)

- Polyuria, polydipsia, and dehydration
- Dehydration → ↑ HR, hypotension, dry mucous membranes, ↓ skin turgor
- Nausea, vomiting, abdominal pain (either due to intra-abdominal process or DKA), ileus
- Kussmaul's respirations (deep) to compensate for metabolic acidosis with odor of acetone
- Δ MS → somnolence, stupor, coma

Diagnostic studies

- ↑ **anion gap metabolic acidosis**: can later develop nonanion gap acidosis due to urinary loss of ketones (HCO_3 equivalents) and fluid resuscitation with chloride
- **Ketosis**: ⊕ **urine and serum ketones** (acetoacetate measured, but predominant ketone is β-OH-butyrate; urine ketones may be ⊕ in fasting normal individuals)
- ↑ serum glucose
- ↑ BUN and Cr (dehydration ± artifact due to ketones interfering with some Cr assays)
- Pseudohyponatremia: corrected Na = measured Na + [(2.4 × (measured glucose - 100)]
- ↓ or ↑ K (but even if serum K is elevated, usually *total body K depleted*); ↓ total body phos
- Leukocytosis, ↑ amylase (even if no pancreatitis)

Typical DKA "Flow sheet" Setup											
Time	VS	UOP	pH	HCO₃	AG	Ketones	Glc	K	PO₄	IVF	Insulin

Note: Main ketone produced is β-OH-butyrate (βOHB), but ketone measured is acetoacetate (Ac-Ac).
As DKA is treated, βOHB → Ac-Ac, ∴ AG can decrease while measured ketones can increase.

Treatment of DKA	
Rule out possible precipitants	Infection, intra-abdominal process, MI, etc.
Aggressive hydration	NS 10-14 ml/kg/h, tailor to dehydration & CV status
Insulin	10 U IV push followed by 0.1 U/kg/h
	Continue insulin drip until AG normal
	If glc <250 and AG still high → add dextrose to IVF
	and continue insulin to metabolize ketones
	AG normal → SC insulin (overlap IV & SC 2-3 h)
Electrolyte repletion	K: add 20-40 mEq/L IVF if serum K <4.5
	insulin promotes K entry into cells → ↓ serum K
	careful K repletion in Pts with renal failure
	HCO₃: replete if pH <7 or if cardiac instability
	PO₄: replete if <1

HYPEROSMOLAR HYPERGLYCEMIC STATE

Definition, Precipitants, Pathophysiology (Diabetes Care 2003;26:S33)
- Extreme hyperglycemia (w/o ketoacidosis) + hyperosm. + Δ MS in DM2 (typically elderly)
- Precip same as for DKA, but also include dehydration and renal failure
- Hyperglycemia → osmotic diuresis → dehydration → prerenal azotemia → ↑ glc, etc.

Clinical manifestations & Diagnostic studies
- Dehydration and Δ MS
- ↑ **serum glc** (usually >600 mg/dl) and ↑ **serum osmolality** (usually >350 mOsm/L)
- No ketoacidosis; usually ↑ BUN & Cr; [Na] depends on hyperglycemia & dehydration

Treatment (r/o possible precipitants; ~15% mortality due to precipitating factors)
- **Aggressive hydration**: initially NS, average fluid loss up to 8-10 L
- **Insulin** (eg, 10 U IV followed by 0.05-0.1 U/kg/h)

GLYCEMIC CONTROL IN CRITICALLY ILL PATIENTS (NEJM 2006;355:1903)

- Tight glycemic control w/ IV insulin (glc 80-110) confers survival benefit in critically ill surgical Pts; in MICU Pts, some benefit on morbidity and a mortality benefit for those in ICU >3 d (NEJM 2001;345:1359 & 2006;354:449)
- Benefit of normoglycemia in acute MI less well-established
- Goal for ICU and acute MI Pts is maintaining glc <140 w/ avoidance of hypoglycemia and resultant adrenergic surge; standardized insulin infusion protocols should be used

HYPOGLYCEMIA

Etiologies in diabetics
- Excessive insulin, oral hypoglycemics, missed meals, renal failure (↓ insulin & SU clearance), hypothyroidism
- β-blockers can mask symptoms of hypoglycemia

Etiologies in nondiabetics
- ↑ **insulin**: exogenous insulin, sulfonylureas, insulinoma, anti-insulin antibodies
- ↓ **glucose production**: hypopituitarism, adrenal insufficiency, glucagon deficiency, hepatic failure, renal failure, alcoholism, sepsis
- Postprandial, especially postgastrectomy: excessive response to glucose load
- Low glc w/o sx can be normal, espec. in woman

Clinical manifestations (glucose < ~55 mg/dl)
- **CNS**: headache, visual Δs, Δ MS, weakness (neuroglycopenic sx)
- **Autonomic**: diaphoresis, palpitations, tremor (adrenergic sx)

Evaluation (NEJM 1995;332:1144)
- BUN, Cr, LFTs, TFTs
- 72-h fast with monitored blood glucoses; stop for neuroglycopenic sx
- At end of fast, give 1 mg glucagon IV and measure response of plasma glc before feeding
- *At time of hypoglycemia*: insulin, C peptide (↑ with insulinoma and sulfonylureas, ↓ with exogenous insulin), β-OH-butyrate, sulfonylurea levels, and IGF-II

Treatment
- Glucose paste, fruit juice are first-line Rx for Pts who can take POs
- If IV access available, give 25-50 g of D₅₀ (50% dextrose)
- If no IV, can give glucagon 0.5–1 mg IM or SC (side effect: N/V)

LIPID DISORDERS

Measurements
- Lipoproteins = lipids (cholesteryl esters & triglycerides) + phospholipids + proteins include: chylomicrons, VLDL, IDL, LDL, HDL, Lp(a)
- Measure after 12-h fast; LDL is calculated = TC − HDL − (TG/5) (if TG >400, order direct LDL measurement as calc. LDL inaccurate). Lipid levels stable up to 24 h after ACS and other acute illnesses, then ↓ and may take 6 wks to return to nl.
- Metabolic syndrome (≥3 of following): waist ≥40" in man or ≥35" in woman; TG ≥150; HDL <40 mg/dl in man or <50 mg/dl in woman; BP ≥130/85 mmHg; fasting glc ≥130 mg/dl

Secondary Dyslipidemias	
Category	**Disorders**
Endocrinopathies	Type 2 diabetes (↑ TG, ↓ HDL)
	Hypothyroidism (↑ LDL, ↑ TG); hyperthyroidism (↓ LDL)
	Cushing's syndrome & exogenous steroids (↑ TG)
Renal diseases	Renal failure (↑ TG); nephrotic syndrome (↑ LDL)
Hepatic diseases	Cholestasis, PBC (↑ LDL); liver failure (↓ LDL); acute hepatitis (↑ TG)
Lifestyle	Obesity (↑ TG, ↓ HDL); sedentary lifestyle (↓ HDL); alcohol (↑ TG, ↑ HDL); tobacco (↓ HDL)
Medications	Thiazides (↑ LDL); β-blockers (↑ TG, ↓ HDL)
	Estrogens (↑ TG, ↑ HDL); protease inhibitors (↑ TG)

Primary dyslipidemias
- Familial hypercholesterolemia (FH, 1:500): defective LDL receptor; ↑↑ chol, nl TG; ↑ CAD
- Familial defective apoB100 (FDB, 1:1000): similar to FH
- Familial combined hyperlipidemia (FCH, 1:200): polygenic; ↑ chol, ↑ TG, ↓ HDL; ↑ CAD
- Familial dysbetalipoproteinemia (FDBL, 1:10,000): apoE ε2/ε2 + DM, obesity, renal disease, etc.; ↑ chol and TG; tuberoeruptive and palmar striated xanthomas; ↑ CAD
- Familial hypertriglyceridemia (FHTG, 1:500): ↑ TG, ± ↑ chol, ↓ HDL, pancreatitis

Physical examination findings
- Tendon xanthomas: seen on Achilles, elbows, and hands; imply LDL >300 mg/dl
- Eruptive xanthomas: pimplelike lesions on extensor surfaces; imply TG >1000 mg/dl
- Xanthelasma: yellowish streaks on eyelids seen in various dyslipidemias
- Corneal arcus: common in older adults, imply hyperlipidemia in young Pts

Treatment
- Every 1 mmol (39 mg/dl) ↓ LDL → 21% ↓ major vascular events (CV death, MI, stroke, revasc) in individuals w/ & w/o CAD (Lancet 2005;366:1267)
- Fewer clinical data, but TG <400 and HDL >40 are additional reasonable targets

NCEP Guidelines	
Clinical risk	**LDL Goal**
High: CHD, CVD, PAD, AAA, DM, or ≥2 RFs & 10-y risk >20%	<100 mg/dl or <70 if very high risk (ACS, CAD + multiple RFs or + met syndrome)
Mod high: ≥2 RFs & 10-y risk 10-20%	<130 mg/dL (optional <100 mg/dl)
Mod: ≥2 RFs & 10-y risk <10%	<130 mg/dl
Lower: 0-1 RFs	<160 mg/dl

RFs: male ≥45 or female ≥55, smoking, HTN, ⊕ FHx, HDL <40. If HDL >60 subtract 1 RF. Framingham 10-y CHD risk score at www.nhlbi.nih.gov/guidelines/cholesterol. (JAMA 2001;285:2486; Circulation 2004;110:227)

Drug Treatment				
Drug	**↓ LDL**	**↑ HDL**	**↓ TG**	**Side effects/comments**
Statins	20-60%	5-10%	10-25%	↑ aminotransferases in 0.5-3%; ✓ LFTs before, at 8-12 wks, and then q6mos; risk dose-depend. Myalgias <10% (not always ↑ CK), myositis 0.5%, rhabdo < 0.1%, risk dose-depend. Doubling of dose → 6% further ↓ LDL
Ezetimibe	15-20%	–	–	Well tolerated; typically w/ statin
Fibrates	5-15%	5-15%	35-50%	Myopathy risk ↑ with statin. Dyspepsia, gallstones
Niacin	10-25%	~30%	40%	Flushing (Rx w/ ASA), pruritis, ↑ glc, gout, nausea, severe hepatitis (rare)
Resins	20%	3-5%	? ↑	Bloating, binds other meds

Figure 8-1 Approach to arthritis

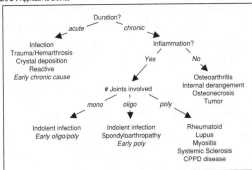

Comparison of Major Arthritides				
Feature	OA	RA	Gout	Spondylo-arthropathy
Onset	gradual	gradual	acute	variable
Inflammation	⊖	⊕	⊕	⊕
Pathology	degeneration	pannus	microtophi	enthesitis
# of joints	poly	poly	mono to poly	oligo or poly
Type of joints	small or large	small	small or large	large
Locations typically involved	hips, knees, spine 1st CMC DIP, PIP	MCP, PIP wrists feet, ankles	MTP feet, ankles knees	sacroiliac spine large peripheral
Special articular findings	Bouchard's nodes Heberden's nodes	ulnar dev. swan neck boutonnière	urate crystals	en bloc spine enthesopathy (eg, Achilles)
Bone changes	osteophytes	osteopenia erosions	erosions	erosions ankylosis
Extra-articular features		SC nodules pulmonary cardiac splenomegaly	tophi olec. bursitis renal stones	uveitis conjunctivitis aortic insuff. psoriasis IBD
Lab data	normal	⊕ RF, anti-CCP	↑ UA	

Analysis of Joint Fluid				
Test	Normal	Noninflammatory	Inflammatory	Septic
Appearance	clear	clear, yellow	clear to opaque yellow-white	opaque
WBC/mm³	<200	<2,000	>2,000	>2,000 usually >50K
Polys	<25%	<25%	≥50%	≥75%
Culture	⊖	⊖	⊖	⊕
Conditions		OA, internal derangement	RA, crystal CTD spondyloarth.	infection

ARTHRITIS 8-1

RHEUMATOID ARTHRITIS (RA)

Definition and epidemiology
- Chronic, symmetric, debilitating and destructive polyarthritis caused by inflammatory, proliferative synovial tissue (pannus) formation in affected joints
- Genetic factors: ↑ incidence in Pts w/ shared epitope on Class II MHC DRB1 and DR4
- Environmental factors: smoking, silica dust exposure
- Greatly increased risk of developing RA in individuals carrying the shared epitope who smoke due to gene–environment interaction (Arth Rheum 2004;50:3085)
- Prevalence = 1% of adults; female:male = 3:1; onset 35-50 y; worldwide

Clinical manifestations (Lancet 2001;358:903)
- **Pain, swelling,** and impaired function of joints (typically PIPs, MCPs, wrists, knees, ankles, MTPs, and cervical spine) with **morning stiffness** for ≥1 h
- Joint immobilization, muscle shortening, bone & cartilage destruction, joint deformities: **ulnar deviation, swan neck** (MCP flexion, PIP hyperextension, DIP flexion) **boutonnière** (PIP flexion, DIP hyperextension), **cock-up deformities** (toes)
- **C1-C2 instability** → myelopathy, ∴ ✓ C-spine flex/ext films prior to elective intubation
- **Rheumatoid nodules** (20-30%; usually in RF ⊕ Pts): SC nodules on extensor surfaces along tendon sheaths and in bursae; also occur in lung, heart, and sclera
- Constitutional symptoms: fever, weight loss, malaise
- Ocular: scleritis, episcleritis, keratoconjunctivitis sicca (associated Sjögren's)
- Pulmonary
  ILD: COP, fibrosis, nodules, Caplan's syndrome (pneumoconiosis + rheumatoid nodules)
  pleural disease: pleuritis, pleural effusions (classically low glucose)
  airway disease: obstruction (cricoarytenoid arthritis), bronchiolitis, bronchiectasis
- Cardiac: pericarditis, myocarditis, nodules can cause valvular and/or conduction disease
- Heme: anemia of chronic disease, leukemia, lymphoma
- Vascular: small nail fold infarcts, palpable purpura, leukocytoclastic vasculitis
- Longstanding seropositive, erosive RA:
  Felty's syndrome (1%): neutropenia, RF ⊕, splenomegaly; ↑ risk of NHL
  large granular lymphocyte syndrome: neutropenia, lymphocytosis blood/marrow
- Remember that rheumatoid joints can become superinfected

Laboratory and radiologic studies
- **RF** (IgM anti-IgG Ab) in 85% of Pts; levels correlate only loosely with disease activity
  nonspecific as also seen in other rheumatic diseases (SLE, Sjögren's), chronic inflammation (SBE, hepatitis, TB), type II cryoglobulinemia, 5% of healthy population
- **Anti-CCP** (Ab to cyclic citrullinated peptide): similar Se (~80%, more Sp (~90%) than RF for RA (Rheum 2006;45:20)
- ↑ ESR and CRP; ⊕ ANA in ~15%; ↑ globulin during periods of active disease
- Radiographs of hands and wrists: periarticular osteopenia, erosions, and deformities

Classification criteria (4 of 7; ~90% Se & Sp; Arth Rheum 1988;31:315)
- **Morning stiffness** ≥1 h × 6 wks
- **Hand joint arthritis** × 6 wks
- **Rheumatoid nodules**
- **Radiographic changes** c/w RA (ie, erosions and periarticular osteopenia)
- **Arthritis** ≥3 joints simultaneously × 6 wks
- **Symmetric joint involvement** × 6 wks
- ⊕ **Rheumatoid factor**

Management (NEJM 2004;350:2591 & 2006;355:704; Lancet 2004;364:263)
- Early dx and Rx w/ frequent follow-up and escalation of Rx as needed → ↓ disease activity and radiographic progression, ↑ physical fxn and quality of life
- Initial therapy
  nonselective NSAIDs (? ↑ CV adverse events) or COX-2 inhibitors (↑ CV adverse events w/ some); sx control as indicated
  glucocorticoids (joint injection or low-dose oral): acutely ↓ inflammation
  physical and occupational therapy
- Start **Disease-Modifying Anti-Rheumatic Drug (DMARD)** therapy w/in 3 mos for any Pt w/ established disease and ongoing inflammation (Annals 2007;146:406)
  monotherapy with methotrexate, sulfasalazine, leflunomide, or hydroxychloroquine **OR**
  combination of DMARD + glucocorticoid or anti-TNF (Arth Rheum 2005;52:3360 & 3371)
  escalation therapy → add medication (usually a biologic) or change DMARD
  biologics: never use 2 biologics concurrently in the same Pt
    anti-TNF (etanercept, infliximab, adalimumab; screen for TB prior to Rx); **IL-1 receptor antagonist** (anakinra); **CTLA4-IgG** (abatacept; NEJM 2005;353:144); **anti-CD20** (rituximab) for anti-TNF nonresponders (NEJM 2006;350:2572)
  other agents: azathioprine, penicillamine, gold, minocycline, cyclosporine

CRYSTAL DEPOSITION ARTHRITIDES

GOUT

Definition
- Urate crystal deposition in joints and other tissues → **acute** and chronic inflammation

Epidemiology
- More common in men than in women; peak incidence 5th decade
- Most common cause of inflammatory arthritis in men over 30
- *Rare* in premenopausal women (estrogens promote renal urate excretion)
- Risk factors: metabolic syndrome, HTN, chronic kidney disease; ↑ intake of meat, seafood, and EtOH (*Lancet* 2004;363:1277; *NEJM* 2004;350:1093)

Etiologies (*Annals* 2005;143:499)
- Uric acid (UA) is end product of purine catabolism and is renally excreted. Serum level reflects balance between production and excretion.

	Overproduction	Underexcretion
Primary hyperuricemia	**Idiopathic** Rare inherited enzyme (HGPRT, PRPP) defic.	**Idiopathic**
Secondary hyperuricemia	↑ **meat, seafood, EtOH intake** **Myelo- & lymphoproliferative dis.** Chronic hemolytic anemia Cytotoxic drugs, psoriasis Severe muscle exertion	**Dehydration** ↓ renal function Drugs: **diuretics**, PZA, EMB, salicylates, CsA Keto- or lactic acidosis

Clinical manifestations
- **Acute arthritis**: sudden onset, **painful monoarticular arthritis**; flares episodic
  location: **MTP of great toe** ("podagra"), feet, ankles, knees; occasionally polyarticular
  overlying skin is warm, tense, dusky red; Pt may be febrile
  precipitants: rapid Δ UA; ↑ purine or alcohol; surgery; infection; diuretics, dehydration
  recovery: subsides in 3–10 d; intercritical period = remission of joint pain between attacks
- **Tophi**: deposits of urate crystals → foreign body rxn and deposition in SC tissue &
  joints; commonly in joints of fingers, wrists, knees; also on pinna, Achilles tendon,
  and pressure areas, eg, ulnar aspect of forearm
- **Bursitis**: olecranon, patellar (must be differentiated from intra-articular effusion)
- **Chronic tophaceous gout**: chronic arthritis from tophus formation → pain, joint erosion
- **Renal**: uric acid stones; urate nephropathy (interstitial deposits)
- **Asymptomatic hyperuricemia**: serum UA > 6.8 mg/dl w/o disease manifestations

Diagnostic studies
- ↑ UA, but can be misleading and does *not* make the diagnosis of acute attack
- Arthrocentesis
  take care not to tap through an infected area thus introducing infections into joint space
  polarized microscopy → **needle-shaped, negatively birefringent crystals** (yellow
  parallel and blue perpendicular to axis marked on polarizer), intra- or extracellular
  WBC 20,000–100,000/mm³, > 50% polys
  infection can coexist with acute attacks, ∴ always check Gram stain and culture
- Radiographs
  early → show soft tissue swelling; useful to exclude chondrocalcinosis or septic changes
  late → bony erosions with overhanging edge, soft tissue calcifications within tophi

Acute Treatment for Gout		
Drug	**Mechanism**	**Comments**
NSAIDs	↓ inflammation	Gastritis; ↓ dose in renal insufficiency
Colchicine (PO or IV)	Inhibits polymerization of microtubules → prevention of chemotaxis and phagocytosis	Nausea, vomiting, and diarrhea IV and high PO doses → bone marrow suppression, myopathy, neuropathy ↓ dose in renal insufficiency
Corticosteroids (PO, IA, or IV) *or* **Corticotropin** (SC, IM, or IV)	↓ inflammation	Highly effective for recalcitrant cases Rule out joint infection first

(*NEJM* 2003;349:1647)

Chronic treatment

- ↓ urate production by ↓ dietary intake of meat and seafood (note: vegetables high in purines are not associated with ↑ risk); ↑ intake of lowfat dairy products; ↓ alcohol (esp. beer); weight control
- Avoid dehydration and hyperuricemic drugs (eg, diuretics, low-dose ASA)
- Prophylaxis if frequent attacks *or* starting antihyperuricemic therapy:
  daily low-dose colchicine (~50% ↓ risk of acute flare; *J Rheum 2004;31:2429*)
  NSAIDs (less evidence of effectiveness; *Ann Rheum Dis 2006;65:1312*)
- **Antihyperuricemic therapy** for tophi, frequent attacks, nephrolithiasis; goal UA <6 mg/dl
  however, do not start w/o prophylaxis and until 2-4 wks after acute attack as Δ in serum UA concentration can precipitate an attack
  allopurinol (xanthine oxidase inhibitor); side effects: hypersensitivity, rash, diarrhea, dyspepsia, headache, renal failure, BM suppression, and hepatitis; CBC monitoring and dose adjustment necessary in Pts concurrently taking AZA
  probenecid or **sulfinpyrazone** (uricosuric agents) for underexcreters (urine UA <600 mg/24 h)
  febuxostat (nonpurine xanthine oxidase inhib. *NEJM 2005;353:2450*) awaiting FDA approval

---

CALCIUM PYROPHOSPHATE DIHYDRATE (CPPD) DEPOSITION DISEASE

Definition

- Deposition of CPPD crystals w/in tendons, ligaments, articular capsules, synovium, cartilage
- Acute inflammation due to CPPD crystals in a joint is termed **pseudogout**
- **Chondrocalcinosis**: calcification of cartilage visible on radiographs, resulting from CPPD deposition in articular cartilage, fibrocartilage, or menisci

Pathogenesis

- ↑ synovial & joint fluid levels of inorganic pyrophosphate produced by articular chondrocytes from ATP hydrolysis in response to a variety of insults or inherited defects favors CPPD crystallogenesis and deposition in the cartilage matrix

Epidemiology

- More common in elderly: 20% over age 60 have CPPD of knee joints in autopsy studies

Etiologies

- Most cases *idiopathic*, but consider search for underlying cause, especially in the young
- **Metabolic**: hypomagnesemia, alkaline phosphatase deficiency, hyperparathyroidism, hypothyroidism, familial hypocalciuric hypercalcemia, gout, Gitelman's syndrome, X-linked hypophosphatemic rickets, hemochromatosis
- Joint injections with hyaluronate can precipitate attacks
- Familial chondrocalcinosis (autosomal dominant disorder)

Clinical manifestations

- Pseudogout: acute mono- or asymmetric oligoarticular arthritis, *indistinguishable from gout except through synovial fluid exam for crystals*
  location: **knees, wrists,** and MCP joints
  precipitants: surgery, trauma, or severe illness
- "PseudoRA": chronic polyarticular arthritis with morning stiffness; ± RF
- Premature OA: destruction of articular cartilage and bony overgrowths → degen. of joints

Diagnostic studies

- Arthrocentesis
  take care not to tap through an infected area thus introducing infxn into joint space
  polarized microscopy → **rhomboid-shaped, weakly positively birefringent crystals** (yellow *perpendicular* and blue parallel to axis marked on polarizer)
  WBC 2000-100,000/mm³, >50% polys
  infection can coexist with acute attacks, ∴ always check Gram stain and culture
- Screen for associated metabolic diseases when dx a new case: ✓ Ca, Mg, TSH, Fe, glc, UA
- **Radiographs**: though not a prerequisite for the diagnosis of CPPD disease, chondrocalcinosis appears as punctate and linear densities in articular cartilage, menisci, triangular fibrocartilage of the wrist, small joints of fingers, and symphysis pubis

Treatment

- Acute therapy for pseudogout: same as for gout, though colchicine not as effective
- Chronic therapy: treat predisposing disease
- Low-dose daily colchicine may be effective prophylaxis in some Pts

SERONEGATIVE SPONDYLOARTHROPATHIES

GENERAL

Definition (*Annals* 2002;136:896)
- A spectrum of systemic inflammatory arthritides w/ predilection for the spine, entheses, sacroiliac, and peripheral joints
- Notable for *absence* of rheumatoid factor or autoantibodies; ± ↑ ESR
- ↑ prevalence of HLA-B27 (⊕ in 50-90% vs. 6-8% of general pop.), but *not* used for dx
- Synovial fluid of affected joints shows an inflammatory, nonseptic picture

ANKYLOSING SPONDYLITIS

Epidemiology
- Onset in teens or mid-20s; onset after age 40 very unusual; male:female ratio = 3:1; HLA-B27 ⊕ in 90%

Clinical manifestations
- Gradual onset of chronic, intermittent bouts of lower back pain and stiffness
- **Morning stiffness** that improves with hot shower and exercise
- Progressive limitation of motion in cervical, thoracic, and/or lumbar spine over time
  ⊕ modified **Wright-Schober test** (<4 cm ↑ in distance between a point at lumbosacral jxn and one 10 cm above, when going from standing to maximum forward flexion)
- **Enthesitis**: inflammation at site of tendon/ligament insertion into bone, eg, Achilles tendinitis, plantar fasciitis, rigidity of spine (bamboo spine by x-ray)
- **Arthritis in peripheral joints can occur**, eg, hips, shoulders, knees
- Acute anterior **uveitis** (25-40% at some time during disease): presents with unilateral blurred vision, lacrimation, and photophobia
- Cardiovascular disease (5%): ascending aortitis, AI, conduction system abnormalities
- Neurologic complications: spinal fractures, C1/2 subluxation, or cauda equina syndrome

Imaging studies
- Radiographs of spine to assess progression of disease:
  Sacroiliac joint disease with erosions and sclerosis
  Calcification of spinal ligaments with bridging syndesmophytes ("bamboo spine")
  Squaring and generalized demineralization of vertebral bodies, "shiny corners"
- MRI spine to assess inflammation in sacroiliac joint

Treatment (*Lancet* 2007;369:1379)
- Supportive: physical therapy, NSAIDs, steroid injection
- Anti-TNF shown to improve symptoms and function (*Ann Rheum Dis* 2006; 65:423)
- Sulfasalazine and methotrexate: somewhat effective for peripheral arthritis, but little or no effect on spinal symptoms

REACTIVE ARTHRITIS

Epidemiology
- Ages 20-40; male:female ratio = 5:1; more common in Caucasians

Pathogenesis
- Immune-mediated aseptic synovitis in a genetically susceptible host post-GU or GI infxn
- Bacteria associated with disease
  GU: *Chlamydia* and *Ureaplasma urealyticum*
  GI: *Shigella, Salmonella, Yersinia, Campylobacter, C. difficile*

Clinical presentation
- Originally described as a triad of **seronegative arthritis, nongonococcal urethritis, and noninfectious conjunctivitis** ("Reiter's syndrome")
- **Arthritis**: 10-30 d post–inciting infection → mild constitutional sx, low back pain, asymmetric, mono- or oligoarticular arthritis of primarily large joints (knees, ankles, feet), enthesopathy, and sacroiliitis. Can develop *sausage digits* (dactylitis) of extremities.
- **Urethritis/cervicitis**: usually *Chlamydia* infection preceding arthritis, but also can see sterile urethritis in postdysenteric reactive arthritis
- **Conjunctivitis**: noninfectious, unilateral or bilateral and ± uveitis, iritis, and keratitis

- Cutaneous manifestations (may go unnoticed by Pt)
  circinate balantitis: shallow, painless ulcers of glans penis and urethral meatus
  keratoderma blenorrhagica: hyperkeratotic skin lesions on soles of feet, scrotum, palms, trunk, scalp
  stomatitis and superficial oral ulcers
- GI: diarrhea and abdominal pain either w/ or w/o infectious agent
- CV: AI from inflammation and scarring of aorta and valve; conduction defects

Radiographs
- Early: **soft tissue swelling and effusions** around affected joints
- Late: asymmetric proliferation of bone at site of inflammation
- **Asymmetric sacroiliitis** in 70% Pts

Diagnostic studies
- PCR of urine or genital swab for *Chlamydia*, stool cultures, *C. difficile* toxin, etc., but ⊖ studies do not rule out

Treatment and prognosis
- NSAIDs, steroid injection for mono- or oligoarthritis, sulfasalazine if inflammation persists
- Antibiotics if evidence of active or antecedent infection, as cx may be ⊖
- Arthritis may persist for months to years and recurrences are common

---

PSORIATIC ARTHRITIS

Epidemiology
- Seen in >10% of Pts w/ psoriasis (and not necessarily those with severe skin disease)
- Arthritis may *precede* onset of skin disease, even by years
- 20-40% of Pts with psoriatic arthritis have spinal or sacroiliac involvement
- Men and women are affected equally and most Pts in 30s and 40s

Clinical manifestations
- Several clinical patterns of arthritis:
  monoarticular/oligoarticular (eg, large joint, DIP joint, dactylitic digit): most common initial manifestation
  polyarthritis (small joints of the hands and feet, wrists, ankles, knees, elbows): indistinguishable from RA
  arthritis mutilans: severe destructive arthritis with bone resorption
  axial disease: similar to ankylosing spondylitis ± peripheral arthritis
- Enthesopathies, tendinitis
- Fingernails: pitting, transverse depressions, onycholysis, subungal hyperkeratosis
- Eye inflammation (30%): conjunctivitis, iritis, episcleritis and keratoconjunctivitis sicca
- Psoriatic skin lesions

Radiographs
- **"Pencil-in-cup"** deformity seen at DIP joints, erosive changes
- Spinal involvement, sacroiliitis

Treatment
- Symptom control: NSAIDs; intra-articular glucocorticoid injections
- Anti-TNF (etanercept, infliximab, adalimumab) ↓ progression of disease
- Sulfasalazine: only DMARD shown to improve sx, but not progression of disease
- Other: gold, MTX, CsA, AZA, leflunomide, PUVA, antimalarials, penicillamine

---

ENTEROPATHIC (IBD-ASSOCIATED)

Epidemiology
- Seen in 20% of Pts w/ IBD; more frequently seen in Crohn's than UC

Clinical manifestations
- **Peripheral, migratory, asymmetric, non-deforming oligoarthritis**: abrupt onset, large joints, course *parallels* GI disease
- **Spondylitis**: associated more strongly with HLA-B27, course does *not* parallel GI disease
- **Sacroiliitis**
- Erythema nodosum, pyoderma gangrenosum (= neutrophilic dermatosis → painful ulcers w/ violaceous border; Ddx incl. idiopathic, IBD, RA, myelogenous leukemia), anterior uveitis

Treatment
- 5-ASA compounds, etc. for underlying IBD (see "IBD")

INFECTIOUS ARTHRITIS

DIAGNOSIS AND EMPIRIC TREATMENT

Diagnosis
- **Arthrocentesis** should be performed as soon as suspected
- *Take care not to tap through an infected area thus introducing infxn into joint space*
- Send fluid for cell count, gram stain, bacterial culture
  WBC >50,000 with poly predominance suspicious for bacterial infection
  (crystals do *not* rule out septic arthritis!)

Initial therapy
- Prompt empiric antibiotics guided by gram stain
- If gram stain negative, empiric coverage w/ **ceftriaxone + nafcillin or vancomycin**
- Modify antibiotics based on culture results and clinical course

Common microbes		Population	Initial antibiotic regimen
GPC	S. aureus (most common)	Normal joints Prosthetic joints Damaged joints	Nafcillin or Vancomycin if suspect MRSA (eg, hospitalized Pt)
	S. epidermidis	Prosthetic joints Post–joint procedure	Nafcillin or Vancomycin if suspect MRSA (eg, hospitalized Pt)
	Streptococci	Healthy adults Splenic dysfunction	Penicillin G or Ampicillin
GN	Diplococci: N. gonorrhea	Sexually active young adults	Ceftriaxone
	Rods: E. coli, Pseudomonas, Serratia	IVDA GI infection Immunocompromised	Ceftriaxone + antipseudomonal aminoglycoside if suspect IVDA

BACTERIAL (NONGONOCOCCAL)

Epidemiology and risk factors
- **Immunocompromised host** (eg, diabetics, HIV, elderly, SLE)
- **Damaged joints**: RA, OA, gout, trauma, prosthetic, prior arthrocentesis (rare)
- **Bacterial seeding**
  bacteremia secondary to IVDA, endocarditis, or skin infection
  direct inoculation or spread from contiguous focus (eg, cellulitis, septic bursitis, osteo)

Clinical manifestations
- Acute onset of **monoarticular arthritis** (>80%) with pain, swelling, and warmth
- Location: **knee** (most common), hip, wrist, shoulder, ankle. In IVDA, tends to involve other areas, eg, sacroiliac joint, symphysis pubis, sternoclavicular and manubrial joints.
- **Constitutional symptoms**: fevers, chills, sweats, malaise, myalgias, pain
- Infection can track from initial site to form fistulae, abscesses, or osteomyelitis
- Septic bursitis must be differentiated from septic intra-articular effusion

Additional diagnostic studies
- Synovial fluid: **WBC usually >100,000** (but can be as low as 1000), **>90% polys**
  gram stain ⊕ in ~75% of Staph, ~50% of GNR; culture ⊕ in >90% of cases
- **Leukocytosis** with left shift
- **Blood cultures** ⊕ in >50% of cases
- Conventional radiographs usually normal until after ~2 wks of infection when bony erosions, joint space narrowing, osteomyelitis, periostitis can be seen
- **CT and MRI** useful especially for suspected hip infection or epidural abscess

Definitive treatment
- **Antibiotics**
- **Surgical drainage**/lavage indicated in many cases, especially for larger joints
- Prognosis: 10-50% mortality depending on virulence of organism, time to Rx, host

DISSEMINATED GONOCOCCAL INFECTION (DGI)

Epidemiology
- Most frequent type of infectious arthritis in sexually active young adults
- Caused by *Neisseria gonorrhea*
- **Normal host** as well as Pts w/ deficiencies of terminal components of complement
- Female:male ratio = 4:1. ↑ incidence during menses, pregnancy and postpartum period. ↑ incidence in homosexual males. Rare after age 40.

Clinical manifestations
- Preceded by **mucosal infection** (eg, endocervix, urethra, or pharynx) that is often asx
- Usually presents as two distinct syndromes:
  Joint localized: purulent arthritis (40%) usually of knees, wrists, hands, or ankles
  Bacteremia: triad of polyarthritis, tenosynovitis, skin lesions
    prodrome: fever, malaise, **migratory polyarthralgias** (wrist, knees, ankles, elbows)
    acute onset of **tenosynovitis** (60%) in wrists, fingers, ankles, toes
    rash (>50%): gunmetal gray pustules with erythematous base on extremities & trunk
- Rare complications: Fitz-Hugh Curtis (perihepatitis), pericarditis, meningitis, myocarditis, osteomyelitis

Additional diagnostic studies
- **Leukocytosis** with left shift; ↑ ESR
- Synovial fluid: **WBC >50,000** (but can be <10,000), **poly predominant**
  Gram stain ⊕ in ~25% of cases
  culture ⊕ in up to 50% of cases if culture anaerobically on Thayer-Martin media
  PCR for gonococcal DNA can improve Se (not yet widely available)
- Blood culture: more likely ⊕ in tenosynovitis; rarely in joint localized disease
- Gram stain and culture of skin lesions occasionally ⊕
- Cervical, urethral, pharyngeal, rectal cultures on Thayer-Martin media indicated; check for *Chlamydia*

Treatment
- Ceftriaxone × 7 d w/ empiric doxycycline for possible concurrent *Chlamydia*
- Joint aspiration or arthroscopy/lavage may be required for Pts with purulent arthritis

% Autoantibodies in Patients with Rheumatic Diseases										
Disease	ANA & Pattern	RF	dsDNA	Sm	Ro	La	Scl-70	Cent	Jo	RNP
SLE	95-99 D, S, N	20	50-70	30	35	15	0	0	0	30-50
RA	15-35 D	85	<5	0	10	5	0	0	0	10
Sjögren's	>90 D, S	75	<5	0	55	40	0	0	0	15
Diffuse SSc	>90 N, S, D	30	0	0	5	1	40	<5	0	30
Limited SSc	>90 S, N, D	30	0	0	5	1	<5	70	0	30
PM-DM	75-95	33	0	0	0	0	10	0	25	0
MCTD	95-99 S, D	50	0	0	<5	<5	0	0	0	100

(D = diffuse or homogeneous, S = speckled, N = nucleolar; *Primer on the Rheumatic Diseases*, 12th ed., 2001)

- Autoantibody testing is directed by clinical findings, as autoantibodies themselves do not define a particular connective tissue disease
- Overlap syndromes encompassing more than one connective tissue disorder may be reflected serologically by the presence of multiple autoantibodies

see "Systemic Lupus Erythematosus" and "Rheumatoid Arthritis" for those diseases

SYSTEMIC SCLEROSIS AND SCLERODERMA DISORDERS

Definition and epidemiology
- **Scleroderma** refers to the presence of tight, thickened skin.
- Anatomic distribution of sclerodermatous skin defines subtypes and disease associations
  localized scleroderma: *morphea* (plaques of fibrotic skin), *linear* (fibrotic bands), *"en coup de saber"* (linear scleroderma on one side of scalp and forehead ≈ saber scar)
  systemic sclerosis (SSc): multiorgan involvement
    SSc with *diffuse cutaneous* disease (incl. proximal extremities & trunk)
    SSc with *limited cutaneous* disease (CREST syndrome)
    SSc *sine scleroderma* (visceral disease without skin involvement)
- Peak onset of SSc between **ages 30-50**; more common in **women** than men
- 1-2/100,000 annual incidence of systemic disease in the U.S.
- Stimulatory autoantibodies against PDGF receptor activating collagen gene expression proposed as pathogenic mechanism for development of fibrosis (*NEJM 2006;354:2667*)

Classification criteria (1 major or 2 minor; 97% Se, 98% Sp; *Arth Rheum 1980;23:581*)
- *Major*: **skin findings extend** *proximal* **to MCP or MTP joints**
- *Minor*: **sclerodactyly** (skin findings limited to the fingers)
  digital pitting scars from loss of substance on the finger pad
  bibasilar **pulmonary fibrosis**
- Proposed additions to the above criteria include the presence of Raynaud's phenomenon, findings on nailfold capillaroscopy (eg, dropout and dilatation), and serologies
- **Other causes** of thickened skin: diabetes (scleredema ≠ scleroderma), hypothyroidism, nephrogenic fibrosing dermopathy, eosinophilic fasciitis, amyloidosis, GVHD, drug or toxin

Diagnostic studies
- Autoantibodies
  ⊕ **anti-Scl-70** (anti-topoisomerase 1): 40% of diffuse, 15% of limited
  ⊕ **anti-centromere**: 60-80% of limited, <5% of diffuse
  ⊕ ANA (>90%), ⊕ RF (30%)
- If renal involvement → ↑ BUN and Cr, proteinuria
- If pulmonary involvement → interstitial pattern on CXR/chest CT, restriction and/or ↓ D_LCO on PFTs; PHT revealed by echocardiography
- Skin bx not routine, but helpful to assess other possible causes for skin thickening

	Clinical Manifestations of Systemic Sclerosis	
Organ	**Involvement**	
Skin	Tightening and thickening of extremities, face, and trunk "Puffy" hands, carpal tunnel syndrome, sclerodactyly Nailfold capillary dilatation & dropout Immobile, pinched, "mouselike" facies and "purse-string" mouth Calcinosis cutis (subcutaneous calcification) Telangiectasias	
Arteries	Raynaud's phenomenon (80%); digital or visceral ischemia	
Renal	Scleroderma renal crisis = sudden onset severe HTN, RPGN, MAHA Crescentic GN (rare) with ⊕ p-ANCA (J Rheum 2006;33:1886)	
GI	GERD and erosive esophagitis Esophageal dysmotility → dysphagia, odynophagia, aspiration Gastric dysmotility → early satiety and gastric outlet obstruction Small intestinal dysmotility → bloating, diarrhea, malabsorption	
Musculoskel	Polyarthralgias & joint stiffness; muscle weakness, tendon friction rubs	
Cardiac	Myocardial fibrosis, pericarditis; conduction abnormalities	
Pulmonary	Pulmonary fibrosis; pulmonary hypertension	
Endocrine	Amenorrhea and infertility common; thyroid fibrosis ± hypothyroidism	

Systemic Sclerosis		
	Limited	**Diffuse**
Skin	Thickening on distal extremities and face only	Thickening on extremities (incl. digits), face, *and* trunk
Nails	Capillary dropout ± dilatation	Capillary dropout & *dilatation*
Pulmonary	PHT > fibrosis	Fibrosis > PHT
GI	GERD, hypomotility *Primary biliary cirrhosis*	GERD, hypomotility
Renal		Renovascular HTN
Cardiac		Restrictive cardiomyopathy
Other	**CREST syndrome =** **C**alcinosis, **R**aynaud's **E**sophageal dysmotility **S**clerodactyly, **T**elangiectasias	
Antibodies	Anticentromere (70%)	Anti-Scl 70 (40%)
Prognosis	Survival >70% at 10 y	Survival 40-60% at 10 y

Treatment (organ-based approach)
- Pulmonary
  fibrosis: **cyclophosphamide** (NEJM 2006;354:2653), steroids
  PHT: pulmonary **vasodilators** (see "Pulmonary Hypertension")
- Renal: monitor BP monthly, intervene early to avoid HTN crisis; dipstick for protein
  ACE inhibitors (not ARB) for HTN crisis (poor prognosis w/ 50% mortality)
- GI: PPI and/or H2-blockers for GERD; antibiotics for malabsorption
  hypomotility: metoclopramide or erythromycin; nonoperative Rx of pseudoobstruction
- Cardiac: NSAIDs or steroids for pericarditis
- Arthritis: acetaminophen, NSAIDs, PT
- Myositis: MTX, AZA, steroids
- Skin: PUVA for morphea; emollients or oral steroids (caution can precip HTN renal crisis)
  for pruritis; immunosuppressives offer only minimal to modest benefit for fibrosis

INFLAMMATORY MYOPATHIES

Definition and epidemiology (Lancet 2003;362:971)
- **Polymyositis** (PM): *T cell-mediated muscle injury* → skeletal muscle inflam. & weakness
- **Dermatomyositis** (DM): *immune complex deposition in blood vessels with complement activation* → skeletal muscle inflam. & weakness + *skin manifestations*
- **Inclusion body myositis** (IBM): *T cell-mediated muscle injury, vacuole formation with amyloid deposition* → skeletal muscle inflam. & weakness
- PM/DM: onset typically 40s and 50s; more common in women than men
  ↑ risk of cancer (especially ovarian) in PM (~10% of Pts) and DM
- IBM: onset after age 50; men >women; often *misdiagnosed as polymyositis*

Clinical manifestations
- **Muscle weakness**: gradual, progressive, often painless, symmetric, and *proximal*; typically difficulty climbing stairs, arising from chairs, brushing hair; ± tenderness of affected areas; *asymmetry and distal weakness more common in IBM* than PM/DM
- **Dermatologic**
  erythematous rash on sun-exposed skin: neck & shoulders (shawl sign), face, chest
  heliotrope rash (purplish discoloration) over upper eyelids ± periorbital edema
  Gottron's papules (*pathognomonic*): violaceous often scaly areas symmetrically over dorsum of PIP and MCP joints, elbows, patellae, medial malleoli
  subungal erythema, cuticular telangiectases, "**mechanic's hands**" (skin cracks on digits)
- Polyarthralgias or polyarthritis
- Vasculitis of skin, muscle, GI tract and eyes; Raynaud's (30%, usu. DM and overlap CTD)
- Visceral involvement
  pulmonary: acute alveolitis, chronic ILD, weakness of respiratory muscles
  cardiac (33%): myocarditis, pericarditis, arrhythmias
  GI: dysphagia

Diagnostic studies
- ↑ **CK**, aldolase, SGOT, and LDH; ± ↑ ESR & CRP
- Autoantibodies: ⊕ ANA (>75%), ⊕ RF (33%)
  ⊕ **anti-Jo-1** (25%), associated with nonerosive polyarthritis, Raynaud's, ILD
  ⊕ **anti-Mi-2** (5-10%), more common with DM, may have better prognosis
- **EMG**: ↑ spontaneous activity, ↓ amplitude, polyphasic potentials with contraction
- **Muscle biopsy**: all with muscle fiber necrosis, degeneration & regeneration
  PM: endomysial inflam. (CD8 T cells) surrounds non-necrotic fibers, ↑ MHC class I
  DM: perimysial, perivascular inflam. (B & CD4 T cells), complement in vessels
  IBM: same as PM with eosinophilic inclusions and rimmed vacuoles (EM)

Classification criteria (*NEJM 1975;292:344*; revision under way to reclassify, include IBM)
- Polymyositis = 4 criteria; Dermatomyositis = 3 criteria + derm features
1. Symmetrical weakness   4. EMG evidence
2. Muscle biopsy evidence   5. Dermatologic features
3. Elevation of muscle enzymes

Treatment (PM and DM, no effective treatment for IBM)
- **High-dose steroids**
- DMARDs (eg, MTX and AZA) are 2nd line
  cyclophosphamide if resistant, ILD or vasculitis; IVIg for resistant DM ± PM or for life-threatening esophageal or respiratory muscle involvement
- √ for occult malignancy; monitor respiratory muscle strength with spirometry

Myosides, Myopathies, and Myalgias					
Disease	Weakness	Pain	↑ CK	↑ ESR	Biopsy
DM/PM	⊕	⊖	⊕	±	as above
IBM	⊕	⊖	⊕	⊖	as above
Hypothyroidism	⊕	±	⊕	⊖	mild necrosis inflammation atrophy
Steroid-induced	⊕	⊖	⊖	⊖	atrophy
PMR	⊖ (limited by pain)	⊕	⊖	⊕	normal
Fibromyalgia	⊖ (limited by pain)	⊕ (tender points)	⊖	⊖	normal

---

SJÖGREN'S SYNDROME

Definition and epidemiology
- Chronic dysfunction of **exocrine glands** due to lymphoplasmacytic infiltration
- Can be primary or secondary (associated with RA, scleroderma, SLE, PM, HIV)
- More prevalent in women than in men; typically presents between 40-60 y of age

Clinical manifestations
- **Dry eyes** (keratoconjunctivitis sicca): ↓ tear production; burning, scratchy sensation
- **Dry mouth** (xerostomia): difficulty speaking/swallowing; dental caries; xerotrachea
- **Parotid gland enlargement** or intermittent swelling (bilateral)

- Other manifestations: chronic arthritis; interstitial nephritis (40%), type I RTA (20%); vasculitis (25%); vaginal dryness/dyspareunia; pleuritis; pancreatitis
- ↑ risk of lymphoproliferative disorders (~50× ↑ risk of lymphoma and WM in 1° Sjögren's)

Diagnostic studies

- Autoantibodies: ⊕ ANA (95%), ⊕ RF (75%)
  Primary Sjögren's: ⊕ **anti-Ro** (anti-SS-A, 56%) and ⊕ **anti-La** (anti-SS-B, 30%)
- **Schirmer test**: filter paper in palpebral fissures to assess tear production
- **Rose-Bengal** staining: dye which reveals devitalized epithelium of cornea/conjunctiva
- **Biopsy** (minor salivary, labial, lacrimal, or parotid gland): lymphoplasmacytic infiltration

Classification criteria (4 of 6 has 94% Se & 94% Sp; *Arthritis Rheum* 1993;36:340)
1. Dry eyes
2. Dry mouth
3. ⊕ Schirmer test or Rose-Bengal staining
4. Inflammatory foci on minor salivary gland bx
5. Objective ↓ in salivary gland function
6. Ab to Ro/SS-A or La/SS-B

Treatment

- Ocular: artificial tears, **cyclosporine eyedrops**
- Oral: sugarfree gum, lemondrops, saliva substitute, hydration, cholinergic Rx
- Systemic: NSAIDs, steroids, DMARDs; treat underlying disease (secondary Sjogren's)

MIXED CONNECTIVE TISSUE DISEASE (MCTD)

Definition

- MCTD Pts have features of **SLE, systemic sclerosis**, and/or **polymyositis**, often evolving a dominant phenotype of SLE or systemic sclerosis

Clinical manifestations

- **Raynaud's phenomenon** typical presenting symptom
- Hand edema: "puffy hands", sclerodactyly, RA-like **arthritis** without erosions
- Pulmonary involvement (85%) with **pulmonary hypertension**, fibrosis
- GI dysmotility (70%)
- Low risk for renal HTN crisis or glomerulonephritis; if either, reconsider diagnosis of MCTD

Diagnostic studies

- ⊕ ANA (95-99%), ⊕ RF (50%)
- **Anti-U1-RNP** present by definition in MCTD, but *not* specific (seen in up to 50% SLE Pts)

Treatment

- As per specific rheumatic diseases detailed above

RAYNAUD'S PHENOMENON

Clinical manifestations (NEJM 2002;347:1001)

- Episodic, reversible digital ischemia, in response to cold or stress, classically: **blanching** (ischemia) → **cyanosis** (venule dilatation) → **rubor** (resolution with reactive hyperemia); color change usually well demarcated; affects fingers, toes, ears, nose
- Associated sx include cold, numbness, & paresthesias → throbbing & pain

Primary = Raynaud's disease (50%; excluded all secondary causes)
- Onset age 20-40 y, female:male = 5:1
- Clinical: mild, symmetric episodic attacks; no evidence of peripheral vascular disease, **no tissue injury**, normal nailfold capillary examination, ⊖ ANA, normal ESR

Secondary = Raynaud's phenomenon (50%)
- Collagen vascular disease: SSc, SLE, RA, PM-DM (*abnormal nailfold exam*) exaggerated vascular reactivity ultimately leads to **tissue ischemia & injury**
- Arterial disease: peripheral atherosclerosis, thromboangiitis obliterans (*abnormal pulses*)
- Hematologic: cryoglobulinemia, Waldenström's, antiphospholipid syndrome
- Trauma (vibration or repetitive motion injury) & drugs (ergot alkaloids)

Treatment

- Avoid cold, maintain warmth of digits & body; avoid cigarettes, drugs, and trauma
- Long-acting CCB, α-blockers, ARBs, PO fish oil (primary RP only; *Am J Med* 1989;86:158), topical nitrates, fluoxetine, ASA; bosentan or sildenafil for mod-severe RP espec. w/ PHT; IV prostaglandins (acutely) or digital sympathectomy for severe ischemia

SYSTEMIC LUPUS ERYTHEMATOSUS (SLE)

Multisystem inflammatory autoimmune disease with a broad spectrum of clinical manifestations in association with antinuclear antibody (ANA) production

Epidemiology
- Prevalence 15-50/100,000; predominantly affects women 2nd to 4th decade
- Female:male ratio = 8:1; African American:Caucasian ratio = 4:1
- Complex genetics; some HLA assoc.; rare c1q & c2 defic.

Classification Criteria and Other Clinical Manifestations of SLE		
Organ System	**Am. Coll. Rheum. Criteria**	**Other Features**
Constitutional (84%)		Fever, malaise, anorexia, weight loss
Cutaneous (81%)	1. **Malar rash** 2. **Discoid rash** (erythematous papules w/ keratosis & plugging) 3. **Photosensitivity** 4. **Oral/nasopharyngeal ulcers**	Alopecia Vasculitis Subacute cutaneous lupus Panniculitis (lupus profundus) Urticaria
Musculoskeletal (85%)	5. **Nonerosive arthritis**: episodic, oligoarticular, symmetrical, migratory	Arthralgias and myalgias Avascular necrosis of bone
Cardiopulmonary (33%)	6. **Serositis**: pleuritis (37%) or pleural effusion, pericarditis (29%) or pericardial effusion	Pneumonitis, IPF, PAH Myocarditis, CAD (*NEJM 2003;349:2399, 2407*) Libman-Sacks endocarditis

Renal (77%)	7. **Proteinuria** (>500 mg/dl or 3+ on dipstick) or **urinary cellular casts**	Nephrotic syndrome
		 Lupus nephritis (ISN/RPS):
		   I = min. mesangial;
		   II = mesangial prolif;
		   III = focal (active/chronic);
		   IV = diffuse;
		   V = membranous;
		   VI = advanced sclerotic

Neurologic (54%)	8. **Seizures or psychosis** without other cause	Organic brain syndrome, PML Cranial or periph. neuropathies
Gastrointestinal (~30%)		Serositis (peritonitis, ascites) Vasculitis (bleeding, perf.) Abdominal pain Hepatitis, pancreatitis
Hematologic	9. **Hemolytic anemia** (DAT ⊕) or **leukopenia** (< 4000/mm³), or **lymphopenia** (< 1500/mm³), or **thrombocytopenia** (< 100,000/mm³)	Anemia of chronic disease Antiphospholipid syndrome (VTE w/ ⊕ ACL Ab or ⊕ LAC) Splenomegaly Lymphadenopathy
Other		Sicca syndrome Conjunctivitis or episcleritis Raynaud's (20%) Nailfold capillary changes
Serologies	10. ⊕ **ANA** 11. ⊕ **anti-ds-DNA, anti-sm, or antiphospholipid Abs**	↓ complement (during flare), ↑ ESR, ↑ CRP, ⊕ anti-Ro or anti-RNP, ⊕ RF, ⊕ anti-CCP

If ≥4 of 11 criteria met, Se & Sp for SLE >95%. However, Pt may have SLE but not have 4 criteria at a given point in time. (*Arth Rheum 1982;25:1271 & 1997;40:1725; NEJM 1994;330:1871; Annals 1995;122:940 & 123:42; J Am Soc Neph 2004;15:241; Lancet 2007;369:587*)

- **Drug-induced lupus (DLE)**
   drugs: procainamide, hydralazine, pencillamine, minocycline, INH, methyldopa, quinidine, chlorpromazine, diltiazem, anti-TNF
   clinical: milder disease with predominantly arthritis and serositis
   laboratory: ⊕ anti-histone (95%); ⊖ anti-ds-DNA & anti-Sm; normal complement levels
   course: usually reversible w/in 4-6 wks

Autoantibodies in SLE

AutoAb	Frequency (approx)	Clinical Associations	Timeline
ANA	95-99% if active disease 90% if in remission Homogeneous or speckled	Any or all of the broad spectrum of clinical manifestations Sensitive but not specific	May appear yrs before overt disease
Ro **La**	15-35% ⊕ anti-Ro in ANA ⊖ SLE	Sjögren's/SLE overlap Neonatal lupus Photosensitivity Subacute cutaneous lupus	
ds-DNA	70%; very specific for SLE Titers parallel disease activity, especially renal disease	Lupus nephritis Vasculitis	Appears mos before or at diagnosis
Sm	30%; very specific for SLE	Lupus nephritis	
U1-RNP	40%	MCTD; Raynaud's Tend *not* to have nephritis	
histone	DLE (90%), SLE (80%)	Mild arthritis and serositis	At diagnosis

(*NEJM* 2003;349:1526)

Workup
- Detailed history and exam to assess for signs and symptoms of disease
- Autoantibodies: ANA, if ⊕ → ✓ anti-ds-DNA, anti-Sm, anti-Ro, anti-La, anti-U1-RNP
- Electrolytes, BUN, Cr, U/A, urine sediment, 24-h urine for CrCl and protein
- CBC, Coombs' test, PTT, anticardiolipin and lupus anticoagulant, complement levels

Treatment of SLE

Drug	Indication	Adverse Effects
NSAIDs	Arthralgias/arthritis, myalgias Mild serositis	Gastritis, UGIB Renal failure
Hydroxychloroquine	Mild disease complicated by serositis, arthritis, skin Δs	Macular damage Stevens-Johnson syndrome Myopathy
Corticosteroids	Low doses for mild disease unresponsive to hydroxychloroquine High doses for major manifestations including renal and hematologic	Adrenal suppression Immunosuppression Infection Osteopenia Avascular necrosis of bone Myopathy
Mycophenolate	Nephritis *(induction and/or maintenance)*	Myelosuppression Infection
Cyclophosphamide	Severe nephritis, vasculitis or CNS disease *(induction ± maintenance)*	Myelosuppression Myeloproliferative disorders Immunosuppression Hemorrhagic cystitis, bladder cancer Infertility, teratogen
Azathioprine (AZA)	Mild nephritis (2nd line) Steroid-sparing agent	Myelosuppression Hepatotoxicity Lymphoproliferative disorders
Methotrexate (MTX)	Skin and joint disease Serositis	Myelosuppression Hepatotoxicity Pneumonitis ± fibrosis Alopecia, stomatitis
Cyclosporine (CsA)	Renal disease	Hyperplastic gums, HTN Hirsutism Renal impairment, anemia
Rituximab	Refractory to other agents	B-cell depletion; PML (?)

Prognosis
- 5-y survival rate >90%, 10-y survival rate >80%
- Leading causes of morbidity and mortality: **infection**, **renal failure**, neurologic and cardiovascular events; thrombotic complications (*Medicine* 2003;82:299)

SLE 8-14

LARGE-VESSEL VASCULITIS

Takasu's arteritis ("pulseless disease")
- Systemic granulomatous vasculitis involving aorta and its branches
- Most common in **Asia** and in **young women** of reproductive age
- Clinical manifestations

    Phase I: inflammatory period with **fever, arthralgias**, weight loss

    Phase II: vessel pain and tenderness, ↓ **and unequal pulses in extremities, bruits,** limb claudication, renovascular hypertension (>50%), neurogenic syncope

    most often affects the **subclavian and innominate arteries** (>90%), with carotid renal, pulmonary (~50%), and coronary arteritis and aortitis also commonly seen

    Phase III: burnt out, fibrotic period
- Dx studies: ↑ ESR (75%), CRP; **arteriography** → occlusion, stenosis, irregularity and aneurysms; carotid Doppler studies; MRI/MRA; pathology → focal panarteritis, cellular infiltrate with granulomas and giant cells
- Classification criteria (3 of 6 is 90.5% Se & 97.8% Sp; *Arth Rheum* 1990;33:1129)
    1. age ≤40 y
    2. claudication of the extremities
    3. decreased brachial artery pulse
    4. systolic BP difference >10 mmHg between arms
    5. bruit over subclavian arteries or aorta
    6. arteriogram abnormality (Ao, primary branches, or prox. large arteries in extremities)
- Treatment: steroids, methotrexate, antiplatelet therapy

Giant cell arteritis (GCA) (*NEJM* 2003;349:160)
- Vasculitis affecting cranial branches of aortic arch, especially temporal artery (thus also called "temporal arteritis"), but can cause aortitis as well
- Pts **older than 50** (90% older than 60); female:male ratio = 2:1
- Clinical manifestations (*JAMA* 2002;287:92)

    constitutional symptoms: **low-grade fevers, fatigue**, weight loss, myalgias, anorexia

    headache (2/3); tender temporal arteries and scalp and absent temporal artery pulsation

    ophthalmic artery (20%) → optic neuritis, diplopia, amaurosis fugax and blindness

    facial arteries → **jaw claudication**

    Raynaud's phenomenon; intermittent claudication of extremities; thoracic Ao aneurysm
- Dx studies: ↑ ESR (though in ~5% ESR <40 even before Rx); ↑ CRP

    ESR related to fgbn & Ig in blood; Ddx for >100: infxn, rheum, ESRD, malig

    temporal artery bx (3-5 cm sample length); vasculitis, granulomas)
- Classification criteria (3 of 5 is 93.5% Se & 91.2% Sp; *Arth Rheum* 1990;33:1122)
    1. age ≥50 y
    2. new headache
    3. temp artery tenderness or ↓ pulsation
    4. ↑ ESR >50 mm/h
    5. biopsy → vasculitis & granulomas
- **Polymyalgia rheumatica** (seen in 50% GCA Pts; 15% of Pts w/ PMR develop GCA)

    no universal or validated diagnostic criteria exist; most follow general guidelines:

    age ≥50 y; ESR >40 mm/h (and/or elevated CRP)

    bilateral aching and morning stiffness (>30 min × ≥1 mo), involving 2 of the following 3 areas: neck or torso, shoulders or prox. arms, hips or prox. thighs

    exclude other causes of sx (eg, RA); CK should be normal
- Treatment: **steroids** (if vision threatened *do not await path results* before starting Rx); 40-60 mg/d for GCA; 10-20 mg/d for PMR; follow clinical status and ESR

MEDIUM-VESSEL VASCULITIS

Polyarteritis nodosa ("classic" PAN) (*JAMA* 2002;288:1632)
- Acute or chronic systemic necrotizing vasculitis, typically of renal and other visceral arteries, *without granuloma formation*
- More common in *men*; average age of onset ~ 50 y; strongly **associated with HBV**
- Clinical manifestations (Cupps and Fauci. *The Vasculitides*. Philadelphia: Saunders, 1981)

    constitutional symptoms: **weight loss**, fevers, fatigue

    musculoskeletal (64%): **myalgias**, arthralgias, arthritis

    renal involvement (60%) with **active urinary sediment, hypertension, renal failure**

nervous system (51%): **peripheral neuropathies**, mononeuritis multiplex, stroke
gastrointestinal (44%): **abdominal pain**, GI bleeding/infarction, cholecystitis
cutaneous lesions (43%): **livedo reticularis**, **purpura**, nodules, Raynaud's
cardiac (36%): coronary arteritis, cardiomyopathy, pericarditis
GU (25%): ovarian or **testicular pain**
- Dx studies
  angiogram (mesenteric vessels) → microaneurysms and focal vessel narrowings
  MRA may not be adequate to make the diagnosis
  biopsy (sural nerve or skin) → vasculitis with fibrinoid necrosis *without granulomas*
  ↑ ESR, ↑ WBC, rare eosinophilia, ⊕ HBsAg (30%), p-ANCA (<20%)
- Classification criteria (3 of 10 criteria is 82% Se & 87% Sp; *Arth Rheum* 1990;33:1088)
    1. weight loss ≥ 4 kg
    2. livedo reticularis
    3. testicular pain/tenderness
    4. myalgias, weakness, leg tenderness
    5. mononeuropathy or polyneuropathy
    6. diastolic BP >90 mmHg
    7. elevated BUN >40 mg/dl or Cr >1.5 mg/dl
    8. Hepatitis B virus
    9. Arteriographic abnormality (aneurysms, occlusion of visceral arteries)
    10. Biopsy → vasculitis of small or medium-sized vessel
- Treatment: **steroids**, cyclophosphamide; antiviral therapy for HBV-related PAN

ANCA-ASSOCIATED SMALL-VESSEL VASCULITIS

Disease	Gran.	Renal	Pulm.	Asthma	ANCA Type*	ANCA ⊕
Wegener's granulomatosis	⊕	80%	90%	–	c-ANCA (anti-PR3)	90%
Microscopic polyangiitis	–	90%	50%	–	p-ANCA (anti-MPO)	70%
Churg-Strauss syndrome	⊕	45%	70%	⊕	p-ANCA (anti-MPO)	50%

*Predominant ANCA type; either p- or c-ANCA can be seen in all three diseases. (*NEJM* 1997;337:1512)

Differential diagnosis of ANCA
- **c-ANCA (anti-PR3)**: Wegener's granulomatosis, Churg-Strauss, microscopic polyangiitis
- **p-ANCA (anti-MPO)**: microscopic polyangiitis, Churg-Strauss, PAN, Wegener's granulomatosis, drug-induced vasculitis, nonvasculitic rheumatic diseases
- **atypical ANCA patterns**: drug-induced vasculitis, nonvasculitic rheumatic diseases, ulcerative colitis, primary sclerosing cholangitis, endocarditis, cystic fibrosis

Wegener's granulomatosis
- Necrotizing granulomatous inflammatory disease with systemic vasculitis, particularly involving the upper and lower respiratory tract, and kidney
- Can occur at any age, but ↑ incidence in young and middle-aged adults
- Clinical manifestations
  pulmonary (90%)
    upper: sinusitis, otitis, rhinitis, nasal mucosal ulceration, saddle-nose deformity
    lower: pleurisy, pulmonary infiltrate, nodules, hemorrhage, hemoptysis
  renal (80%): hematuria, **RPGN** (pauci-immune)
  ocular (50%): episcleritis, uveitis and proptosis from orbital granulomas
  neurologic: cranial and peripheral neuropathies, mononeuritis multiplex
  hematologic: ↑ **incidence DVT/PE** (20x) when disease active (*Annals* 2005;142:620)
- Dx studies: **90% ⊕ ANCA** (80-95% c-ANCA, remainder p-ANCA)
  CXR or CT → nodules, infiltrates, cavities; **sinus CT** → sinusitis
  ↑ BUN & Cr, **proteinuria, hematuria**; sediment w/ **RBC casts, dysmorphic RBCs**
  biopsy → **necrotizing granulomatous inflammation** of arterioles, capillaries, veins
- Classification criteria (2 of 4 criteria is 88% Se & 92% Sp; *Arth Rheum* 1990;33:1101)
    1. nasal or oral inflammation: oral ulcers, purulent or bloody nasal discharge
    2. CXR showing nodules, fixed infiltrates, or cavities
    3. microscopic hematuria or urinary red cell casts
    4. granulomatous inflammation on biopsy

- Treatment (*Annals* 1992;116:488; *NEJM* 2003;349:36)

  cyclophosphamide PO (2 mg/kg/d × 3-6 mos) & **prednisone** (1-2 mg/kg/d taper over 6 mos)

  when prednisone ≤20mg/d, begin **maintenance with MTX or AZA** (× additional 18 mos)

  for mild disease MTX/prednisone may be adequate for induction

  disease relapses: *match aggressive disease with aggressive Rx as needed*

  TMP-SMX may prevent upper airway disease relapse incited by respiratory infections

  consider plasmapheresis for dialysis-dependent renal disease

Microscopic polyangiitis (MPA)

- Necrotizing small-vessel vasculitis → **glomerulonephritis, pulmonary capillary alveolitis,** & dermal leukocytoclastic venulitis. Similar to Wegener's but w/o granulomas.
- *Not* associated with HBV (unlike classic PAN)
- Clinical manifestations

  constitutional symptoms: **weight loss, fevers,** fatigue, myalgias

  renal: hematuria, **RPGN** (pauci-immune)

  pulmonary: cough and/or hemoptysis

  neurologic: mononeuritis multiplex
- Dx studies: **70% ⊕ ANCA** (almost all p-ANCA), **biopsy → necrotizing, pauci-immune inflammation** of arterioles, capillaries, & venules

  w/o granulomas or eosinophilic infiltrates

  urine sediment and CXR findings similar to those seen in Wegener's
- Treatment: as for Wegener's → **cyclophosphamide**; high dose **corticosteroids**; AZA for maintenance; plasmapheresis in some cases

Churg-Strauss syndrome

- Eosinophil-rich granulomatous inflammation involving **lung, peripheral nerves, heart,** kidneys, and skin
- Rare condition that can present at any age, but typically 30-40
- Clinical manifestations

  asthma and allergic rhinitis (new asthma in an adult raises suspicion)

  eosinophilic infiltrative disease or eosinophilic pneumonia

  systemic small-vessel vasculitis with

  neuropathy, coronary arteritis, and myocarditis frequent and severe

  glomerulonephritis and serositis less frequent and less severe
- Dx studies: **50% ⊕ ANCA** (c-ANCA or p-ANCA), **eosinophilia** (80%), biopsy → **microgranulomas,** fibrinoid necrosis and thrombosis of small arteries and veins with **eosinophilic infiltrates**; CXR may show shifting pulmonary infiltrates
- Classification criteria (4 of 6 criteria is 85% Se & 99.7% Sp; *Arth Rheum* 1990;33:1094)

  1. asthma
  2. eosinophilia >10%
  3. mono- or polyneuropathy
  4. migratory or transitory pulm- infiltrates
  5. paranasal sinus abnormality
  6. extravascular eosinophils on biopsy
- Treatment: high-dose **corticosteroids** (+ cyclophosphamide or other DMARDs if nec.)

IMMUNE COMPLEX–ASSOCIATED SMALL-VESSEL VASCULITIS

Henoch-Schönlein purpura (HSP)

- Most common systemic vasculitis in children. Rare in adults (*Semin Arthritis Rheum* 1994;37:187)
- Begins after an upper respiratory tract infection or drug exposure; IgA-mediated
- Clinical manifestations: **palpable purpura** on extensor surfaces & buttocks; non-deforming **polyarthralgias** especially involving hips, knees, and ankles; colicky **abdominal pain** ± GIB or intussusception; nephritis ranging from **microscopic hematuria** and proteinuria to ESRD; many have **fever**
- Diagnostic studies: normal plt count; **skin bx → leukocytoclastic vasculitis with IgA** and C3 deposition in vessel wall; renal bx → mesangial IgA deposition
- Criteria for classification (2 of 4 is 87% Se and 88% Sp; *Arth Rheum* 1990;33:1114)

  1. palpable purpura
  2. age ≤20 y at disease onset
  3. bowel angina
  4. biopsy showing granulocytes in the walls of arterioles or venules
- Treatment: supportive; steroids ± DMARDs for renal or severe disease

Cryoglobulinemic vasculitis: see "Cryoglobulinemia"

Connective tissue disease-associated vasculitis

- Vasculitis associated with **RA**, **SLE**, or **Sjögren's syndrome**
- Clinical manifestations

  distal arteritis: digital ischemia, livedo reticularis, palpable purpura, cutaneous ulceration

  visceral arteritis: pericarditis and mesenteric ischemia

  peripheral neuropathy
- Diagnostic studies: skin and sural nerve biopsies, angiography, EMG
- Treatment: steroids, cyclophosphamide, MTX (other DMARDs)

Cutaneous leukocytoclastic angiitis

- Heterogeneous group of clinical syndromes due to **immune complex deposition** in capillaries, venules, and arterioles; includes *hypersensitivity vasculitis*
- Overall the most common type of vasculitis
- Etiologies

  drugs: penicillin, aspirin, amphetamines, thiazides, chemicals, immunizations

  infections: strep throat, bacterial endocarditis, TB, hepatitis, staphylococcal infections

  tumor antigens

  foreign proteins (serum sickness)
- Clinical manifestations: abrupt onset of **palpable purpura**, **cutaneous ulceration** and **transient arthralgias** after exposure to the offending agent, variably accompanied by fever, arthralgias and other organ involvement; peripheral neuropathy
- Dx studies: ↑ ESR, ↓ **complement levels**, eosinophilia; **skin biopsy →** **leukocytoclastic vasculitis with neutrophils**, nuclear fragments 2° to karyorrhexis, Ig + complement deposition on direct immunofluorescence *w/o IgA present*, perivascular hemorrhage and fibrinoid deposits *w/o cryoglobulin deposition*
- Classification criteria (3 of 5 criteria is 71% Se & 84% Sp; Arth Rheum 1990;33:1108)
  1. age > 16 y
  2. medication taken at disease onset
  3. palpable purpura
  4. maculopapular rash
  5. biopsy showing granulocytes in a perivascular or extravascular location
- Treatment: withdrawal of offending agent ± rapid prednisone taper

Behçet's syndrome

- Multisystem vasculitis that may involve small-, medium- and large-sized vessels, characterized by recurrent oral and genital ulcers with variable manifestations affecting the skin, eye, CNS, and musculoskeletal system
- Associated with HLA B51, highest prevalence on the old Silk Road (Turkey) and other Asian countries
- Classification criteria (#1 + ≥2 others is 91% Se & 96% Sp; Lancet 1990;335:1078)
  1. recurrent **oral aphthous ulceration** (at least 3 times in one year)
  2. recurrent **genital ulceration**
  3. eye lesions: uveitis (with hypopyon), scleritis, retinal vasculitis, optic neuritis
  4. skin lesions: **pustules**, papules, folliculitis, **erythema nodosum**
  5. ⊕ pathergy test (prick forearm with sterile needle → pustule)
- Other clinical manifestations

  arthritis: mild, symmetric, chronic and nondestructive, involving knees and ankles

  neurologic: focal deficits, pleocytosis, inflammatory infiltrates *w/o vasculitis*

  vascular: superficial or deep vein thrombosis (25%); arterial stenosis, occlusion, and aneurysm can also occur
- Evaluation: ulcer bx, cerebral angio (rarely necessary); slit lamp exam and funduscopy
- Treatment (Arth Rheum 1997;40:769)

  azathioprine *early helps prevent ocular disease, ulcerations and improves prognosis*

  mucocutaneous: steroids, colchicine, dapsone, thalidomide (males), etanercept

  ocular: steroids, AZA, IFN-α2a, infliximab, CsA, cyclophosphamide, chlorambucil

  CNS disease: oral/IV steroids, methotrexate, CsA, cyclophosphamide, chlorambucil

  arthritis: steroids, colchicine, IFN-α2a

CRYOGLOBULINEMIA

Definition (Arth Rheum 1999;42:2507)
- **Proteins that precipitate on exposure to the cold,** characterized by their composition
- **Type 1 (monoclonal)**: *monoclonal Ig (usually IgM or IgG)*
- **Type 2 (mixed)**: *monoclonal IgM usu. with RF activity* + *polyclonal IgG*
- **Type 3 (polyclonal)**: *polyclonal immunoglobulins*

Epidemiology
- Female predominance
- Age of onset ~50 y

Etiologies
- **Lymphoproliferative disorders**: multiple myeloma, Waldenström's macroglobulinemia, CLL, B-cell NHL. Usually associated with *Type 1* cryoglobulinemia.
- **HCV infection**: >80% of Pts with *Type 2* cryoglobulinemia are HCV RNA ⊕ (NEJM 1992;327:1490)
- **Autoimmune syndromes**: usually associated with *Type 3* cryoglobulinemia
- Infections: viral (EBV, CMV), bacterial (endocarditis), and parasitic infections
- Essential (idiopathic)
- Renal transplant recipients, w/ or w/o HCV infection

Pathophysiology
- Chronic immune stimulation and/or lymphoproliferation → immune complex (IC) formation
- Defective/insufficient IC clearance → IC deposition with complement activation
- Promotes: *platelet aggregation* → small vessel thromboses, *inflammation* → vasculitis

Clinical manifestations
- General: **weakness**, low-grade fever
- Dermatologic: lower extremity **purpura**, **livedo reticularis**, leg ulcers, Raynaud's phenomenon, leukocytoclastic vasculitis
- Rheumatologic: symmetric, migratory **arthralgias** of small or medium joints
- Renal (50%): **glomerulonephritis** (proteinuria, hematuria, ARF, hypertension, edema)
- Hematologic: anemia, thrombocytopenia
- GI: abdominal pain, hepatosplenomegaly, abnormal LFTs
- Neurologic: peripheral neuropathy and mononeuritis multiplex

Diagnostic studies
- ⊕ **cryocrit** (amount not necessarily associated with disease activity), **cryoglobulin electrophoresis**
- ⊕ rheumatoid factor (RF)
- ↓ **C4 levels,** variable C3 levels, ↑ ESR
- If blood sample not kept at 37° C → cryoprecipitation → loss of RF and ↓↓ complement
- In Type 2 cryoglobulinemia: ⊕ HCV RNA, ⊖ anti-HCV Ab
- Biopsy of affected area (skin, kidney)

Treatment
- Treat underlying disorder:
  chemotherapy and/or radiation for lymphoproliferative disorders
  antiviral therapy and/or rituximab for HCV (Rhem 2006;45:8427)
  DMARDs for rheumatic disease
- NSAIDs for control of mild symptoms
- Prednisone + other immunosuppressants (eg, cyclophosphamide) for major organ involvement
- Plasmapheresis in severe disease

AMYLOIDOSIS

Accumulation of insoluble fibrillar proteins that form β-pleated sheets

Classification of Amyloidosis			
Type	**Precursor**	**Causative diseases**	**Organ systems**
AL ("Primary") Most common	Ig light chain (monoclonal)	MM Light chain disease ($\lambda > \kappa$) MGUS, WM	**Renal, cardiac, GI, neuro, cutaneous,** hepatic, pulmonary, musculoskel, heme
AA ("Secondary")	Serum amyloid (SAA)	Chronic infections: osteo, TB, empyema, leprosy Inflam: RA, IBD, FMF Neoplasms: renal, HD	**Renal, GI, hepatic,** neuro, cutaneous
Hereditary	Transthyretin (TTR), et al.	Mutant proteins	**Neurologic,** cardiac
Senile	TTR, ANP	*Normal* proteins; 2° aging	**Cardiac,** aorta, GI
Aβ₂M	β₂-microglobulin	Dialysis-associated β2m (normally renally excreted)	Musculoskeletal
Organ-specific	β-amyloid protein Peptide hormones et al.	Localized production and processing	Neurologic Endocrine et al.

(Adapted from *NEJM* 1997;337:898 & 2003;349:583)

Clinical Manifestations of Amyloidosis		
System	**Manifestations**	**Amyloid**
Renal	Proteinuria or nephrotic syndrome	AL, AA
Cardiac	Cardiomyopathy (restrictive & dilated) ↓ QRS amplitude, conduction abnormalities, AF Orthostatic hypotension	AL, hereditary, senile, organ-specific
GI	Diarrhea, malabsorption, protein loss Ulceration, hemorrhage, obstruction Macroglossia → dysphonia and dysphagia	all systemic
Neurologic	Peripheral neuropathy with painful paresthesias Autonomic neuro → impotence, dysmotility, ↓ BP Carpal tunnel syndrome	hereditary, AL, organ-specific, Aβ₂m
Cutaneous	Waxy, nonpruritic papules; periorbital ecchymoses "Pinch purpura" = skin bleeds with minimal trauma	AL
Hepatic & Splenic	Hepatomegaly, usually *without* dysfunction Splenomegaly, usually *without* leukopenia or anemia	all systemic
Endocrine	Deposition with rare hormonal insufficiency	organ-specific
Musculoskel	Arthralgias and arthritis	AL, Aβ₂m
Pulmonary	Airway obstruction	AL, AA
Hematologic	Factor X deficiency	AL

Diagnostic studies
- Abdominal SC fat pad or rectal biopsy → apple-green birefringence on Congo red stain
- If suspect AL → ✓ SPEP, SIEP, UPEP, ± BM bx
- If suspect renal involvement: ✓ U/A (proteinuria)
- If suspect cardiac involvement: ✓ ECG (↓ voltage, conduction abnormalities) & echocardiogram (biventricular thickening with "*granular sparkling*" appearance)
- Genetic testing for hereditary forms

Treatment
- AL: melphalan + prednisone (*NEJM* 1997;336:1202), ? iododoxorubicin, ? stem cell transplant
- AA: treatment of underlying disease
  Familial Mediterranean Fever: colchicine (*NEJM* 1986;314:1001)
- For hereditary amyloidoses in which amyloid precursor protein is produced by the liver (eg, TTR), liver transplantation may prevent further deposition
- Heart, kidney, and liver transplantation may be considered in those with advanced disease

Prognosis
- AL amyloid: median survival ~12-18 mos; if cardiac involvement, median survival ~6 mos

CHANGE IN MENTAL STATUS

Definitions (nb, description of state better than imprecise use of terms)
- **Confusion** (encephalopathy): unable to maintain coherent thought process
- **Delirium**: waxing & waning confusional state w/ additional sympathetic signs
- **Drowsiness**: ↓ level of consciousness, but rapid arousal to verbal or noxious stimuli
- **Stupor**: impaired arousal to noxious stimuli, but some preserved purposeful movements
- **Coma**: sleep-like state of unresponsiveness, with no purposeful response to stimuli

Etiologies	
Primary Neurologic	**Systemic** (especially in elderly)
Stroke	Cardiac: severe CHF, HTN encephalopathy
Seizure (postictal, status, nonconvulsive)	Pulmonary: ↓ P_aO_2, ↑ P_aCO_2
Infection: meningoencephalitis, abscess	GI: liver failure, constipation, Wilson's
Epidural/subdural hematoma	Renal: uremia, hypo- and hypernatremia
Concussion	Endocrine: ↓ glc, DKA, HHNS, ↑ Ca, hypo-
Hydrocephalus	or hyperthyroidism, Addisonian crisis
Complicated migraine	ID: pneumonia, UTI, sepsis
Venous thrombosis	Hypo- and hyperthermia
Cholesterol or fat emboli	Medications (espec. opiates & sedatives)
CNS vasculitis	Alcohol & toxins
TTP	

Initial evaluation
- **History** (typically from others): previous or recent illnesses, including underlying dementia or psychiatric disorders; head trauma; meds, drug or alcohol use
- **General physical examination** including signs of trauma, stigmata of liver disease, embolic phenomena, signs of drug use, nuchal rigidity (may be present in meningitis or subarachnoid hemorrhage, but *do not test* if question of trauma/cervical spine fracture)
- **Neurologic examination**
  Observation for spontaneous movements, response to stimuli, papilledema
  Cranial nerves: eye position at rest, response to visual threat, corneal reflex, facial grimace to nasal tickle, cough/gag (with ET tube manipulation if necessary)
  Pupil size & reactivity: pinpoint → opiates; midposition & fixed → midbrain lesion; fix & dilated → severe anoxic encephalopathy, herniation
  Intact oculocephalic ("doll's eyes," eyes move opposite head movement) or oculovestibular ("cold calorics," eyes move toward lavaged ear) imply brainstem intact
  Look for signs of ↑ ICP: H/A, vomiting, HTN, ↓ HR, papilledema, unilateral dilated pupil
  Motor response in the extremities to noxious stimuli – noting purposeful vs. posturing
  Deep tendon reflexes, Babinski response

Glasgow Coma Scale			
Eye opening	**Best verbal response**	**Best motor response**	**Points**
		Follows commands	6
	Oriented	Localizes pain	5
Spontaneous	Confused	Withdraws from pain	4
To voice	Inappropriate words	Flexor response	3
To painful stimuli	Unintelligible sounds	Extensor response	2
None	None	None	1
Sum points from each of the 3 categories to calculate the score			

Initial treatment
- Control airway, monitor vital signs, IV access
- Immobilization of C-spine if concern for cervical trauma
- Thiamine (100 mg IV) *prior to dextrose* to prevent exacerb. of Wernicke encephalopathy
- Dextrose (50 g IV push)
- Naloxone 0.01 mg/kg if opiates suspected; flumazenil 0.2 mg IV if benzos suspected
- If concern for ↑ ICP and herniation: ↑ head of bed; osmotherapy with mannitol; hyperventilation; dexamethasone; consider emergent surgical decompression

Diagnostic studies
- Head CT; radiographs to r/o C-spine fracture; CXR to r/o PNA (in elderly)
- Laboratory: electrolytes, BUN, Cr, ABG, LFTs, CBC, PT, PTT, tox screen, TSH, U/A
- Lumbar puncture to r/o meningitis
- EEG to r/o nonconvulsive seizures

ANOXIC BRAIN INJURY

Prevalence
- Pts w/ at least 5 min of cerebral hypoxia at risk
- 1.5 million cardiac arrests per yr in U.S.; 30% survive, but only 10-20% return to independence

Initial evaluation
- Neuro exam: focus on coma exam → cranial nerves, motor response to pain
- Imaging: usually not informative w/in first day after arrest, but should be done prior to initiating hypothermia if patient found down or witnessed to hit head

Induced hypothermia *(NEJM 2002;346:549, 559)*
- Indications: comatose w/in 6 h following cardiac arrest (not isolated resp. arrest). Only fully studied in VT/VF, but acceptable to perform after asystole or PEA arrest.
- Contraindications: active bleeding, including cerebral; known sepsis; recent surgery or trauma (relative); CV instability; clear improvement in neurological exam (purposeful movements, vocalizations)
- Method: target temperature 32-34°C × 24 h (from time of initiation of cooling)
  cold saline infusions; ice packs to the head, neck and torso; cooling blankets
  may use cooling vest or endovascular catheter if available
- Complications
  cardiac dysrhythmias (bradycardia most common): if significant dysrhythmia or
    hemodynamic instability, d/c cooling and *actively* rewarm patient (this is only
    circumstance in which active rewarming should be performed; o/w rewarm at no
    faster than 0.5°C per h)
  coagulopathy: Pts can receive fibrinolytics, GP IIb/IIIa inhibitors, etc. and still undergo
    cooling. ✓ PT and PTT.
  infection: ✓ surveillance blood cultures during cooling
  hyperglycemia
  hypokalemia during cooling, hyperkalemia w/ rewarming; keep K 4-5 mEq/L

Ongoing evaluation
- Neuro exam: daily focus on coma exam, cranial nerves, GCS score. Pt needs to be off sedation for adequate time to evaluate (depends on doses used, duration of Rx, metabolic processes in the individual Pt)
- Imaging: noncontrast CT 24 h after arrest, if unrevealing, MRI around day 3-5
- EEG: should be performed in any Pt w/ seizures or myoclonus (to r/o status epilepticus); should be considered in all unresponsive Pts (to r/o nonconvulsive seizures)
- Somatosensory evoked potentials (SSEP): helpful for prediction of poor outcome if absent cortical responses bilaterally; should not be performed earlier than 48 h after arrest (72 h if cooled)

Prognosis
- Uniformly poor prognosis can be predicted at 72 h only in Pts who have absent pupillary and corneal reflexes, and no motor response to pain; also with absent SSEPs at 48 h
- Otherwise, requires multifactorial approach, considering neuro exam, age and comorbid diseases, and ancillary data (neuroimaging, EEG, SSEP)
- When in doubt, err on the side of giving more time (especially in younger Pts)

SEIZURES

Definitions (*NEJM* 2003;349:1257)
- **Seizure** = abnormal, paroxysmal, excessive discharge of CNS neurons; occurs in 5-10% of the population; clinical manifestations can range from dramatic to subtle
- **Epilepsy** = recurrent seizures due to an underlying cause; 0.5-1.0% of population
- **Generalized seizures** (involves brain diffusely)
  Tonic-clonic (grand mal): tonic phase (10-20 sec) with contraction of muscles (causing expiratory moan, cyanosis, pooling of secretions, tongue biting) → clonic phase (~30 sec) with intermittent relaxing and tensing of muscles
  Absence (petit mal): transient lapse of consciousness w/o loss of postural tone
  Myoclonic (infantile spasms & juvenile myoclonic epilepsy): sudden, brief contraction
- **Partial or focal seizures** (involves discrete areas, implies a focal, structural lesion)
  Simple: without impairment of consciousness; may be motor, sensory, or autonomic
  Complex: with impairment of consciousness ± automatisms or psychogenic features
  Partial with secondary generalization: starts focal, becomes diffuse

Ddx
- **Syncope:** lacks true aura (although Pt may describe feeling unwell w/ diaphoresis, nausea, and tunneling of vision), motor manifestations <30 sec (convulsive activity for <10 sec may occur with transient cerebral hypoperfusion), and w/o postictal disorientation, muscle soreness, or sleepiness; skin pallor & clamminess support syncope
- **Psychogenic seizure:** may see side-to-side head turning, asymmetric large amplitude limb movements, diffuse twitching w/o LOC, and crying/talking during event
- **Other:** metabolic disorders (eg, alcoholic blackouts, hypoglycemia); migraines; TIAs; narcolepsy; nonepileptic myoclonus

Etiologies
- **A**lcohol withdrawal, illicit drugs, meds (eg, β-lactams, meperidine, CsA, antidep., clozapine)
- **B**rain tumor or penetrating trauma
- **C**erebrovascular disease, including subdural hematomas, hypertensive encephalopathy
- **D**egenerative disorders of the CNS (eg, Alzheimer's)
- **E**lectrolyte (hyponatremia) & other metabolic (eg, uremia, liver failure, hypoglycemia)

Clinical manifestations
- **Aura** (sec to mins): premonition consisting of abnormal smells/tastes, unusual behavior, oral or appendicular automatisms
- **Ictal period** (sec to mins): tonic and/or clonic movements of head, eyes, trunk or extrem.
- **Postictal period** (mins to h): slowly resolving period of confusion, disorientation, and lethargy. May be accompanied by focal neurological deficits ("Todd's paralysis").
- **Status epilepticus**: continuous tonic-clonic seizure ≥30 mins, or repeated seizures such that there is no resolution of postictal periods. Complications include neuronal death, rhabdomyolysis, and lactic acidosis.
- **Nonconvulsive status epilepticus** alteration of awareness (ranging from confusion to coma) w/o motor manifestations. Dx with EEG.

Clinical evaluation
- Seizure: patient usually w/o recollection, must talk to witnesses
  unusual behavior before seizure (ie, an aura)
  type & pattern of abnl movements, incl. head turning & eye deviation (gaze preference *away* from seizure focus)
  loss of responsiveness
- HPI: recent illnesses/fevers, head trauma
- PMH: prior seizures or ⊕ FHx, prior meningitis/encephalitis, prior stroke or head trauma
- Medications, alcohol, and illicit drug use
- General physical exam should include the skin, looking for neuroectodermal disorders (eg, neurofibromatosis, tuberous sclerosis) that are associated with seizures
- Neurological exam should look for focal abnormalities → underlying structural abnormality

Diagnostic studies
- Laboratory: full electrolytes, BUN, Cr, glc, LFTs, tox screen, medication levels
- EEG
  frequent seizures: can confirm by demonstrating repetitive rhythmic activity (nb, generalized seizures will always have abnormal EEG; partial seizures may not)
  infrequent seizures: may show interictal epileptiform activity (eg, spikes or sharp waves), but such patterns seen in up to 2% of normal population
  sleep deprivation ↑ dx yield of EEG; video monitoring may help w/ psychogenic seizures

- MRI to r/o structural abnormalities; ↑ Se w/ fine coronal cuts of frontal & temporal lobes
- Lumbar puncture (after ruling out space-occupying lesion): if suspect meningitis or encephalitis and in *all* HIV ⊕ patients

Treatment *(NEJM 2001;344:1145; Lancet 2006;367:1087 & 2007;369:1000, 1016)*
- Treat any underlying causes, including CNS infections, intoxication or withdrawal, etc.
- Antiepileptic drug (AED) therapy is usually reserved for Pts w/ underlying structural abnormality or an idiopathic seizure *plus* (1) status epilepticus on presentation, (2) focal neurologic exam, (3) postictal Todd's paralysis, or (4) abnormal EEG
- For Pts w/ infrequent seizures, early (vs. delayed) intervention w/ AED ↑ time to seizure recurrence, but has no effect on long-term seizure-free status *(Lancet 2005;365:2007)*
- Generalized tonic-clonic: valproic acid, phenytoin, topiramate, lamotrigine
- Partial (w/ or w/o 2° generalization): carbamazepine, oxcarbazepine, lamotrigine, phenytoin, valproic acid
- Absence: ethosuximide, valproic acid
- Secondary agents: leviteracitam, gabapentin, clonazepam, phenobarbital
- Introduce gradually, monitor carefully
- May consider withdrawal if seizure-free (typically for at least 1 y) and normal EEG
- Individual state laws mandate seizure-free duration before being allowed to drive

Antiepileptic Drugs and Side Effects			
Medication	**Avg daily dose**	**Side effects**	
		Neurologic	Systemic
Phenytoin	300-400 mg		Gum hyperplasia, ↓ Ca, ↑ K
Carbamazepine	600-1800 mg	Dizziness Ataxia Diplopia Confusion Drowsiness	Aplastic anemia Leukopenia Hepatotoxicity Hyponatremia
Valproic acid	750-2000 mg		Hepatotoxicity, ↑ NH₃ Thrombocytopenia
Phenobarbital	60-180 mg		Rash
Ethosuximide	750-1250 mg		Rash Bone marrow suppression
Gabapentin	900-2400 mg		GI upset
Leviteracitam	1500-3000 mg	Drowsiness Emotional lability	GI upset (rare)

(JAMA 2004;291:605, 615)

Status epilepticus (consult neurology)
- Place Pt in semiprone position to ↓ risk of aspiration
- Oral airway or, if prolonged, endotracheal intubation
- IV access, start normal saline infusion
- STAT labs including glc, Na, Ca, serum & urine toxicology screen, anticonvulsant levels
- Thiamine (100 mg IV) *prior to dextrose* to prevent exacerb. of Wernicke's encephalopathy
- Dextrose (50 g IV push)
- Na or Ca repletion as needed

Treatment of Status Epilepticus			
(proceed to next step if seizures continue)			
Step	Antiepileptic	Dosing regimen	Typical adult dose
1	**Lorazepam** or **Diazepam**	0.1 mg/kg at 2 mg/min 0.2 mg/kg at 5 mg/min	Successive 2-4 mg IV pushes Successive 5-10 mg IV pushes
	Lorazepam marginally slower onset of action (3 vs. 2 min) but at least as efficacious (success 65%) & longer duration of effect (12-24 h vs. 15-30 min)		
2	**Phenytoin** or **Fosphenytoin**	20 mg/kg at 50 mg/min 20 mg PE/kg at 150 mg/min + 5-10 mg/kg if still seizing	1.0-1.5 g IV over 20 min 1.0-1.5 g PE IV over 5-10 min + 500 mg IV if still seizing
	Subsequent steps typically mandate intubation, EEG monitoring, and ICU admission		
3	Phenobarbital	20 mg/kg at 50-75 mg/min + 5-10 mg/kg if still seizing	1.0-1.5 g IV over 30 min + 500 mg IV if still seizing
4	General anesthesia with midazolam, pentobarbital, or propofol		

(JAMA 1983;249:1452; NEJM 1998:338:970 & 339:792)

ISCHEMIC (~70%)

Etiologies
- Embolic (~ 75%): artery → artery, cardioembolic, paradoxical, or cryptogenic
- Thrombotic (~ 25%): lacunar (arteriolar, seen in HTN & DM) or large vessel
- Other: dissection, vasculitis, vasospasm, hyperviscosity, watershed

Clinical Manifestations	
Embolic: rapid onset, sx maximum at onset	
Thrombotic: progression of sx over h to days with stuttering course	
Artery	**Deficits**
ICA/Ophth	Amaurosis fugax (transient monocular blindness)
ACA	Hemiplegia (leg > arm) Confusion, abulia, urinary incontinence, primitive reflexes
MCA	Hemiplegia (arm & face > leg); hemianesthesia; homonymous hemianopia Aphasia if dom. hemisphere: sup. div. → expressive; inf. → receptive Apraxia and neglect if nondominant hemisphere Drowsiness & stupor seen later (due to brain swelling)
PCA	Thalamic syndromes with contralateral hemisensory disturbance, aphasia Macular-sparing homonymous hemianopia
Vertebral	Wallenberg's syndrome = numbness of ipsilateral face and contralateral limbs, diplopia, dysarthria, ipsilateral Horner's
Basilar	Pinpoint pupils, long tract signs (quadriplegia and sensory loss), cranial nerve abnormalities, cerebellar dysfunction
Cerebellar	Vertigo, nausea/vomiting, diplopia, nystagmus, ipsilateral limb ataxia
Lacunar	Pure hemiplegia, pure hemianesthesia, ataxic hemiparesis, or dysarthria + clumsy hand

Transient ischemia attacks (TIAs) are sudden neurologic deficits caused by cerebral ischemia that resolve w/in 24 h (usually w/in 1 h) and are a harbinger of stroke. Ddx: seizure, migraine, syncope, anxiety.

Physical examination
- General including rhythm, murmurs, carotid & subclavian bruits, signs of peripheral emboli
- Neurologic including NIH stroke scale (NIHSS)

Diagnostic studies
- Laboratory: electrolytes, Cr, glc, CBC, PT, PTT, LFTs, tox screen; hypercoagulable w/u (consider in young Pts; send once stable & ideally before anticoag)
- ECG
- **Urgent CT** is usually the initial imaging study because of its rapidity and availability
  first, noncontrast CT to r/o hemorrhage (Se for ischemic Δs is <20% w/in 12 h)
  then, CT angio to evaluate cerebrovascular anatomy & patency
  consider CT perfusion for areas of reversible ischemia
- MRI offers superior imaging but may not identify acute hemorrhage (although recent data suggests may be equivalent; *JAMA 2004;292:1823*) and may be falsely ⊖ for small brainstem strokes w/in 1st 3 h; should be avoided if Pt is unstable or will delay therapy
- Carotid Doppler U/S, transcranial Doppler (TCD)
- Holter monitoring to assess for paroxysmal AF
- Echocardiography w/ bubble study to r/o PFO or atrial septal aneurysm (confer ~4× ↑ risk of stroke; *NEJM 2001;345:1740*), cardiac thrombus, valvular vegetations

Treatment of TIA (*NEJM 2002;347:1687*)
- **Heparin IV → warfarin** for known or presumptive cardioembolic TIAs; use as bridge to mechanical intervention (CEA, stenting) for large vessel atherothrombotic disease
- **Antiplatelet therapy** with ASA, clopidogrel, or ASA + dipyridamole
- Carotid revascularization if sx >70% ipsilateral stenosis (see below)

Risk of progression of TIA to stroke (*Lancet 2007;369:283*)
- **$ABCD^2$:** Age ≥60 y (+1); BP ≥140/90 (+1); Clinical features: unilateral weakness (+2), speech impairment w/o weakness (+1); Duration ≥60 min (+2) or 10-59 min (+1); Diabetes (+1)
- Risk of stroke at 2 d: low risk (0-3) = 1.0%; moderate (4-5) = 4.1%; high (6-7) = 8.1%

Treatment of ischemic stroke (Lancet 2003;362:1211)

- **Thrombolysis (IV)**: 0.9 mg/kg (max 90 mg), w/ 10% as bolus over 1 min, rest over 1 h
  consider if onset w/in 3 h, large deficit, ∅ hemorrhage, and ∅ contraindication to lysis
  12% absolute ↑ in excellent functional outcome, 5.8% absolute ↑ ICH, 4% absolute ↓
  mortality (p = NS) (NINDS rt-PA Stroke Study, NEJM 1995;333:1381)
- Intra-arterial therapy with thrombolysis (PROACT II, JAMA 1999;282:2003) or catheter-based
  techniques promising (66% rate of recanalization) but still experimental
  currently reserved for occlusion of a major vessel (ICA, MCA, basilar)
- Anticoagulation with UFH of no proven benefit with ↑ risk of hemorrhagic transformation
  consider infusion w/o bolus if Pt not thrombolysed and having progressive sx
  long-term warfarin if embolic stroke; no role in nonembolic stroke (NEJM 2001;345:1444)
- **Antiplatelet therapy**
  ASA ↓ death & recurrent stroke (Stroke 2000;31:1240) and is superior to warfarin alone (NEJM 2005;352:1305)
  dipyridamole + ASA superior to ASA alone (J Neurol Sci 1996;143:1; Lancet 2006;367:1665)
  clopidogrel + ASA not more effective than ASA alone and ↑ bleeding (Lancet 2004;364:331)
- BP should *not* be lowered unless severe (SBP >200) or evidence of MI or CHF
  if considering thrombolysis, then lower to <180/110 with nitrates or labetalol
- DVT prophylaxis: enoxaprin 40 mg SC qd more efficacious than UFH 5000 U SC q12h
  (Lancet 2007;369:1347)
- Cerebral edema peaks at 3-4 d poststroke → ↑ ICP requiring
  elevated head of bed >30°
  intubation and hyperventilation to P_aCO_2 ~30 (transient benefit)
  osmotherapy with mannitol IV 1 gm/kg → 0.25 g/kg q6h; ± hypertonic saline
  surgical decompression
- Statin → ↓ in recurrent stroke & ↓ MACE (HPS, Lancet 2002;360:7; SPARCL, NEJM 2006;355:549)

Carotid revascularization

- Carotid endarterectomy (*if* institutional morbidity & mortality ≤6%) indicated for:
  symptomatic stenosis ≥70% (? 50-69% if male, age ≥75 y, or recent sx) → 65% ↓
  stroke (NASCET, NEJM 1991;325:445; Lancet 2004;363:915)
  asx stenosis ≥70% & <75 y → ~50% ↓ stroke (ACST, Lancet 2004;363:1491)
- Superiority and even noninferiority of carotid *stenting* remains controversial (NEJM 2004;351:1493; Lancet 2006;368:1239; NEJM 2006;355:1660)

HEMORRHAGIC (~30%)

Etiologies

- Intracerebral (ICH, ~90%): HTN, AVM, amyloid angiopathy, anticoagulation/thrombolysis, venous thrombosis
- Subarachnoid (SAH, ~10%; Lancet 2007;369:306): ruptured aneurysm, trauma

Clinical manifestations

- ICH: sudden impairment in level of consciousness
  vomiting ± headache
  may cause progressive focal neurologic deficit depending on site of hemorrhage
- SAH: severe headache, nausea, & vomiting
  nuchal rigidity and other signs of meningeal irritation
  impairment in level of consciousness

Diagnostic studies

- CT or ? MRI (JAMA 2004;292:1823)
- Angiography (CT or conventional) to determine the source of bleeding (aneurysm, AVM)
- LP to ✓ for xanthochromia if no evidence of hemorrhage on CT and suspicious for SAH

Treatment

- Reverse any coagulopathies
- Recombinant activated Factor VII is currently investigational, but may ↓ hematoma
  expansion and mortality at the expense of ↑ risk of adverse thromboembolic events
  (NEJM 2005;352:777)
- Strict BP control w/ goal SBP <140, unless risk for hypoperfusion b/c critical carotid sten.
- ICH: surgical decompression for large hemorrhage with clinical deterioration
- SAH: nimodipine to ↓ risk of vasospasm, phenytoin for seizure prophylaxis, endovascular
  (Lancet 2005;366:783) or surgical correction of aneurysm/AVM to prevent rebleeding
- Cerebral venous thrombosis: paradoxically, requires anticoagulation with IV heparin

Feature	Upper Motor Neuron	Lower Motor Neuron	Myopathy
Distribution of weakness	Regional	Distal, segmental	Proximal
Atrophy	None	Severe	Mild
Fasciculations	None	Common	None
Tone	↑	↓	Normal or ↓
DTRs	+ + + +	0 / +	+ / + +
Babinski	Present	Absent	Absent

PERIPHERAL NEUROPATHIES

Etiologies
- **Mononeuropathy** (one nerve): entrapment, compression, trauma, DM, Lyme
- **Mononeuropathy multiplex** (multiple, noncontiguous, separate nerves)
  Axonal: vasculitis, sarcoidosis, diabetes, hereditary neuropathy with pressure palsies
- **Polyneuropathy** (multiple symmetric nerves)
  Demyelinating
    acute: acute inflammatory demyelinating polyneuropathy (AIDP) = Guillain-Barré
    subacute: CIDP, meds (taxol)
    chronic: diabetes, hypothyroidism, toxins, paraneoplastic, paraproteinemia, hereditary
  Axonal
    acute: porphyria, vasculitis
    subacute: meds (cisplatin, taxol, vincristine, INH, ddI), alcohol, B_{12} defic., sepsis
    chronic: diabetes, uremia, lead, arsenic, Lyme, HIV, paraneoplastic, paraproteinemia

Clinical manifestations
- Motor and/or sensory dysfunction with weakness and/or dysesthesias
- Depressed or absent DTRs

Diagnostic studies
- Electrolytes, BUN, Cr, Glc, HbA_{1C}, CBC, TSH, LFTs, ANA, ESR, SPEP
- HIV, Lyme titers, heavy metal screening as indicated by clinical history
- EMG, NCS, nerve biopsy; MRI if possible radiculopathy or plexopathy

GUILLAIN-BARRÉ SYNDROME (GBS)

Definition and epidemiology
- Acute inflammatory demyelinating polyneuropathy (AIDP)
- Incidence 1-2 per 100,000
- Precipitants: viral illness (EBV, CMV, HSV, HIV), URI (*Mycoplasma*), gastroenteritis (*Campylobacter*), surgery, older immunizations

Clinical manifestations
- Ascending paralysis over hours to days
- *Hypoactive or absent reflexes*
- Sensory dysesthesias are often first symptoms, back pain is also common
- Respiratory compromise requiring ventilatory assistance occurs in 30%; autonomic instability and arrhythmias occur in 50%

Diagnostic studies
- Lumbar puncture: albuminocytologic dissociation = ↑ protein w/o pleocytosis (<20 lymphs)
- EMG & NCS: ↓ nerve conduction velocity and conduction block
- FVC & NIF: to assess for risk of respiratory failure

Treatment
- Plasma exchange (*Neurology* 1985;35:1096) or IVIg (*NEJM* 1992;326:1123)
  no additional benefit with both (*Lancet* 1997;349:225)
- Supportive care with monitoring in ICU setting if rapid progression or resp. failure
- Watch for autonomic dysfunction: labile BP, dysrhythmias (telemetry)

MYASTHENIA GRAVIS

Definition and epidemiology
- Autoimmune disorder with Ab directed against acetylcholine receptor (AChR) in NMJ
- Prevalence 1 in 7500
- Occurs at all ages; peak for women in 20s-30s; peak for men in 60s-70s

Clinical manifestations
- Weakness and *fatigability* with weakness worse with repetitive use, relieved by rest
- Cranial muscles involved early → ocular (ptosis, diplopia) in 50%; bulbar (difficulty chewing, dysarthria, dysphagia) in 15%
- Limb weakness proximal > distal; DTRs preserved
- Exacerbations triggered by stressors such as URI, surgery, pregnancy, meds (eg, aminoglycosides, procainamide, phenytoin); prednisone can *worsen* acutely
- Myasthenic crisis = exacerbation → need for respiratory assistance
- Cholinergic crisis = weakness due to *overtreatment* with anticholinesterase medications; may have excessive salivation, abdominal cramping and diarrhea; rare at normal doses

Diagnostic studies, etc.
- Bedside tests: timing of sustained upgaze, forced mouth closure on tongue blade, etc.
- Edrophonium (Tensilon) test: temporary ↑ strength; false ⊕ & ⊖ occur; atropine at bedside
- EMG: ↓ response with repetitive nerve stimulation (vs. ↑ response in Lambert-Eaton)
- Anti-AChR Ab: Se 80%, 50% if ocular disease only; Sp >90%; muscle specific receptor tyrosine Kinase (MuSK) may account for some AchR Ab-negative cases
- CT or MRI of thorax to evaluate thymus (65% hyperplasia, 10% thymoma)

Treatment
- Anticholinesterase medications (eg, pyridostigmine)
- Thymectomy: mandatory if thymoma; also leads to improvement in 85% Pts w/o thymoma
- Immunosuppression: prednisone, azathioprine, cyclophosphamide
- Myasthenic crisis: treat precipitant
  consider d/c anticholinesterase if suspect cholinergic crisis
  aggressive immunosuppression with glucocorticoids (but watch for initial worsening)
  IVIg, plasmapheresis
  ICU if rapid or severe (follow FVC, NIF)

MYOPATHIES (ALSO SEE RHEUMATOLOGY)

Etiologies
- Hereditary: Duchenne, Becker, limb-girdle, myotonic
- Endocrine: hypothyroidism, hyperparathyroidism, Cushing syndrome
- Toxic: statins, fibrates, glucocorticoids, zidovudine, alcohol, cocaine, antimalarials, colchicine
- Polymyositis and dermatomyositis

Clinical manifestations
- Progressive weakness, proximal > distal
- ± Myalgias
- Eventual muscle atrophy

Diagnostic studies
- CK (↑ in inflammatory myopathies)
- EMG/NCS
- Muscle biopsy

Primary headache syndromes
- Tension: associated with muscle contraction in neck or lower head
- Migraine: *see below*
- Cluster: periodic, paroxysmal, brief, sharp, orbital headache that may awaken from sleep
  ± lacrimation, rhinorrhea, conjunctival injection, or unilateral Horner's syndrome

Secondary causes of headaches
- Vascular: stroke, intracerebral hemorrhage, SAH, subdural hematoma
  AVM, unruptured aneurysm, arterial hypertension, venous thrombosis
- Infection: meningitis, encephalitis, abscess
- Brain tumor
- CSF disorder: ↑ (hydrocephalus) or ↓ (s/p LP)
- Trigeminal neuralgia
- Extracranial: sinusitis, TMJ syndrome, temporal arteritis

Clinical evaluation (*JAMA* 2006;296:1274)
- History: quality, severity, location, duration, time of onset, precipitants/relieving factors
- Associated symptoms (visual Δs, nausea, vomiting, photophobia)
- Focal neurologic symptoms
- Head or neck trauma, constitutional symptoms
- Medications, substance abuse
- General and neurologic examination
- *Warning signs that should prompt neuroimaging:*
  worst ever, worsening over days, wakes from sleep
  vomiting, aggravated by exertion or Valsalva
  fever, abnl neurologic exam, aura, cluster-type headache

MIGRAINE

Epidemiology
- Affects 15% of women and 6% of men; onset usually by 30 y

Clinical manifestations (*Lancet* 2004;363:381; *JAMA* 2006;296:1274)
- Unilateral or bilateral, retro-orbital, throbbing or pulsatile headache; lasts 4-72 h
- Often accompanied by nausea, vomiting, photophobia
- "POUNDing": <u>P</u>ulsatile; duration 4-72 h<u>O</u>urs; <u>U</u>nilateral; <u>N</u>ausea & vomiting; <u>D</u>isabling
  LR 3.5 if 3 criteria are met, LR 24 if ≥4 criteria are met
- Classic (18%) = visual aura (scotomata with jagged or colored edge) precede
  headache
- Common (64%) = headache without aura
- Complicated = accompanied by stereotypical neurologic deficit that may last hrs
- Precipitants: stress, hunger, foods (cheese, chocolate) and food additives (MSG), fatigue,
  alcohol, menstruation, exercise

Treatment (*NEJM* 2002;346:257)
- Eliminate precipitants
- Prophylaxis: TCA, βB, CCB, valproic acid, topiramate (*JAMA* 2004;291:965)
- Abortive therapy
  ASA, acetaminophen, caffeine, high-dose NSAIDs
  metoclopramide IV, prochlorperazine IM or IV
  5-HT$_1$ agonists ("triptans"); contraindic. in Pts w/ complicated migraine, CAD, prior stroke
  combination of triptan + NSAID more efficacious than either single agent alone (*JAMA* 2007;297:1443)
  ergotamine, dihydroergotamine; use with caution in Pts with CAD

BACK AND SPINAL CORD DISEASE

Ddx of back pain
- **Musculoskeletal**
  strain (experienced by up to 80% of the population at some time)
  osteoarthritis, vertebral compression fracture, ankylosing spondylitis
- **Disk herniation syndromes** (see below)
- **Metastatic**: lung, breast, prostate, multiple myeloma, lymphoma
- **Infectious**: vertebral osteomyelitis or epidural abscess (see ID section)
- **Visceral disease with referred pain**
  PUD, cholelithiasis
  pancreatitis, pancreatic cancer
  pyelonephritis, nephrolithiasis
  uterine or ovarian cancer, salpingitis
  leaking aortic aneurysm

Initial evaluation
- **History**: location, radiation, neurologic symptoms, infection, malignancy
- **General physical examination**: local tenderness, ROM, signs of infection or malignancy,
  Spurling sign (cervical radicular pain w/ neck extension & lateral rotation *toward*
  affected side)
  Straight leg raise (⊕ = radicular pain at <60°),
  ipsilateral: 95% Se, 40% Sp; crossed (contralateral): 25% Se, 90% Sp
- **Neurologic examination**: full motor (including sphincter tone), sensory (including
  perineal region), and reflexes including anal (S4) and cremasteric (L2)
- **Laboratory** (depending on suspicions): CBC, ESR, Ca, PO4, Aφ
- **Neuroimaging** (depending on suspicions): x-rays, CT or CT myelography, MRI, bone scan
- EMG/NCS may be useful to distinguish root/plexopathies from peripheral neuropathies

DISC HERNIATION SYNDROMES

Clinical manifestations
- Back pain aggravated by activity (esp. bending, straining, and coughing), relieved by
  resting on unaffected side with affected leg in flexed posture
- "Sciatica" = aching pain that radiates from the buttocks down the lateral aspect of the leg,
  often to the knee or lateral calf ± numbness and paresthesias radiating to lateral foot

Cervical and Lumbar Disk Herniation Patterns				
Disc	Root	Pain / Paresthesias	Sensory loss	Motor loss	Reflex loss
C4-C5	C5	Neck, shoulder upper arm	Shoulder	Deltoid, biceps, infraspinatus	Biceps
C5-C6	C6	Neck, shoulder, lat. arm, radial forearm, thumb & index finger	Lat. arm, radial forearm, thumb & index finger	Biceps, brachioradialis	Biceps, brachio-radialis, supinator
C6-C7	C7	Neck, lat. arm, ring & index fingers	Radial forearm, index & middle fingers	Triceps, extensor carpi ulnaris	Triceps, supinator
C7-T1	C8	Ulnar forearm and hand	Ulnar half of ring finger, little finger	Intrinsic hand muscles, wrist extensors, flexor dig profundus	Finger flexion
L3-L4	L4	Anterior thigh, inner shin	Anteromedial thigh and shin, inner foot	Quadriceps	Patella
L4-L5	L5	Lat. thigh and calf, dorsum of foot, great toe	Lat. calf and great toe	Extensor hallucis longus, ± foot dorsiflexion, invers. & evers.	None
L5-S1	S1	Back of thigh, lateral posterior calf, lat. foot	Posterolat. calf, lat. and sole of foot, smaller toes	Gastrocnemius ± foot eversion	Achilles

(Nb, lumbar disk protrusion tends to compress the root corresponding to the level of the vertebra below it.)

Treatment
- Conservative: avoid bending/lifting; NSAIDs
- Spinal epidural steroid injections: radicular pain refractory to medical management
- Surgery: cord compression or cauda equina syndrome (see below); progressive loss of motor function; bowel or bladder dysfunction; failure to respond to conservative therapy
  (*NEJM* 2007;356:2245)

CORD COMPRESSION

Clinical manifestations
- Flaccid paraparesis and absent reflexes if acute
- Spastic paraparesis and hyperactive reflexes if subacute to chronic
- Posterior column dysfunction in legs (loss of vibratory sense or proprioception)
- Bilateral Babinski responses
- *Conus medullaris syndrome*: symmetric saddle anesthesia, bladder & bowel dysfunction (urinary retention, ↓ anal tone), absent bulbocavernosus and anal reflexes
- *Cauda equina syndrome*: severe back pain, leg weakness and/or sensory loss, ± ↓ reflexes in lower extremities, relative sparing of bowel & bladder function (but occurs)

Evaluation and treatment
- STAT MRI and neurology consultation
- Empiric dexamethasone 10 mg IV or methylprednisolone 30 mg/kg IVB over 15 min → 5.4 mg/kg/h starting 45 min after bolus and continuing for 23 h
- Emergent radiation therapy ± surgery for compression due to metastatic disease
- Emergent neurosurgical consultation

SPINAL STENOSIS

Clinical manifestations
- Neurogenic claudication = back or buttocks pain induced by walking or prolonged standing, relieved by bending forwards and by rest
- ± Focal weakness, sensory loss, diminished reflexes
- Unlike claudication: max discomfort in anterior thighs, preserved lower extremity pulses
- Unlike disk herniation: pain relieved by sitting

Evaluation
- MRI

Treatment
- Conservative: avoid bending/lifting; NSAIDs
- Surgical decompression if failure to respond to conservative therapy
  (*NEJM* 2007;356:2257)

Figure 10-1 ACLS VF/pulseless VT, asystole & PEA algorithms

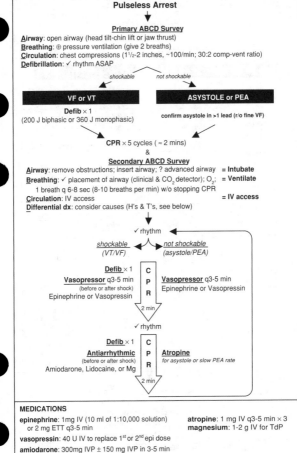

Pulseless Arrest

↓

Primary ABCD Survey

Airway: open airway (head tilt-chin lift or jaw thrust)
Breathing: ⊕ pressure ventilation (give 2 breaths)
Circulation: chest compressions (1½-2 inches, ~100/min; 30:2 comp-vent ratio)
Defibrillation: ✓ rhythm ASAP

shockable / *not shockable*

VF or VT	**ASYSTOLE or PEA**
Defib × 1 (200 J biphasic or 360 J monophasic)	confirm asystole in >1 lead (r/o fine VF)

CPR × 5 cycles (≈ 2 mins)
&
Secondary ABCD Survey

Airway: remove obstructions; insert airway; ? advanced airway = Intubate
Breathing: ✓ placement of airway (clinical & CO₂ detector); O₂; 1 breath q 6-8 sec (8-10 breaths per min) w/o stopping CPR = Ventilate
Circulation: IV access = IV access
Differential dx: consider causes (H's & T's, see below)

✓ rhythm

shockable (VT/VF) / *not shockable (asystole/PEA)*

Defib × 1
Vasopressor q3-5 min
(before or after shock)
Epinephrine or Vasopressin

C P R 2 min

Vasopressor q3-5 min
Epinephrine or Vasopressin

✓ rhythm

Defib × 1
Antiarrhythmic
(before or after shock)
Amiodarone, Lidocaine, or Mg

C P R 2 min

Atropine
for asystole or slow PEA rate

MEDICATIONS

epinephrine: 1mg IV (10 ml of 1:10,000 solution) or 2 mg ETT q3-5 min

vasopressin: 40 U IV to replace 1st or 2nd epi dose

amiodarone: 300mg IVP ± 150 mg IVP in 3-5 min

lidocaine: 1.0-1.5 mg/kg IVP (~100 mg) then 0.5-0.75 mg/kg (~50 mg) q5-10 min, max 3 mg/kg

atropine: 1 mg IV q3-5 min × 3
magnesium: 1-2 g IV for TdP

Treatment of reversible causes of PEA & asystole

Hypovolemia: volume infusion	Toxins/Tablets: med-specific
Hypoxia: oxygenate	Tamponade: pericardiocentesis
Hydrogen ions (acidosis): NaHCO₃	Tension PTX: needle decompression
Hypokalemia: KCl	Thrombosis (ACS): PCI (or lysis), IABP
Hyperkalemia: Ca, NaHCO₃, insulin/glc	Thrombosis (PE): lysis, thrombectomy
Hypoglycemia: glucose	Trauma (hypovol, ↑ ICP): per ATLS
Hypothermia: warming	

(Adapted from ACLS 2005 Guidelines, *Circ* 2005;112(Suppl I):IV-58)

Figure 10-2 ACLS tachycardia algorithm

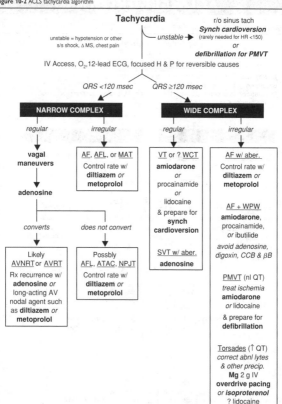

Tachycardia

Tachycardia

unstable = hypotension or other s/s shock, Δ MS, chest pain

→ *unstable* →

r/o sinus tach
Synch cardioversion (rarely needed for HR <150)

or

defibrillation for PMVT

IV Access, O₂,12-lead ECG, focused H & P for reversible causes

QRS <120 msec | *QRS ≥120 msec*

NARROW COMPLEX

regular | *irregular*

regular:
vagal maneuvers
↓
adenosine

irregular:
AF, AFL, or MAT
Control rate w/ **diltiazem** or **metoprolol**

converts | *does not convert*

converts:
Likely AVNRT or AVRT
Rx recurrence w/ **adenosine** or long-acting AV nodal agent such as **diltiazem** or **metoprolol**

does not convert:
Possbly AFL, ATAC, NPJT
Control rate w/ **diltiazem** or **metoprolol**

WIDE COMPLEX

regular | *irregular*

regular:
VT or ? WCT
amiodarone or procainamide or lidocaine & prepare for **synch cardioversion**

SVT w/ aber.
adenosine

irregular:
AF w/ aber.
Control rate w/ **diltiazem** or **metoprolol**

AF + WPW
amiodarone, procainamide, or ibutilide
avoid adenosine, digoxin, CCB & βB

PMVT (nl QT)
treat ischemia
amiodarone or lidocaine
& prepare for **defibrillation**

Torsades (↑ QT)
correct abnl lytes & other precip.
Mg 2 g IV
overdrive pacing or **isoproterenol**
? lidocaine

CARDIOVERSION

Ancillary equipment
O₂ sat monitor
suction device
IV line
intubation equipment

Premedicate
call anesthesia service
midazolam 1-5 mg
fentanyl 100-300 µg
titrate to effect

Synchronized cardioversion
100, 200, 300, 360 J
or biphasic equivalent

MEDICATIONS

adenosine: 6 mg *rapid IVP* then 20 cc NS bolus, 12 mg IVP q2 min × 2 if needed

amiodarone: 150 mg IV over 10 min

diltiazem: 15-20 mg IV over 2 min, 20-25 mg 15 min later if needed, 5-15 mg/h

ibutilide: 1 mg over 10 min, repeat × 1 if needed

lidocaine 1-1.5 mg/kg IVP, repeat in 5-10 min

metoprolol 5 mg IV q5 min × 3

procainamide 17 mg/kg at 50 mg/min (*avoid if EF↓*)

verapamil 2.5-5 mg IV over 2 min, 5-10 mg 15-30 min later if needed

(Adapted from ACLS 2005 Guidelines, *Circ* 2005;112(Suppl I):IV-67)

ACLS 10-2

Figure 10-3 ACLS bradycardia algorithms

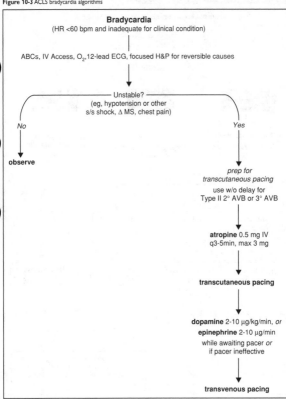

Bradycardia
(HR <60 bpm and inadequate for clinical condition)

ABCs, IV Access, O₂, 12-lead ECG, focused H&P for reversible causes

Unstable?
(eg, hypotension or other
s/s shock, Δ MS, chest pain)

No

Yes

observe

*prep for
transcutaneous pacing*
use w/o delay for
Type II 2° AVB or 3° AVB

atropine 0.5 mg IV
q3-5min, max 3 mg

transcutaneous pacing

dopamine 2-10 μg/kg/min, *or*
epinephrine 2-10 μg/min
while awaiting pacer *or*
if pacer ineffective

transvenous pacing

(Adapted from ACLS 2005 Guidelines, *Circ* 2005;112(Suppl I):IV-67)

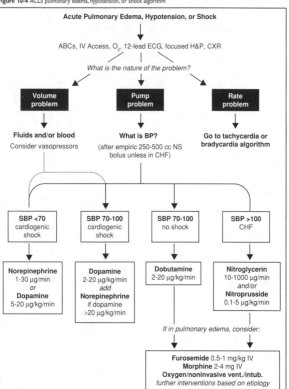

Figure 10-4 ACLS pulmonary edema, hypotension, or shock algorithm

Acute Pulmonary Edema, Hypotension, or Shock

ABCs, IV Access, O₂, 12-lead ECG, focused H&P, CXR

What is the nature of the problem?

| **Volume problem** | **Pump problem** | **Rate problem** |

Volume problem
Fluids and/or blood
Consider vasopressors

Pump problem
What is BP?
(after empiric 250-500 cc NS bolus unless in CHF)

Rate problem
Go to tachycardia or bradycardia algorithm

SBP <70
cardiogenic shock

Norepinephrine
1-30 µg/min
or
Dopamine
5-20 µg/kg/min

SBP 70-100
cardiogenic shock

Dopamine
2-20 µg/kg/min
add
Norepinephrine
if dopamine
>20 µg/kg/min

SBP 70-100
no shock

Dobutamine
2-20 µg/kg/min

SBP >100
CHF

Nitroglycerin
10-1000 µg/min
and/or
Nitroprusside
0.1-5 µg/kg/min

If in pulmonary edema, consider:

Furosemide 0.5-1 mg/kg IV
Morphine 2-4 mg IV
Oxygen/noninvasive vent./intub.
further interventions based on etiology

(Adapted from ACLS 2005 Guidelines)

Drug	Class	Dose	
		per kg	average
Pressors, Inotropes, and Chronotropes			
Phenylephrine	α_1	10-300 µg/min	
Norepinephrine	$\alpha_1 > \beta_1$	1-40 µg/min	
Vasopressin	V_1	0.01-0.1 U/min (usually <0.04)	
Epinephrine	$\alpha_1, \alpha_2, \beta_1, \beta_2$	2-20 µg/min	
Isoproterenol	β_1, β_2	0.1-10 µg/min	
Dopamine	D	0.5-2 µg/kg/min	50-200 µg/min
	β, D	2-10 µg/kg/min	200-500 µg/min
	α, β, D	>10 µg/kg/min	500-1000 µg/min
Dobutamine	$\beta_1 > \beta_2$	2-20 µg/kg/min	50-1000 µg/min
Milrinone	PDE	50 µg/kg over 10 min then 0.375-0.75 µg/kg/min	3-4 mg over 10 min then 20-50 µg/min
Inamrinone	PDE	0.75 mg/kg over 3 min then 5-15 µg/kg/min	40-50 mg over 3 min then 250-900 µg/min
Vasodilators			
Nitroglycerin	NO	10-1000 µg/min	
Nitroprusside	NO	0.1-10 µg/kg/min	5-800 µg/min
Nesiritide	BNP	2 µg/kg IVB then 0.01 µg/kg/min	
Labetalol	α_1, β_1, and β_2 blocker	20 mg over 2 min then 20-80 mg q10min or 10-120 mg/h	
Fenoldopam	D	0.1-1.6 µg/kg/min	10-120 µg/min
Epoprostenol	vasodilator	2-20 ng/kg/min	
Enalaprilat	ACE	0.625-2.5 mg over 5 min then 0.625-5 mg q6h	
Hydralazine	vasodilator	5-20 mg q20-30min	
Antiarrhythmics			
Amiodarone	K et al. (Class III)	150 mg over 10 min, then 1 mg/min × 6h, then 0.5 mg/min × 18h	
Lidocaine	Na channel (Class IB)	1-1.5 mg/kg then 1-4 mg/min	100 mg then 1-4 mg/min
Procainamide	Na channel (Class IA)	17 mg/kg over 60 min then 1-4 mg/min	1 g over 60 min then 1-4 mg/min
Ibutilide	K channel (Class III)	1 mg over 10 min, may repeat × 1	
Propranolol	β blocker	0.5-1 mg q5min then 1-10 mg/h	
Esmolol	$\beta_1 > \beta_2$ blocker	500 µg/kg then 25-300 µg/kg/min	20-40 mg over 1 min then 2-20 mg/min
Verapamil	CCB	2.5-5 mg over 1-2 min repeat 5-10 mg in 15-30 min prn 5-20 mg/h	
Diltiazem	CCB	0.25 mg/kg over 2 min reload 0.35 mg/kg × 1 prn then 5-15 mg/h	20 mg over 2 min reload 25 mg × 1 prn then 5-15 mg/h
Adenosine	purinergic	6 mg rapid push if no response: 12 mg → 12-18 mg	

Drug	Class	Dose	
		per kg	average
Sedation			
Morphine	opioid	1-unlimited mg/h	
Fentanyl	opioid	50-100 μg then 50-unlimited μg/h	
Thiopental	barbiturate	3-5 mg/kg over 2 min	200-400 mg over 2 min
Etomidate	anesthetic	0.2-0.5 mg/kg	100-300 mg
Propofol	anesthetic	1-3 mg/kg then 0.3-5 mg/kg/h	50-200 mg then 20-400 mg/h
Diazepam	BDZ	1-5 mg q1-2h then q6h prn	
Midazolam	BDZ	0.5-2 mg q5min prn or 0.5-4 mg then 1-10 mg/h	
Ketamine	anesthetic	1-2 mg/kg	60-150 mg
Haloperidol	antipsychotic	2-5 mg q20-30min	
Naloxone	opioid antag.	0.4-2 mg q2-3min to total of 10 mg	
Flumazenil	BDZ antag.	0.2 mg over 30 sec then 0.3 mg over 30 sec if still lethargic may repeat 0.5 mg over 30 sec to total of 3 mg	
Paralysis			
Succinylcholine	depolar. paralytic	0.6-1.1 mg/kg	70-100 mg
Tubocurare	nACh	10 mg then 6-20 mg/h	
Pancuronium	nACh	0.08 mg/kg	2-4 mg q30-90'
Vecuronium	nACh	0.08 mg/kg then 0.05-0.1 mg/kg/h	5-10 mg over 1-3 min then 2-8 mg/h
Cisatracurium	nACh	5-10 μg/kg/min	
Miscellaneous			
Aminophylline	PDE	5.5 mg/kg over 20 min then 0.5-1 mg/kg/h	250-500 mg then 10-80 mg/h
Insulin		10 U then 0.1 U/kg/h	
Glucagon		5-10 mg then 1-5 mg/h	
Octreotide	somatostatin analog	50 μg then 50 μg/h	
Phenytoin	antiepileptic	20 mg/kg at 50 mg/min	1-1.5 g over 20-30 min
Fosphenytoin	antiepileptic	20 mg/kg at 150 mg/min	1-1.5 g over 10 min
Phenobarbital	barbiturate	20 mg/kg at 50-75 mg/min	1-1.5 g over 20 min
Mannitol	osmole	1.5-2 g/kg over 30-60 min repeat q6-12h to keep osm 310-320	

ANTIBIOTICS

The following tables of spectra of activity for different antibiotics are generalizations. Sensitivity data at your own institution should be used to guide therapy.

Penicillins

Generation	Properties	Spectrum
Natural	Some GPC, GPR, GNC, most anaerobes (except *Bacteroides*)	Group A streptococci Enterococci, *Listeria* *Pasteurella* *Actinomyces*, Syphilis
Anti-Staph	Active vs. PCNase-producing Staph Little activity vs. Gram $\ominus$	Staphylococci (except MRSA) Streptococci
Amino	Penetrates porin channel of Gram $\ominus$ Not stable against PCNases	*E. coli, Proteus, H. influenzae Salmonella, Shigella* Enterococci, *Listeria*
Extended	Penetrates porin channel of Gram $\ominus$ More resistant to PCNases	Most GNR incl. *Enterobacter, Pseudomonas, Serratia*
Carbapenem	Resistant to most β-lactamases	Most gram $\oplus$ and $\ominus$ bacteria incl. anaerobes (except MRSA and VRE)
Monobactams	Active vs. Gram $\ominus$ but not Gram $\oplus$	Gram $\ominus$ bacterial infxn in Pt w/ PCN or Ceph allergy
β-lact. Inhib.	Inhib. plasma-mediated β-lactamases	Adds Staph, *B. fragilis* and some GNR (*H. influenzae, M. catarrhalis*, some *Klesiella*)

Cephalosporins

Resistant to most β-lactamases. No activity vs. MRSA or enterococci.

Gen.	Spectrum	Indications
First	Most GPC (incl. Staph & Strep) Some GNR (incl. *E. coli, Proteus, Klebsiella*)	Used for surgical prophylaxis & skin infxns
Second	↓ activity vs. GPC, ↑ vs. GNR. 2 subgroups: Respiratory: ↑ activity vs. *H. influenzae* & *M. catarrhalis* GI/GU: ↑ activity vs. *B. fragilis*	PNA/COPD flare Abdominal infxns
Third	Broad activity vs. GNR and some anaerobes Ceftazidime active vs. *Pseudomonas*	PNA, sepsis, meningitis
Fourth	↑ resistance to β-lactamases (incl. of Staph and *Enterobacter*)	Similar to 3rd gen. MonoRx for nonlocalizing febrile neutropenia

Other Antibiotics

Antibiotic	Spectrum
Vancomycin	Gram $\oplus$ bacteria incl. MRSA, PCNase-producing pneumococci and enterococci (except VRE)
Linezolid Daptomycin Quinopristin/ Dalfopristin	GPC incl. MRSA & VRE
Quinolones	Enteric GNR & atypicals. 3rd & 4th gen. ↑ activity vs. Gram $\oplus$.
Aminoglycosides	GNR. Synergy w/ cell-wall active abx (β-lactam, vanco) vs. GPC. ↓ activity in low pH (eg, abscess). No activity vs. anaerobes.
Macrolides	GPC, some respiratory Gram $\ominus$, atypicals
TMP-SMZ	Some enteric GNR, PCP, *Nocardia, Toxoplasma*, most community-acquired MRSA
Clindamycin	Gram $\oplus$ (except enterococci) & anaerobes (incl. *B fragilis*)
Metronidazole	Anaerobes (incl. *B fragilis*)
Doxycycline	*Rickettsia, Ehrlichia, Chlamydia, Mycoplasma, Nocardia*, Lyme

Penicillins				
Antibiotic	Normal dose	Dose in renal failure (by GFR)		
		>50	10-50	<10
Natural penicillins				
Penicillin G	0.4-4 MU IM/IV q4h	NC	NC	1-2 MU q4h
Penicillin V	250-500 mg PO q6h	NC	NC	NC
Anti-staphylococcal				
Dicloxacillin	250-500 mg PO q6h	NC	NC	NC
Nafcillin	1-2 g IM/IV q4h	NC	NC	NC
Oxacillin	1-2 g IM/IV q4h	NC	NC	NC
Aminopenicillins				
Amoxicillin	250-500 mg PO q8h	NC	250-500 mg q8-12h	250 mg q12h
Amox-clav	250-500 mg PO q8h	NC	250-500 mg q8-12h	250 mg q12h
Ampicillin	1-2 g IM/IV q4h	NC	1-2 g q8h	1-2 g q12h
Amp-sulbact	1.5-3 g IM/IV q6h	NC	1.5-3 g q12h	1.5-3 g q24h
Extended-spectrum penicillins				
Piperacillin	2-4 g IM/IV q4-6h	NC	2-4 g q8h	2-4 g q12h
Pip-tazo	3.375 g IV q6h	NC	2.25 g q6h	2.25 g q8h
Ticarcillin	2-4 g IM/IV q4h	NC	2-3 g q6h	2 g q12h
Ticar-clav	3.1 g IV q4h	NC	3.1 g q6h	2 g q12h
Other β-lactams				
Aztreonam	1-2 g IM/IV q8h	NC	1 g q8h	0.5 g q8h
Ertapenem	1 g IV/IM q24h	NC	0.5 g q24h (if CrCl <30)	
Imipenem	250-500 mg IV q6h	NC	250-500 mg q8-12h	250-500 mg q12h
Meropenem	1 g IV q8h	NC	0.5-1 g IV q12h	0.5 g IV q24h

Macrolides				
Antibiotic	Normal dose	Dose in renal failure (by GFR)		
		>50	10-50	<10
Azithromycin	500 mg IV qd 500 mg PO on d 1, then 250 mg PO qd	NC	NC	NC
Clarithromycin	250-500 mg PO bid	?↓	?↓	?↓
Erythromycin	0.5-1 g IV q6h 250-500 mg PO qid	NC	NC	250-500 mg IV or 250 mg PO q6h
Telithromycin*	800 mg PO qd	NC	600 mg qd (if CrCl <30)	

*Ketolide (ketone derivative of macrolide nucleus)

Tetracyclines				
Antibiotic	Normal dose	Dose in renal failure (by GFR)		
		>50	10-50	<10
Doxycycline	100 mg PO/IV q12-24h	NC	NC	NC
Tigecycline	100 mg IV × 1 then 50 mg q12h	NC	NC	NC

Cephalosporins				
Antibiotic	**Normal dose**	**Dose in renal failure** (by GFR)		
		>50	10-50	<10
1st generation				
Cefadroxil	0.5-1 g PO q12h	NC	0.5 g q12-24h	0.5 g q36h
Cefazolin	1 g IM/IV q8h	NC	1 g q12h	1 g q24h
Cephalexin	250-500 mg PO q6h	NC	NC	NC
2nd generation				
Cefaclor	250-500 mg PO q8h	NC	NC	NC
Cefotetan	1-2 g IM/IV q12h	NC	1-2 g q24h	1 g q24h
Cefoxitin	1-2 g IM/IV q4h	1-2 g q6h	1-2 g q8h	1 g q12h
Cefprozil	250-500 mg PO q12-24h	NC	NC	250 mg q12h
Cefuroxime	750-1500 mg IM/IV q6h	NC	750-1500 mg q8h	750 mg q24h
Loracarbef	200-400 mg PO q12h	NC	200 mg q12h	200 mg q3-5d
3rd generation				
Cefdinir	600 mg PO qd	NC	NC	300 mg qd
Cefditoren	200-400 mg PO bid	NC	200 mg bid	200 mg qd
Cefixime	400 mg PO q24h	NC	300 mg q24h	200 mg q24h
Cefoperazone	1-3 g IV q8h	NC	NC	NC
Cefotaxime	1-2 g IM/IV q6h	NC	NC	1-2 g q12h
Cefpodoxime	100-400 mg PO q12h	NC	NC	400 mg q24h
Ceftazidime	1-2 g IV q8h	NC	1-2 g q12h	1 g q24h
Ceftibuten	400 mg PO qd	NC	200 mg qd	100 mg qd
Ceftizoxime	1-2 g IV q6h	NC	1 g q12h	0.5 g q12h
Ceftriaxone	1-2 g IM/IV q12-24h	NC	NC	NC
4th generation				
Cefepime	1-2 g IM/IV q12h	NC	1-2 g q16-24h	1-2 g q24-48h

Fluoroquinolones				
Antibiotic	**Normal dose**	**Dose in renal failure** (by GFR)		
		>50	10-50	<10
1st generation				
Nalidixic acid	1 g PO qid	n/a	n/a	n/a
2nd generation				
Ciprofloxacin	500-750 mg PO q12h 200-400 mg IV q12h	NC	250-500 mg q12h	250-500 mg q24h
Lomefloxacin	400 mg PO qd	NC	200-400 mg qd	200 mg qd
Norfloxacin	400 mg PO q12h	NC	400 mg q12-24h	400 mg q24h
Ofloxacin	200-400 mg PO/IV q12h	NC	400 mg q24h	200 mg q24h
3rd generation				
Levofloxacin	250-500 mg PO/IV q24h	NC	250 mg q24h	250 mg q48h
4th generation				
Gatifloxacin	400 mg PO/IV qd	NC	200 mg qd	200 mg qd
Gemifloxacin	320 mg PO qd	NC	160 mg qd	
Moxifloxacin	400 mg PO qd	NC	NC	NC

Aminoglycosides				
Antibiotic	**Normal dose**	**Dose in renal failure** (by GFR)		
		>50	10-50	<10
Gentamicin	1-1.7 mg/kg q8h	60-90% q8-12h	30-70% q12-18h	20-30% q24-48h
Tobramycin		or ~1-1.7 mg/kg q(8 × serum Cr)h		
Amikacin	5 mg/kg q8h	60-90% q8-12h	30-70% q12-18h	20-30% q24-48h
		or ~5 mg/kg q(8 × serum Cr)h		

Other Antibiotics				
Antibiotic	**Normal dose**	**Dose in renal failure** (by GFR)		
		>50	10-50	<10
Chloramphenicol	0.5-1 g IV/PO q6h	NC	NC	NC
Clindamycin	600 mg IV q8h 150-300 mg PO qid	NC	NC	NC
Daptomycin	4 mg/kg IV q24h	NC	4 mg/kg q48h (if CrCl <30)	
Linezolid	400-600 mg IV/PO q12h	NC	NC	NC
Metronidazole	1000 mg load then 500 mg IV/PO q6h	NC	NC	NC
Nitrofurantoin	50-100 mg PO qid	NC	avoid	avoid
Quinopristin/ Dalfopristin	7.5 mg/kg IV q8-12h	NC	NC	NC
TMP-SMX*	2-5 mg TMP/kg PO/IV q6h	NC	2-5 mg TMP/kg q12h	avoid
Vancomycin	1 g IV q12h	NC	1 g q24-72h ✓ trough (goal 5-10, ? <15 for some infxns) adjust dose & interval	

(*single strength table = 1 ampule = 80 mg of TMP + 400 mg SMX)

CARDIOLOGY

Hemodynamic parameters	Normal value
Mean arterial pressure (MAP) $= \dfrac{SBP + (DBP \times 2)}{3}$	70-100 mmHg
Heart rate (HR)	60-100 bpm
Right atrial pressure (RA)	≤ 6 mmHg
Right ventricular (RV)	systolic 15-30 mmHg diastolic 1-8 mmHg
Pulmonary artery (PA)	systolic 15-30 mmHg mean 9-18 mmHg diastolic 6-12 mmHg
Pulmonary capillary wedge pressure (PCWP)	≤ 12 mmHg
Cardiac output (CO)	4-8 L/min
Cardiac index (CI) $= \dfrac{CO}{BSA}$	2.6-4.2 L/min/m^2
Stroke volume (SV) $= \dfrac{CO}{HR}$	60-120 ml/contraction
Stroke volume index (SVI) $= \dfrac{CI}{HR}$	40-50 ml/contraction/m^2
Systemic vascular resistance (SVR) $= \dfrac{MAP - mean\ RA}{CO} \times 80$	800-1200 dynes $\times$ sec/cm^5
Pulmonary vascular resistance (PVR) $= \dfrac{mean\ PA - mean\ PCWP}{CO} \times 80$	120-250 dynes $\times$ sec/cm^5

("Rule of 6s" for PA catheter-measured pressures: RA ≤ 6, RV $\leq 30/6$, PA $\leq 30/12$, WP ≤ 12)
(1 mmHg = 1.36 cm water or blood)

Fick cardiac output

Oxygen consumption (L/min) = CO (L/min) $\times$ arteriovenous (AV) oxygen difference
CO = oxygen consumption / AV oxygen difference
Oxygen consumption must be measured (can estimate w/ 125 ml/min/m^2, but inaccurate)
AV oxygen difference = Hb (g/dl) $\times$ 10 (dl/L) $\times$ 1.36 (ml O_2/g of Hb) $\times$ (S_aO_2-S_vO_2)
  S_aO_2 is measured in any arterial sample (usually 93-98%)
  S_vO_2 (mixed venous O_2) is measured in RA, RV, or PA (assuming no shunt) (normal ~75%)

$$\therefore \textbf{Cardiac output (L/min)} = \frac{Oxygen\ consumption}{Hb\ (g/dl) \times 13.6 \times (S_aO_2 - S_vO_2)}$$

Shunts

$$Q_p = \frac{Oxygen\ consumption}{Pulm.\ vein\ O_2\ sat - Pulm.\ artery\ O_2\ sat} \quad \text{(if no R} \rightarrow \text{L shunt, PV } O_2 \text{ sat} \approx S_aO_2)$$

$$Q_s = \frac{Oxygen\ consumption}{S_aO_2 - mixed\ venous\ O_2\ sat} \quad \text{(MVO}_2 \text{ drawn proximal to potential L} \rightarrow \text{R shunt)}$$

$$\frac{Q_p}{Q_s} = \frac{S_aO_2 - MV\ O_2\ sat}{PV\ O_2\ sat - PA\ O_2\ sat} \approx \frac{S_aO_2 - MV\ O_2\ sat}{S_aO_2 - PA\ O_2\ sat} \quad \text{(if only L} \rightarrow \text{R and no R} \rightarrow \text{L shunt)}$$

Valve area

Gorlin equation: Valve area $= \dfrac{CO/(DEP \text{ or } SEP) \times HR}{44.3 \times constant \times \sqrt{\Delta P}}$ (constant = 1 for AS, 0.85 for MS)

Hakki equation: Valve area $\approx \dfrac{CO}{\sqrt{\Delta P}}$

Coronary artery anatomy

Figure 10-5 Coronary arteries

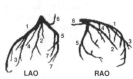

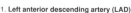

LEFT CORONARY ARTERY	RIGHT CORONARY ARTERY
LAO RAO	LAO RAO

1. **Left anterior descending artery (LAD)**
2. Ramus medianus artery
3. Diagonal branches
4. Septal branches
5. **Left circumflex artery (LCx)**
6. Left atrial circumflex artery
7. Obtuse marginal branches

1. Conus artery
2. SA node artery
3. Acute marginal branches
4. Posterior descending artery (PDA)
5. AV node artery
6. Posterior left ventricular artery (PLV)

(From Grossman WG. *Cardiac Catheterization and Angiography*, 4th ed. Philadelphia: Lea & Febiger, 1991, with permission.)

PULMONARY

Dead space = lung units that are ventilated but not perfused
Intrapulmonary shunt = lung units that are perfused but not ventilated

Alveolar gas equation: $P_AO_2 = [F_1O_2 \times (760 - 47)] - \dfrac{P_aCO_2}{R}$ (where R ≈ 0.8)

$$P_AO_2 = 150 - \dfrac{P_aCO_2}{0.8} \text{ (on room air)}$$

A-a gradient = $P_AO_2 - P_aO_2$ [normal A-a gradient ≈ 4 + (age/4)]
Minute ventilation ($\dot{V}_E$) = tidal volume (V_T) × respiratory rate (RR) (normal 4-6 L/min)
Tidal volume (V_T) = alveolar space (V_A) + dead space (V_D)

Fraction of tidal volume that is dead space $\left(\dfrac{V_D}{V_T}\right) = \dfrac{P_aCO_2 - P_{expired}CO_2}{P_aCO_2}$

$P_aCO_2 = k = \times \dfrac{CO_2 \text{ Production}}{\text{alveolar ventilation}} = k \times \dfrac{\dot{V}_{CO_2}}{RR \times V_T \times \left(1 - \dfrac{V_D}{V_T}\right)}$

NEPHROLOGY

Anion gap (AG) = $Na - (Cl + HCO_3)$ (normal = [alb] × 2.5; typically 12 ± 2 mEq)

Delta-delta ($\Delta\Delta$) = [Δ AG (ie, calc. AG - expected) / Δ HCO$_3$ (ie, 24 - measured HCO$_3$)]

Urine anion gap (UAG) = $(U_{Na} + U_K) - U_{Cl}$

Calculated osmoles = $(2 \times Na) + \left(\dfrac{glc}{18}\right) + \left(\dfrac{BUN}{2.8}\right) + \left(\dfrac{EtOH}{4.6}\right)$

Osmolal gap (OG) = measured osmoles - calculated osmoles   (normal < 10)

Estimated creatinine clearance = $\dfrac{[140 - age(yrs)] \times wt\ (kg)}{serum\ Cr\ (mg/dl) \times 72}$ (× 0.85 in women)

Fractional excretion of Na (FE$_{Na}$, %) = $\left[\dfrac{\dfrac{U_{Na}(mEq/L)}{P_{Na}(mEq/L)} \times 100\%}{\dfrac{U_{Cr}(mg/ml)}{P_{Cr}\ (mg/dl)} \times 100\ (ml/dl)}\right] = \dfrac{U_{Na}}{P_{Na}} \Big/ \dfrac{U_{Cr}}{P_{Cr}}$

Corrected Na in hyperglycemia

estimate in all Pts: corrected Na = measured Na + $\left[2.4 \times \dfrac{(measured\ glc - 100)}{100}\right]$

however, Δ in Na depends on glc (Am J Med 1999;106:399)

Δ is 1.6 mEq per each 100 mg/dl ↑ in glc ranging from 100-440

Δ is 4 mEq per each 100 mg/dl ↑ in glc beyond 440

Total body water (TBW) = 0.60 × IBW (× 0.85 if female and × 0.85 if elderly)

Free H$_2$O deficit = TBW $\times \left(\dfrac{[Na]_{serum} - 140}{140}\right) \approx \left(\dfrac{[Na]_{serum} - 140}{3}\right)$ (in 70 kg Pt)

Trans-tubular potassium gradient (TTKG) = $\dfrac{U_K}{P_K} \Big/ \dfrac{U_{Osm}}{P_{Osm}}$

HEMATOLOGY

Heparin for Thromboembolism	
80 U/kg bolus	
18 U/kg/h	
PTT	**Adjustment**
<40	bolus 5000 U, ↑ rate 300 U/h
40-49	bolus 3000 U, ↑ rate 200 U/h
50-59	↑ rate 100 U/h
60-85	no Δ
86-95	↓ rate 100 U/h
96-120	hold 30 min, ↓ rate 150 U/h
>120	hold 60 min, ↓ rate 200 U/h

(Circ 2001;103:2994)

Heparin for ACS	
STEMI w/ fibrinolysis	
60 U/kg bolus (max 4000 U)	
12 U/kg/h (max 1000 U/h)	
UA/NSTEMI	
60-75 U/kg bolus (max 5000 U)	
12-15 U/kg/h (max 1000 U/h)	
PTT	**Adjustment**
<40	bolus 3000 U, ↑ rate 100 U/h
40-49	↑ rate 50 U/h
50-70	no Δ
71-85	↓ rate 50 U/h
86-100	hold 30 min, ↓ rate 100 U/h
101-150	hold 30 min, ↓ rate 150 U/h
>150	hold 60 min, ↓ rate 300 U/h

(ACC/AHA 2004 Guideline for STEMI)

✓ PTT q6h after every change (half-life of heparin is ~ 90 min)

✓ PTT qd or bid once PTT is therapeutic

✓ CBC qd (to ensure Hct and plt counts are stable)

Warfarin Loading Nomogram					
Day	**INR**				
	<1.5	**1.5-1.9**	**2-2.5**	**2.6-3**	**>3**
1-3	5 mg (7.5 mg if > 80 kg)	2.5-5 mg		0-2.5 mg	0 mg
4-5	10 mg	5-10 mg	0-5 mg		0-2.5 mg
6	Dose based on requirements over preceding 5 days				

(*Annals* 1997;126:133; *Archives* 1999;159:46)

Warfarin-heparin overlap therapy
- Indications: when failure to anticoagulate carries ↑ risk of morbidity or mortality
  (eg, DVT/PE, intracardiac thrombus)
- Rationale: (1) Half-life of factor VII (3-6 h) is shorter than half-life of factor II (60-72 h);
  ∴ warfarin can elevate PT *before achieving a true antithrombotic state*
  (2) Protein C also has half-life less than that of factor II;
  ∴ theoretical concern of *hypercoagulable state* before antithrombotic state
- Method: (1) Therapeutic PTT is achieved using heparin
  (2) Warfarin therapy is initiated
  (3) Heparin continued until INR therapeutic for ≥ 2 d and ≥ 4-5 d of warfarin
  (roughly corresponds to ~ 2 half-lives of factor II or a reduction to ~ 25%)

OTHER

Ideal body weight (IBW) = [50 kg (men) or 45.5 kg (women)] + 2.3 kg/inch over 5 feet

$$\text{Body surface area (BSA, m}^2) = \sqrt{\frac{\text{height (cm)} \times \text{weight (kg)}}{3600}}$$

		Disease	
		present	absent
Test	⊕	a (true ⊕)	b (false ⊕)
	⊖	c (false ⊖)	d (true ⊖)

$$\text{Prevalence} = \frac{\text{all diseased}}{\text{all patients}} = \frac{a + b}{a + b + c + d}$$

$$\text{Sensitivity} = \frac{\text{true positives}}{\text{all diseased}} = \frac{a}{a + c} \qquad \text{Specificity} = \frac{\text{true negatives}}{\text{all healthy}} = \frac{d}{b + d}$$

$$\oplus \text{Predictive value} = \frac{\text{true positives}}{\text{all positives}} = \frac{a}{a + b}$$

$$\ominus \text{Predictive value} = \frac{\text{true negatives}}{\text{all negatives}} = \frac{d}{c + d}$$

$$\text{Accuracy} = \frac{\text{true positives} + \text{true negatives}}{\text{all patients}} = \frac{a + d}{a + b + c + d}$$

$$\oplus \text{Likelihood ratio} = \frac{\text{true positive rate}}{\text{false positive rate}} = \frac{Se}{1 - Sp}$$

$$\ominus \text{Likelihood ratio} = \frac{\text{false negative rate}}{\text{true negative rate}} = \frac{1 - Se}{Sp}$$

$$\text{Odds} = \frac{\text{probability}}{1 - \text{probability}} \qquad \text{Probability} = \frac{\text{odds}}{\text{odds} + 1}$$

Posttest odds = pretest odds × LR

ABBREVIATIONS

5'-NT	5'-nucleotidase	asx	asymptomatic
AAA	abdominal aortic aneurysm	AT	atrial tachycardia
AAD	antiarrhythmic drug	ATII	angiotensin II
Ab	antibody	ATIII	antithrombin III
ABE	acute bacterial endocarditis	ATN	acute tubular necrosis
ABG	arterial blood gas	ATRA	all-*trans*-retinoic acid
abnl	abnormal	AV	atrioventricular
ABPA	allergic bronchopulmonary aspergillosis	AVA	aortic valve area
		AVB	atrioventricular block
abx	antibiotics	AVNRT	AV nodal reentrant tachycardia
AC	assist control	AVR	aortic valve replacement
ACE	angiotensin converting enzyme	AVRT	AV reciprocating tachycardia
ACEI	ACE inhibitor	AZA	azathioprine
ACI	anemia of chronic inflammation	Aφ	alkaline phosphatase
ACL	anticardiolipin antibody	b/c	because
ACLS	advanced cardiac life support	BAL	bronchoalveolar lavage
ACS	acute coronary syndrome	βB	beta-blocker
ACTH	adrenocorticotrophic hormone	BBB	bundle branch block
		BCx	blood culture
ADA	adenosine deaminase	BDZ	benzodiazepines
ADH	antidiuretic hormone	bili.	bilirubin
ADL	activities of daily living	BiPAP	bilevel positive airway pressure
AF	atrial fibrillation	BM	bone marrow
AFB	acid-fast bacilli	BMI	body mass index
AFL	atrial flutter	BNP	B-type natriuretic peptide
AFP	α-fetoprotein	BOOP	bronchiolitis obliterans with organizing pneumonia
AFTP	ascites fluid total protein		
AG	aminoglycoside anion gap	BP	blood pressure
		BPH	benign prostatic hypertrophy
Ag	antigen	BRBPR	bright red blood per rectum
AGN	acute glomerulonephritis	BS	breath sounds
AI	aortic insufficiency	BT	bleeding time
AIDS	acquired immunodeficiency syndrome	BUN	blood urea nitrogen
		bx	biopsy
AIHA	autoimmune hemolytic anemia	C'	complement
AIN	acute interstitial nephritis	c/w	compared with consistent with
ALL	acute lymphocytic leukemia		
ALS	amyotrophic lateral sclerosis	CABG	coronary artery bypass grafting
ALT	alanine aminotransferase	CAD	coronary artery disease
AMA	anti-mitochondrial antibody	CALLA	common ALL antigen
AMI	anterior myocardial infarction	CAPD	chronic ambulatory peritoneal dialysis
AML	acute myelogenous leukemia		
AMM/MF	agnogenic myeloid metaplasia/myelofibrosis	CBC	complete blood count
		CBD	common bile duct
ANA	antinuclear antibody	CCB	calcium channel blocker
ANCA	antineutrophilic cytoplasmic antibody	CCl₄	carbon tetrachloride
		CCP	cyclic citrullinated peptide
angio	angiogram	CCS	Canadian Cardiovascular Society
AoV	aortic valve		
APC	activated protein C	CD	Crohn's disease
APS	antiphospholipid antibody syndrome	CEA	carotid endarterectomy
		ceph.	cephalosporin
ARB	angiotensin receptor blocker	CF	cystic fibrosis
ARDS	acute respiratory distress syndrome	CFU	colony forming units
		CHB	complete heart block
ARF	acute renal failure	CHD	congenital heart disease
ARVD	arrhythmogenic RV dysplasia	CHF	congestive heart failure
AS	aortic stenosis	CI	cardiac index
ASA	aspirin	CIARF	contrast-induced acute renal failure
ASD	atrial septal defect		
AST	aspartate aminotransferase		

CKD	chronic kidney disease
CLL	chronic lymphocytic leukemia
CML	chronic myelogenous leukemia
CMML	chronic myelomonocytic leukemia
CMP	cardiomyopathy
CMV	cytomegalovirus
CO	carbon monoxide
	cardiac output
COP	cryptogenic organizing pneumonitis
COPD	chronic obstructive pulmonary disease
COX	cyclooxygenase
CP	chest pain
CPAP	continuous positive airway pressure
CPPD	calcium pyrophosphate dihydrate
Cr	creatinine
CRC	colorectal cancer
CrCl	creatinine clearance
CRI	chronic renal insufficiency
CRT	cardiac resynchronization therapy
CsA	cyclosporine A
CSF	cerebrospinal fluid
CSM	carotid sinus massage
CT	computed tomogram
CTA	CT angiogram
CTD	connective tissue disease
CV	cardiovascular
CVA	cerebrovascular accident
CVD	cerebrovascular disease
	collagen vascular disease
CVP	central venous pressure
CVVH	continuous veno-venous hemofiltration
CW	chest wall
CXR	chest radiograph
d	day
D	death
d/c	discharge
	discontinue
Δ MS	change in mental status
DA	dopamine
DAT	direct antiglobulin test
DBP	diastolic blood pressure
DCIS	ductal carcinoma in situ
DCMP	dilated cardiomyopathy
Ddx	differential diagnosis
DFA	direct fluorescent antigen detection
DI	diabetes insipidus
DIC	disseminated intravascular coagulation
diff.	differential
DIP	desquamative interstitial pneumonitis
	distal interphalangeal
DKA	diabetic ketoacidosis
DL$_{CO}$	diffusion capacity of the lung
DLE	drug induced lupus
DM	dermatomyositis
	diabetes mellitus

DM1	diabetes mellitus type 1
DM2	diabetes mellitus type 2
DMARD	disease-modifying anti-rheumatic drug
DOE	dyspnea on exertion
DRE	digital rectal exam
DSE	dobutamine stress echo
DTRs	deep tendon reflexes
DU	duodenal ulcer
DVT	deep vein thrombosis
dx	diagnosis
EAD	extreme axis deviation
EAV	effective arterial volume
EBV	Epstein-Barr virus
ECG	electrocardiogram
echo	echocardiogram
ECMO	extracorporeal membrane oxygenation
ED	emergency department
EDP	end-diastolic pressure
EDV	end-diastolic volume
EEG	electroencephalogram
EF	ejection fraction
EGD	esophagogastroduodenoscopy
EIA	enzyme-linked immunoassay
ELISA	enzyme-linked immunosorbent assay
EOM	extraocular muscles
EP	electrophysiology
Epo	erythropoietin
EPS	electrophysiology study
ERCP	endoscopic retrograde cholangiopancreatography
ERV	expiratory reserve volume
ESP	end-systolic pressure
ESR	erythrocyte sedimentation rate
ESRD	end-stage renal disease
ESV	end-systolic volume
ET	endotracheal tube
	essential thrombocytosis
EtOH	alcohol
ETT	endotracheal tube
	exercise tolerance test
FDP	fibrin degradation product
FEV$_1$	forced expiratory volume in 1 second
FFP	fresh frozen plasma
FHx	family history
FMD	fibromuscular dysplasia
FMF	familial Mediterranean fever
FNA	fine needle aspiration
FOBT	fecal occult blood testing
FQ	fluoroquinolone
FRC	functional residual capacity
FSGS	focal segmental glomerulosclerosis
FSH	follicle stimulating hormone
FTI	free thyroxine index
FVC	forced vital capacity
G6PD	glucose-6-phosphate dehydrogenase
GBM	glomerular basement membrane

GBS	Guillain-Barré syndrome		IC	inspiratory capacity
GCA	giant cell arteritis		ICa	ionized calcium
G-CSF	granulocyte colony stimulating factor		ICD	implantable cardiac defibrillator
GE	gastroesophageal		ICH	intracranial hemorrhage
gen.	generation		ICP	intracranial pressure
GERD	gastroesophageal reflux disease		ICU	intensive care unit
			IDDM	insulin-dependent diabetes mellitus
GFR	glomerular filtration rate			
GGT	γ-glutamyl transpeptidase		IE	infective endocarditis
GH	growth hormone		IGF	insulin-like growth factor
GIB	gastrointestinal bleed		IIP	idiopathic interstitial pneumonia
GIST	gastrointestinal stromal tumor			
glc	glucose		ILD	interstitial lung disease
GN	glomerulonephritis		IMI	inferior myocardial infarction
GNR	gram negative rods		infxn	infection
GnRH	gonadotropin releasing hormone		INH	isoniazid
			INR	international normalized ratio
GPC	gram positive cocci		IPF	idiopathic pulmonary fibrosis
GPI	glycoprotein IIb/IIIa inhibitor		ITP	idiopathic thrombocytopenic purpura
GRA	glucocorticoid-remediable aldosteronism			
			IVB	intravenous bolus
GU	gastric ulcer		IVC	inferior vena cava
GVHD	graft-versus-host disease		IVDA	intravenous drug abuser
			IVF	intravenous fluids
h	hour		IVIg	intravenous immunoglobulin
h/o	history of			
HA	headache		JVD	jugular venous distention
HAV	hepatitis A virus		JVP	jugular venous pulse
Hb	hemoglobin			
HBIG	hepatitis B immune globulin		LA	left atrium
HBV	hepatitis B virus			lupus anticoagulant
HCC	hepatocellular carcinoma		LABA	long-acting β₂-agonist
HCMP	hypertrophic cardiomyopathy		LAD	left anterior descending coronary artery
Hct	hematocrit			
HCV	hepatitis C virus			left axis deviation
HD	hemodialysis		LAE	left atrial enlargement
HDL	high-density lipoprotein		LAN	lymphadenopathy
HDV	hepatitis D virus		LAP	leukocyte alkaline phosphatase
HELLP	hemolysis, abnormal LFTs, low platelets		LAP	left atrial pressure
			LBBB	left bundle branch block
HEV	hepatitis E virus		LCIS	lobular carcinoma in situ
HF	heart failure		LCx	left circumflex coronary artery
HGPRT	hypoxanthine-guanine phosphoribosyl transferase			
			LDH	lactate dehydrogenase
HHS	hyperosmolar hyperglycemic state		LDL	low-density lipoprotein
			LE	lower extremity
HIT	heparin-induced thrombocytopenia		LES	lower esophageal sphincter
			LFTs	liver function tests
HK	hypokinesis		LGIB	lower gastrointestinal bleed
HL	Hodgkin's lymphoma		LH	luteinizing hormone
HoTN	hypotension		LLQ	left lower quadrant
hpf	high power field		LM	left main coronary artery
HR	heart rate		LMWH	low-molecular-weight heparin
HRT	hormone replacement therapy		LN	lymph node
HS	hereditary spherocytosis		LOC	loss of consciousness
HSCT	hematopoietic stem cell transplantation		LP	lumbar puncture
			lpf	low power field
HSM	hepatosplenomegaly		LQTS	long QT syndrome
HSP	Henoch-Schönlein purpura		LUSB	left upper sternal border
HSV	herpes simplex virus		LV	left ventricle
HTN	hypertension		LVAD	LV assist device
HUS	hemolytic uremic syndrome		LVEDP	LV end-diastolic pressure
			LVEDV	LV end-diastolic volume
			LVH	left ventricular hypertrophy
IABP	intraaortic balloon pump		LVOT	left ventricular outflow tract
IBD	inflammatory bowel disease		LVSD	LV systolic dimension

MAC	mitral annular calcification
	Mycobacterium avium complex
MAHA	microangiopathic hemolytic anemia
MAO	monoamine oxidase
MAP	mean arterial pressure
MAT	multifocal atrial tachycardia
MCD	minimal change disease
MCP	metacarpal phalangeal
MCTD	mixed connective tissue disease
MCV	mean corpuscular volume
MDI	metered dose inhaler
MDS	myelodysplastic syndrome
MEN	multiple endocrine neoplasia
MG	myasthenia gravis
MGUS	monoclonal gammopathy of uncertain significance
MI	myocardial infarction
min	minute
min.	minimal
MM	multiple myeloma
MMEFR	maximal mid-expiratory flow rate
MN	membranous nephropathy
mod.	moderate
mos	months
MPD	myeloproliferative disorder
MPGN	membranoproliferative glomerulonephritis
MR	magnetic resonance
	mitral regurgitation
MRA	magnetic resonance angiography
MRI	magnetic resonance imaging
MRSA	methicillin-resistant *S. aureus*
MS	mitral stenosis
MTb	*Mycobacterium tuberculosis*
MTP	metatarsal phalangeal
MTX	methotrexate
MV	mitral valve
MVA	mitral valve area
MVP	mitral valve prolapse
MVR	mitral valve replacement
Mφ	macrophage
N/V	nausea and/or vomiting
NAC	N-acetylcysteine
NAFLD	non-alcoholic fatty liver disease
NG	nasogastric
NGT	nasogastric tube
NHL	Non-Hodgkin's lymphoma
NIDDM	non-insulin dependent diabetes mellitus
NJ	nasojejunal
nl	normal
NM	neuromuscular
NMJ	neuromuscular junction
NO	nitric oxide
NPJT	non-paroxysmal junctional tachycardia
NPO	nothing by mouth
NPV	negative predictive value
NS	normal saline
NSAID	nonsteroidal anti-inflammatory drug

NTG	nitroglycerin
NVE	native valve endocarditis
O/D	overdose
OA	osteoarthritis
OCP	oral contraceptive pill
OG	osmolal gap
OGT	orogastric tube
OGTT	oral glucose tolerance test
OI	opportunistic infection
OM	obtuse marginal coronary artery
OSA	obstructive sleep apnea
OTC	over-the-counter
p/w	present with
PA	pulmonary artery
PAC	pulmonary artery catheter
PAD	peripheral arterial disease
PAN	polyarteritis nodosa
PASP	pulmonary artery systolic pressure
PAV	percutaneous aortic valvuloplasty
pb	problem
PBC	primary biliary cirrhosis
PCI	percutaneous coronary intervention
PCN	penicillin
PCP	*Pneumocystis jioveci* pneumonia
PCR	polymerase chain reaction
PCWP	pulmonary capillary wedge pressure
PD	peritoneal dialysis
PDA	patent ductus arteriosus
	posterior descending coronary artery
PE	pulmonary embolism
PEA	pulseless electrical activity
PEEP	positive end-expiratory pressure
PEFR	peak expiratory flow rate
PET	positron emission tomography
PFO	patent foramen ovale
PFT	pulmonary function test
PGA	polyglandular autoimmune syndrome
PHT	pulmonary hypertension
PID	pelvic inflammatory disease
PIF	prolactin inhibitory factor
PIP	peak inspiratory pressure
	proximal interphalangeal
PKD	polycystic kidney disease
PM	polymyositis
PMHx	past medical history
PMI	point of maximal impulse
PMN	polymorphonuclear leukocyte
PMV	percutaneous mitral valvuloplasty
PMVT	polymorphic ventricular tachycardia
PNA	pneumonia
PND	paroxysmal nocturnal dyspnea
PNH	paroxysmal nocturnal hemoglobinuria

POTS	postural orthostatic tachycardia syndrome
PPD	purified protein derivative
PPH	primary pulmonary hypertension
PPI	proton pump inhibitors
P_{plat}	plateau pressure
PPM	permanent pacemaker
PPV	positive predictive value
PR	pulmonary regurgitation
PRBCs	packed red blood cells
PRL	prolactin
PRPP	phosphoribosyl-1-pyrophosphate
PRWP	poor R wave progression
PS	pressure support
	pulmonic stenosis
PSA	prostate specific antigen
PSGN	post streptococcal glomerulonephritis
PSHx	past surgical history
PSV	pressure support ventilation
Pt	patient
PT	prothrombin time
PTA	percutaneous transluminal angioplasty
PTH	parathyroid hormone
PTH-rP	parathyroid hormone-related peptide
PTT	partial thromboplastin time
PTX	pneumothorax
PUD	peptic ulcer disease
PV	polycythemia vera
PVD	peripheral vascular disease
PVE	prosthetic valve endocarditis
PVR	pulmonary vascular resistance
qac	before every meal
qhs	every bedtime
QoL	quality of life
Qw	Q wave
r/o	rule out
RA	refractory anemia
	rheumatoid arthritis
	right atrium
RAD	right axis deviation
RAE	right atrial enlargement
RAI	radioactive iodine
RAIU	radioactive iodine uptake
RAS	renal artery stenosis
RBBB	right bundle branch block
RBC	red blood cell
RBF	renal blood flow
RCA	right coronary artery
RCMP	restrictive cardiomyopathy
RCT	randomized controlled trial
RDW	red cell distribution width
RE	reticuloendothelial
RF	rheumatoid factor
RHD	rheumatic heart disease
RI	reticulocyte index
RIBA	recombinant immunoblot assay
RMSF	Rocky Mountain spotted fever
RPGN	rapidly progressive glomerulonephritis

RR	respiratory rate
RT	radiation therapy
RTA	renal tubular acidosis
RUQ	right upper quadrant
RUSB	right upper sternal border
RV	residual volume
	right ventricle
RVAD	RV assist device
RVH	right ventricular hypertrophy
RVOT	RV outflow tract
RVSP	RV systolic pressure
Rx	therapy
s/e	side effect
s/p	status post
s/s	signs and symptoms
SA	sinoatrial
SAAG	serum-ascites albumin gradient
SAH	subarachnoid hemorrhage
SBE	subacute bacterial endocarditis
SBP	spontaneous bacterial peritonitis
	systolic blood pressure
SC	subcutaneous
SCD	sudden cardiac death
SCID	severe combined immunodeficiency
SCLC	small cell lung cancer
Se	sensitivity
sec	second
sev.	severe
SIADH	syndrome of inappropriate antidiuretic hormone
SIEP	serum immunoelectrophoresis
SIMV	synchronized intermittent mandatory ventilation
SLE	systemic lupus erythematosus
SMA	superior mesenteric artery
SMV	superior mesenteric vein
SOS	sinusoidal obstructive syndrome
Sp	specificity
SPEP	serum protein electrophoresis
SR	sinus rhythm
SSCY	Salmonella, Shigella, Campylobacter, Yersinia
SSS	sick sinus syndrome
ST	sinus tachycardia
STD	sexually transmitted disease
STE	ST segment elevation
SV	stroke volume
SVC	superior vena cava
SVR	systemic vascular resistance
SVT	supraventricular tachycardia
sx	symptom(s) or symptomatic
T_3RU	T_3 resin uptake
TAA	thoracic aortic aneurysm
TB	tuberculosis
TBG	thyroid binding globulin
TCA	tricyclic antidepressant
TCD	transcranial Doppler
TdP	torsades de pointes
TdT	terminal deoxynucleotidyl transferase

TEE	transesophageal echo
TFTs	thyroid function tests
TG	triglycerides
TGA	transposition of the great arteries
TIA	transient ischemic attack
TIBC	total iron binding capacity
TIPS	transjugular intrahepatic portosystemic shunt
TLC	total lung capacity
Tn	troponin
TP	total protein
TPN	total parenteral nutrition
Tpo	thrombopoietin
TPO	thyroid peroxidase
TR	tricuspid regurgitation
TRALI	transfusion-related acute lung injury
TRH	thyrotropin releasing hormone
TRS	TIMI risk score
TRUS	transrectal ultrasound
TS	tricuspid stenosis
TSH	thyroid stimulating hormone
TSI	thyroid-stimulating immunoglobulin
TSS	transsphenoidal surgery
TTE	transthoracic echo
TTKG	transtubular potassium gradient
TTP	thrombotic thrombocytopenic purpura
TV	tricuspid valve
TWF	T wave flattening
TWI	T wave inversion
TZD	thiazolidinediones
U/A	urinalysis
U/S	ultrasound
UA	unstable angina
	uric acid
UAG	urine anion gap
UC	ulcerative colitis
UCx	urine culture

UFH	unfractionated heparin
UGIB	upper gastrointestinal bleed
UIP	usual interstitial pneumonitis
ULN	upper limit of normal
UOP	urine output
UPEP	urine protein electrophoresis
UR	urgent revascularization
URI	upper respiratory tract infection
UTI	urinary tract infection
V/Q	ventilation-perfusion
VAD	ventricular assist device
VATS	video-assisted thoracoscopic surgery
VBI	vertebrobasilar insufficiency
VC	vital capacity
VD	vessel disease
VF	ventricular fibrillation
VLDL	very-low-density lipoproteins
VOD	veno-occlusive disease
VSD	ventricular septal defect
V_T	tidal volume
VT	ventricular tachycardia
VTE	venous thromboembolus
vWD	von Willebrand's disease
vWF	von Willebrand's factor
VZV	varicella zoster virus
w/	with
w/o	without
w/u	workup
WCT	wide-complex tachycardia
wk	week
WM	Waldenström's macroglobulinemia
WMA	wall motion abnormality
WPW	Wolff-Parkinson-White syndrome
XRT	radiation therapy